THE PAIN DIARY

Your Guide to Successful
Pain Management

THE PAIN DIARY

Your Guide to Successful Pain Management

The Pain Diary: Your Guide to Successful Pain Management

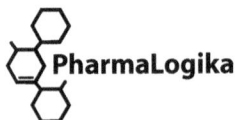

Author: Mindy J. Allport-Settle

Published by PharmaLogika, Inc.

Printed in the United States of America.

ISBN 1-937258-03-3
ISBN-13 978-1-937258-03-0

Acknowledgements

Many chronic pain sufferers are faced with more than just constant pain. They are faced with years of seeking advice from multiple medical professionals in varied disciplines who are not able to find a cause for their pain through the traditional tests and methodology. The patient is left with no answers and — worse — no treatment.

This book was made possible by people who not only believed in the pain and sufferring reported by their patients, but who went beyond the normal practice and found answers and — most importantly — treatments.

While many people helped make this book possible, useful and successful, special thanks go to:

Judy A. McComb, MBA

Linda A. Holliday, MEd

Dr. Wanda L. Radford, MD

Lucia Nixon, MSW, PhD

and

Elisabeth Johnson, RN, NP

CONTENTS

Acknowledgements v

Overview 1

    About this Book 1

    Included Documents and Features 1

Introduction 3

    Instructions for Using this Book 3

EXAMPLES 5

MEDICAL HISTORY 23

MONTHLY SUMMARIES 35

DAILY SUMMARIES 41

About this Book

Receiving appropriate treatment for any medical condition requires providing complete and accurate information to your medical team. Often, it will require more than one visit to more than one medical professional. Each visit requires completing similar forms and each of those professionals will likely ask many of the same questions, but with a slightly different focus.

This book has been designed and tested to help shorten the frequently long and arduous process of diagnosing and successfully managing pain. The needs of the patient, the clinician, and the many supportive members of the medical team (including the patient's family) are perfectly balanced. This book is modeled on the principles of good clinical practices and patient questionnaire requirements for clinical study protocols.

Each page provides a graphic snapshot of critical data and factors related to the many causes of pain, trends over time and treatment effectiveness. It is an invaluable communication tool between the patient and medical team that leads to faster solutions for effective treatment and better treatment compliance for the patient.

Included Documents and Features

- Examples for completing each set of data records

- Comprehensive personal and family medical history section detailing contributing health conditions and possible inherited traits

- Monthly data summaries for easy long term trend analysis

- Daily data records condensing critical information for diagnostic and treatment evaluation and trend analysis

Pain is a *part* of you, but it is not *you*. It is not who you are. It does not define you. It can, however, dictate the choices you make every day. The ability to diagnose the problem and the success of your treatment plan both rely on your ability to accurately report information to your medical team. You are your own best advocate and this book will provide you with the best tool for collaborating with your medical team.

As difficult as pain is to live with, it can also be difficult to diagnose. It's difficult to treat. This book is designed to provide a map of the path your pain takes as well as a means to track the effects of the treatments you use. It will provide your medical team with a comprehensive and concise tool to monitor your response to different treatments and triggers over time so they can best assist you in the management of your pain. By documenting your progress, you will be able to manage your pain more effectively.

Instructions for Using this Book

While it looks like an overwhelming amount of information to document every day, keep in mind that this is meant to be a short term tool designed to help solve a long term problem. This book will make your life, and your medical team's job, easier.

Answer the questions and complete the charts that apply to you. Work with your medical team to determine which tools in the book will help them develop the best treatment plan for you. Typically, just a couple of weeks worth of data will be invaluable in finding the root cause (or causes) of your pain. Additionally, this book should be used as you start new treaments to document how you respond to each form of treatment and quickly steer you toward the best options.

There are two critical directions to keep in mind about this book:

1.) ***Do not become addicted*** to writing in this book and chronicling every second of your day for months on end. Focusing that much on the quantity and quality of your pain can increase the intensity and duration of the pain you experience.

2.) ***Do not become overwhelmed*** by the number of pages in and the amount of information requested in this book. Only fill out the sections that are important to you. Remember that this book is just a tool for you to use in communicating with your medical team.

When you are in pain it is difficult to remember your each aspect of your medical history – but it is the time you need it the most.

The pages in this book are designed to collect comprehensive information. They provide a unique hourly and daily graphical view of your pain scale with exact locations, therapeutic treatments, cognitive and emotional changes, sleep patterns, exercise and activity levels, physiological patterns and changes, and specific drug reactions.

Based on the criteria developed for clinical drug and medical device trials, this graphical interface design documents your pain in a way that is familiar to your medical team so they can quickly recognize patterns and devise an effective treatment plan that will adequately treat your pain.

The following section provides examples of how each page should be completed by you. Take this book with you to your medical appointments so you can discuss the tracked data with your medical team. They might choose to photocopy some of the pages so they can include the tracked data in your chart for later review.

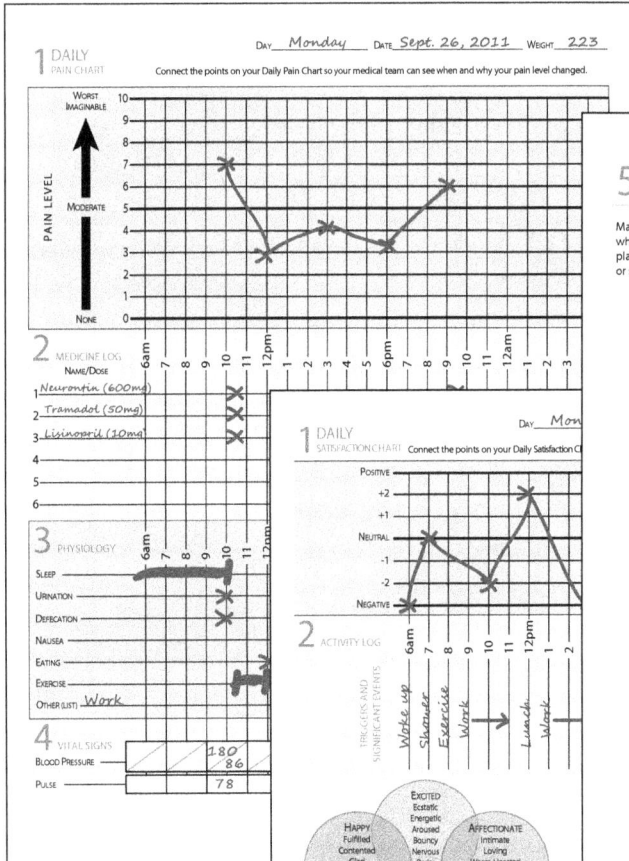

1 DAILY PAIN CHART

Day _Monday_ Date _Sept. 26, 2011_ Weight _223_

Connect the points on your Daily Pain Chart so your medical team can see when and why your pain level changed.

PAIN LEVEL

Worst Imaginable 10
9
8
7
6
Moderate 5
4
3
2
1
None 0

6am 7 8 9 10 11 12pm 1 2 3 4 5 6pm 7 8 9 10 11 12am 1 2 3

2 MEDICINE LOG
Name/Dose
1. Neurontin (600mg)
2. Tramadol (50mg)
3. Lisinopril (10mg)
4.
5.
6.

3 PHYSIOLOGY
Sleep
Urination
Defecation
Nausea
Eating
Exercise
Other (list) _Work_

4 VITAL SIGNS
Blood Pressure 180/86
Pulse 78

1 DAILY SATISFACTION CHART
Day _Mon_
Connect the points on your Daily Satisfaction C

Positive +2
+1
Neutral
-1
-2
Negative

6am 7 8 9 10 11 12pm 1 2

2 ACTIVITY LOG
Time/Hours and Significant Events

Woke up Shower Exercise Work Lunch Work

EXCITED
Ecstatic
Energetic
Aroused
Bouncy
Nervous
Perky
Antsy

HAPPY
Fulfilled
Contented
Glad
Complete
Satisfied
Optimistic
Pleased

AFFECTIONATE
Intimate
Loving
Warm-Hearted
Sympathetic
Touched
Kind
Soft

COMFORTABLE

SAD
Down
Blue
Mopey
Grieved
Dejected
Depressed
Heartbroken

ANGRY
Irritated
Resentful
Miffed
Upset
Mad
Furious
Raging

SCARED
Tense
Nervous
Anxious
Jittery
Frightened
Panic-Stricken
Terrified

____ Increased
____ Decreased
____ Stayed the Same

Did anything unusual happen today?
_____
_____
_____
_____

Describe any changes in your pain:
_____
_____
_____
_____

5 DAILY BODY PAIN DIAGRAM

Mark each place on the diagram where you have had pain today by placing an 'X', circling the location, or shading the area.

Describe the type of pain:

Shooting
Tingling
Numbness
Cold
Surface Pain
Stabbing
Dull
Stinging

Deep
Sharp
Burning / Hot
Aching
Gnawing / Biting
Electrical / Shocks
Other_____

COMMENTS AND MORE INFORMATION:

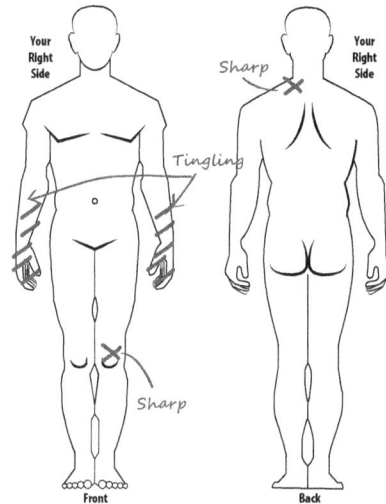

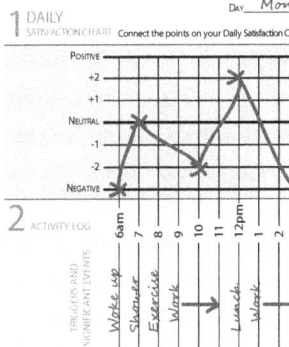

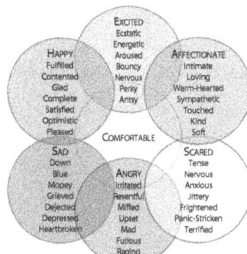

Your Right Side

Sharp

Tingling

Sharp

Front

Back

EXAMPLES

1 PERSONAL
MEDICAL TEAM SUMMARY

NAME	PHONE	FAX	NOTES
Dr. Thomas Darrell	919-552-2292	919-557-7668	Primary Care Physician
ADDRESS			Kathy, Nurse
Fuquay Family Practice			
431 North Judd Parkway NE			
Fuquay-Varina, NC 27526			

NAME	PHONE	FAX	NOTES
Dr. Wanda Radford			OB-Gyn
ADDRESS			Option 5 for Nurse
Wake Women's Health			
Raleigh, NC			

NAME	PHONE	FAX	NOTES
Dr. Kenneth Carnes	919-782-3456		Neurologist
ADDRESS			Medical Record #
Raleigh Neurology			41283367
1540 Sunday Drive			
Raleigh, NC			

NAME	PHONE	FAX	NOTES
ADDRESS			

NAME	PHONE	FAX	NOTES
ADDRESS			

2 CURRENT PERSCRIPTION MEDICATIONS

Drug Name	Dosage	Frequency	Treatment for	Side Effects
Gabapentin	600 mg	2 / day	Neuropathy	Drowsiness
Lisinopril	20 mg	1 / day	High Blood Pressure	None
Tramadol	50 mg	1 / day	Pain	Constipation
Fluoxetine	10 mg	1 / day	Depression	Nausea
Alprazolam	0.5 mg	as needed	Anxiety	Drowsiness

3 CURRENT OVER THE COUNTER MEDICATIONS (ASPIRIN, ETC.)

Drug Name	Dosage	Frequency	Treatment for	Side Effects
Allegra-D		2 / day	Allergies	

4 DRUG ALLERGY SUMMARY

Drug Name (include prescription and other medicines)	Reaction
Erythromycin	Extreme Nausea
Rocephin	Hives, Itching

5 PAIN SURVEY

Place a check (✓) in the appropriate box. ACTIVITY	None	Mild	Moderate	Severe	Unable	HELPFUL TREATMENTS / COMMENTS
Pain when performing the following?						
Bending				✓		
Caring for Infirm Family	✓					N/A
Carrying Groceries		✓				
Changing Position (Sit to Stand)			✓			
Climbing Stairs			✓			
Driving		✓				
Extended Computer Use			✓			
Feeding (Self)		✓				
Household Chores			✓			
Kneeling		✓				
Lifting Children			✓			
Lifting objects			✓			
Pet Care		✓				
Reading (Concentration)	✓					
Self care - Bathing				✓		
Self care - Dressing				✓		
Self care - Shaving				✓		
Sexual Activities					✓	
Sleeping		✓				Ibuprofen & Heating Pad
Sitting (Prolonged)			✓			
Standing (Prolonged)				✓		
Walking				✓		
Yard Work					✓	
Sports / Recreational Activities / Exercise					✓	
List:						
List:						
List:						
List:						
List:						
List any other activities that cause pain:						

6 PERSONAL & FAMILY
HEALTH HISTORY (PAGE 1 OF 3)

Place a check (✓) in the corresponding box for each condition as it applies to you and you relatives.

Condition	You	Your Mother	Your Father	Brother(s)	Sister(s)	Maternal Grandmother	Maternal Grandfather	Maternal Aunt(s)/Uncle(s)	Paternal Grandmother	Paternal Grandfather	Paternal Aunt(s)/Uncle(s)	Comments
Head (Ear, Nose, Throat / Eyes / Jaw):												
Migraine Headaches												
Severe / Frequent Headaches	X											
Jaw Pain / TMJ	X	X				X						
Dizziness or Faintness												
Epilepsy / Seizures or Convulsions												
Near or Farsighted (Glasses)	X	X		X		X	X		X		X	
Glaucoma												
Cataracts												
Blindness												
Recurrent Ear Infecitons												
Deafness / Reduced Hearing						X						
Hay Fever	X	X										
Recurrent Sinusitis												
Overactive Thyroid (Hyperthyroidism)												
Underactive Thyroid (Hypothyroidism)	X						X					
Goiter												
Other:_____												
Psychological:												
Smoking	X											Quit at 35
Alcoholism			X				X					
Chemical Dependency												
Anxiety							X					
Serious Depression												
Post Traumatic Stress Disorder (PTSD)												
Nervous Breakdown												
Suicide / Attempt			X									
Bipolar Disorder				X								
Personality Disorder:_____												
Neurological (Nerves):												
Insomnia	X	X	X	X		X	X	X				
Sleep Apnea												
Peripheral Neuropathy	X					X						
Paralysis												
Orthopedic (Bones, Muscles, etc.):												
Arthritis / Swollen Joints / Rheumatism		X				X	X					
Osteoporosis												
Varicose Veins		X				X						
Connective Tissue Disorder												
Gout												
Broken Bones	X						X					
Cortisone Treatments												
Artificial Joints												
Swollen Feet or Ankles						X	X					
Back Problems / Injury			X									

7 ANNUAL
PERSONAL MEDICAL SUMMARY

By completing this table, you and your medical team will be able to recognize trends and links from your past that will contribute to selecting the best treatment for you. Be brief, but include anything, especially unique or life-changing events and major illnesses or diagnoses, that could be informative.

Year	Age	School Grade	Main Activities / Sports	Occupation	Significant Event	Significant Diagnosis
1971	Born					
1972	1					
1973	2					
1974	3					
1975	4					
1976	5	K	Soccer	Student		
1977	6	1				
1978	7	2				
1979	8	3				
1980	9	4			Got First Dog / Broken Arm	Diabetes
1981	10	5				
1982		6				
1983		7				
1984		8				
1985		9				
1986		10				
1987		11				
1988		12				
1989					Started College	Mononucleosis
1990				Student/Waitress		

3 MENSTRUAL RECORD CHART

MONTH AT A GLANCE: Document each day of your menstrual cycle and the type of flow for each including any spotting between periods. This will provide a means for recognizing patterns over a long period of time.

YEAR 2011

Month	1	2	3	4	5	6	7	8	9	10	11	12	13	14	15	16	17	18	19	20	21	22	23	24	25	26	27	28	29	30	31	No. of days from start of period to beginning of next.	Breast Exam Done (✓)
JAN	▪	▪	X	X	▪	▪	X	X	O	S	S																					27	✓
FEB	O	S	S																						▪	▪	▪	▪	O	S	X	27	✓
MAR	O	S	S		O	O																	X	▪	▪	▪	O	S				26	✓
APR																																	
MAY																																	
JUNE																																	
JULY																																	
AUG																																	
SEPT																																	
OCT																																	
NOV																																	
DEC																																	

TYPE OF FLOW

⊠	NORMAL
◯	EXCEPTIONALLY LIGHT
▪	EXCEPTIONALLY HEAVY
S	SPOTTING

COMMENTS AND MORE INFORMATION: Make notes for and about visits with your healthcare provider, side effects from treatments you may be experiencing, any problems you are having, and more about some of your previous answers or questions.

Extreme cramping starts at least two weeks before period.

4 MEDICATION SIDE EFFECTS

As you and your medical team develop new treatment plans, it will
be especially helpful to record any side effects you experience as
you add new treatments. This can help determine which types of
treatments will work best for you.

Contact your care provider with any side effects.

MEDICATION NAME	DATE STARTED	DATE STOPPED	SIDE EFFECTS / COMMENTS
Gabapentin	2009		Drowsiness
Lisinopril	2010		None
Tramadol	2009	Sept 2011	Constipation
Fluoxetine	Feb 2011		Nausea at 20 mg, dropped to 10 mg
Alprazolam	Sept 2011		Drowsiness → XR felt too drugged
Allegra-D	2005		None / Only take in Spring & Fall
Erythromycin	1992	1992	ALLERGIC / Extreme Nausea
Rocephin	June 2011	June 2011	ALLERGIC / Hives, Itching

1 DAILY
TREATMENT PLAN

As you and your medical team develop new treatment plans, record your plan for the day including new medications, increases or decreases to medications, exercises, physical therapy, or any other treatment efforts.

MEDICATION / TREATMENT	AMOUNT / TIME / COMMENTS
Gabapentin	Increase to 600 mg twice today
Tramadol	Decrease to 50 mg in the morning only
Alprazolam	Take right before going to bed → felt too drugged
Stretching	Increase to twice today

1 DAILY
PAIN CHART

DAY _Monday_   DATE _Sept. 26, 2011_   WEIGHT _223_

Connect the points on your Daily Pain and Satisfaction Charts so your medical team can see when your status changed.

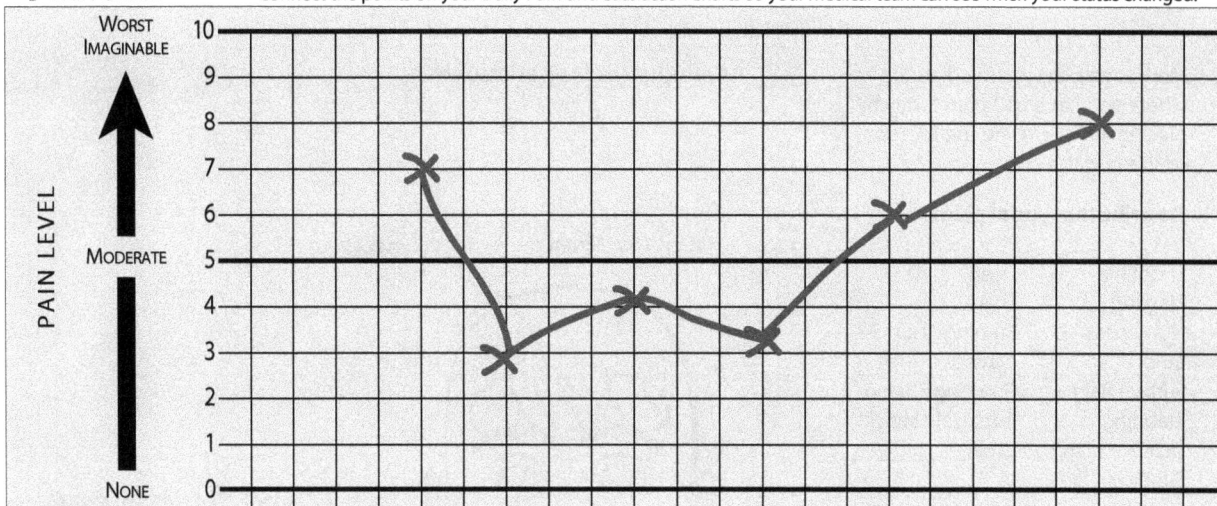

PAIN LEVEL
- WORST IMAGINABLE — 10
- 9
- 8
- 7
- MODERATE — 5
- NONE — 0

2 SATISFACTION

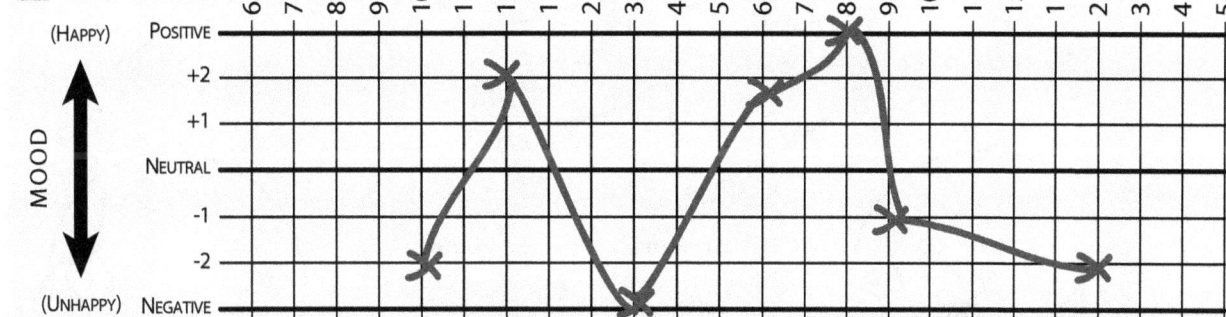

MOOD
- (HAPPY) POSITIVE
- +2
- +1
- NEUTRAL
- -1
- -2
- (UNHAPPY) NEGATIVE

Time axis: 6am 7 8 9 10 11 12pm 1 2 3 4 5 6pm 7 8 9 10 11 12am 1 2 3 4 5

3 PHYSIOLOGY

Time axis: 6am 7 8 9 10 11 12pm 1 2 3 4 5 6pm 7 8 9 10 11 12am 1 2 3 4 5

- SLEEP
- RESTROOM
- NAUSEA / DIZZINESS
- MEAL / SNACK
- EXERCISE
- STRESS / ANXIETY _Work_

MEDICINE NAME / DOSE
1 _Neurontin (600mg)_
2 _Tramadol (50mg)_
3 _All regular pills_

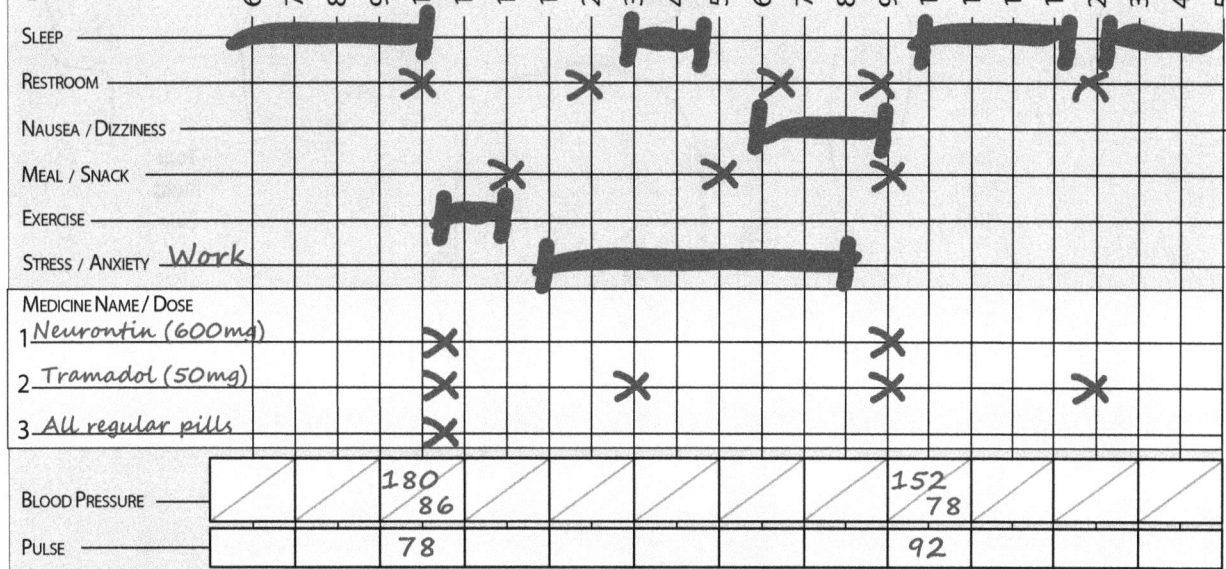

	BLOOD PRESSURE	PULSE
	180/86	78
	152/78	92

4 DAILY HEAD & FACE PAIN DIAGRAM

Mark each place on the diagram where you have had pain today by placing an 'X', circling the location, or shading the area .

COMMENTS AND MORE INFORMATION:

Describe the type of pain:

Shooting	Deep
Tingling	Sharp
Numbness	Burning / Hot
Cold	Aching
Surface Pain	Gnawing / Biting
Stabbing	Electrical / Shocks
Dull	Other_____
Stinging	

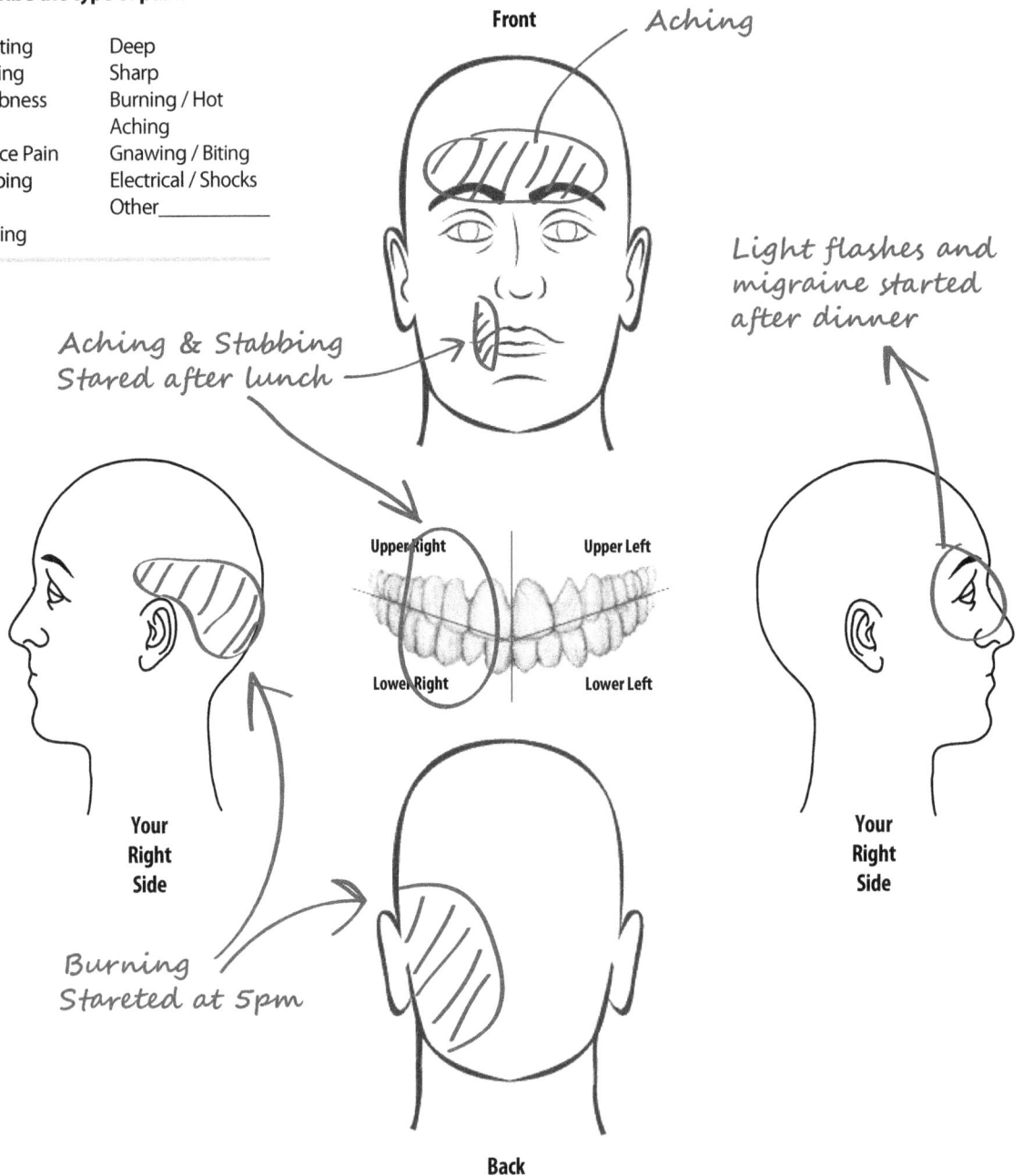

Front

Aching

Light flashes and migraine started after dinner

Aching & Stabbing Stared after lunch

Upper Right   Upper Left

Lower Right   Lower Left

Your Right Side

Your Right Side

Burning Started at 5pm

Back

5 DAILY BODY PAIN DIAGRAM

Mark each place on the diagram where you have had pain today by placing an 'X', circling the location, or shading the area .

Describe the type of pain:

Shooting	Deep
Tingling	Sharp
Numbness	Burning / Hot
Cold	Aching
Surface Pain	Gnawing / Biting
Stabbing	Electrical / Shocks
Dull	Other_____
Stinging	

COMMENTS AND MORE INFORMATION:

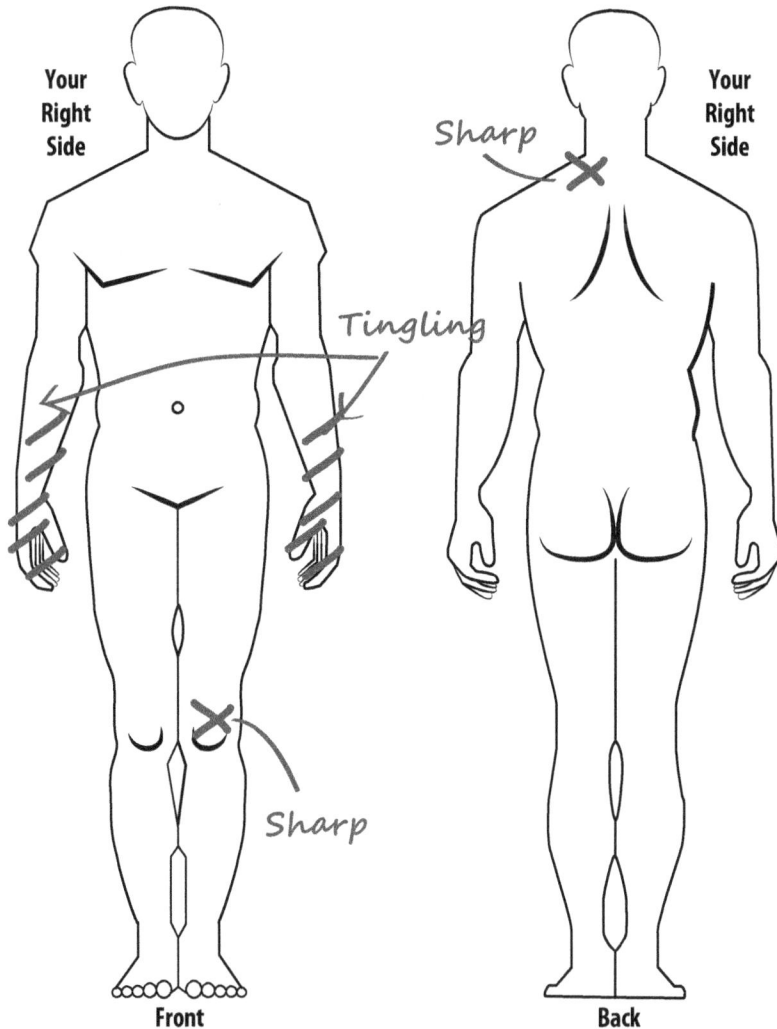

Your Right Side

Sharp

Tingling

Your Right Side

Sharp

Front

Back

6 DAILY PAIN SUMMARY

Were there times during the day that you experienced unrelieved breakthrough pain? ____NO ✔YES

How many times did this happen today?

1 2 3 (4) 5 6 7 8 9 10 more than 10

Did any specific activity start your breakthrough pain?
____NO ✔YES: What activities?

Bending Over

Put an "X" on the body diagram to show each place you've had *BREAKTHROUGH PAIN* today.

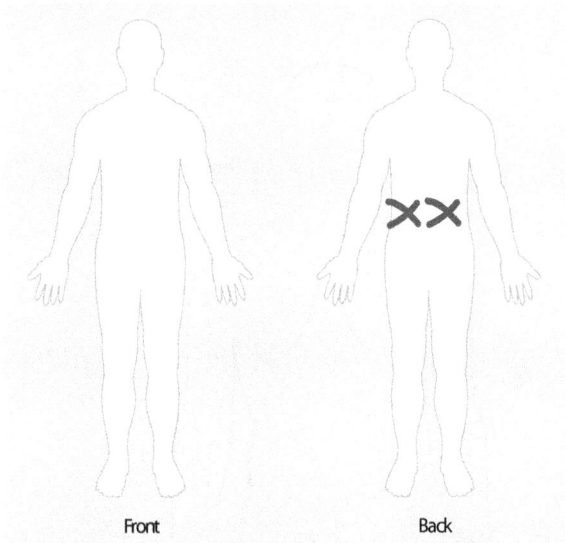

Front   Back

NON-DRUG THERAPIES
(other than prescription or other medicines)
Heating Pad

ACTIVITIES/EXERCISE
Yoga, Weight Lifting

What was your average level of pain today?

0 1 2 3 4 (5) 6 7 8 9 10

Other than prescription medicine, did you do anything else today to relieve the pain? ____NO ✔YES:
(Note any that you used.)
✔ Non-prescription drugs (e.g., acetaminophen, ibuprofen)
____ Herbal remedies
✔ Hot or cold packs
✔ Exercise
✔ Changing position (such as lying down or elevating your legs)
____ Physical therapy
____ Massage
____ Acupuncture
✔ Rest
____ Psychological counseling
____ Talk to trusted friend, family, clergy
____ Prayer, meditation, guided imagery
✔ Relaxation technique (hypnosis, biofeedback)
____ Creative technique (art or music therapy)
____ Other (e.g., specific chiropractic manipulation, osteopathic treatments):
_____

Check any of these common side effects that you've noticed after taking your pain medicine:
____ Drowsiness, sleepiness
____ Nausea, vomiting, upset stomach
✔ Constipation
____ Lack of appetite
✔ Other (describe):
Hallucinations

Did you sleep through the night? ✔NO____YES

If not, how many times was your sleep disrupted? 2

How many hours did you sleep during the night? 6 hrs

COMMENTS AND MORE INFORMATION: Make notes for and about visits with your healthcare provider, side effects from treatments you may be experiencing, any problems you are having coping with your pain, and more about some of your previous answers or questions.
Pain medicine is helping, but I keep seeing shadows move in my peripheral vision.

Is there another medicine that works as well, but without hallucinations?

1 DAILY DIARY

SATISFACTION CHART Connect the points on your Daily Satisfaction Chart so your medical team can see when and why your mental state changed.

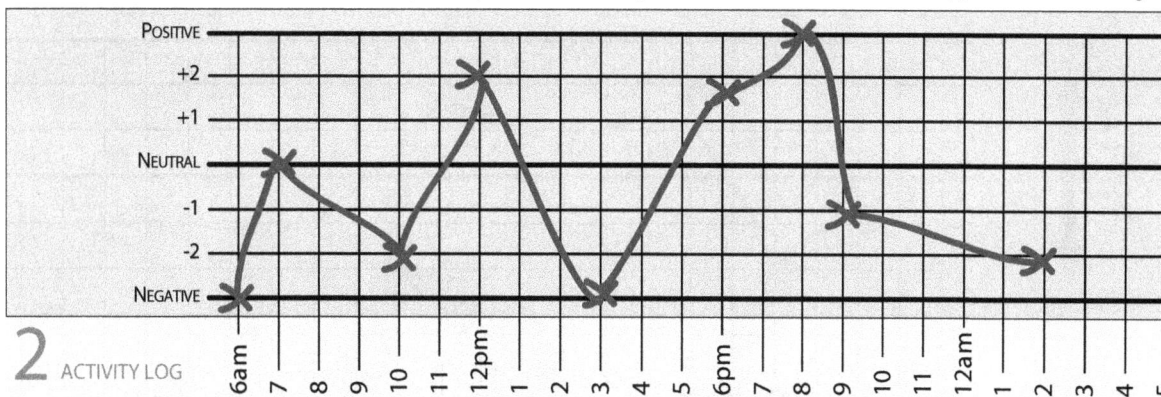

DAY _Monday_ DATE _Sept. 26, 2011_ WEIGHT _223_

POSITIVE
+2
+1
NEUTRAL
-1
-2
NEGATIVE

2 ACTIVITY LOG

6am 7 8 9 10 11 12pm 1 2 3 4 5 6pm 7 8 9 10 11 12am 1 2 3 4 5

TRIGGERS AND SIGNIFICANT EVENTS

Woke up · Shower · Exercise · Work → Lunch · Work → Dinner · Kid's Recital · Watch Scary Movie · Bed · Nightmare

EXCITED
Ecstatic
Energetic
Aroused
Bouncy
Nervous
Perky
Antsy

HAPPY
Fulfilled
Contented
Glad
Complete
Satisfied
Optimistic
Pleased

AFFECTIONATE
Intimate
Loving
Warm-Hearted
Sympathetic
Touched
Kind
Soft

COMFORTABLE

SAD
Down
Blue
Mopey
Grieved
Dejected
Depressed
Heartbroken

ANGRY
Irritated
Resentful
Miffed
Upset
Mad
Furious
Raging

SCARED
Tense
Nervous
Anxious
Jittery
Frightened
Panic-Stricken
Terrified

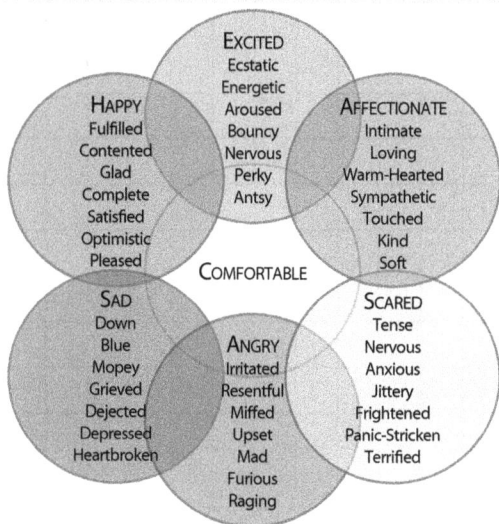

Describe any changes in your pain today:

Back and flank pain got much worse as the day went on.

Did anything unusual happen today?

Argument with a co-worker around 3pm this afternoon.

What did you spend the most time time thinking about today?

Positive Thoughts:

Watching the recital tonight.

Did your pain increase, decrease, or remain the same when you thought about it?

____ Increased
____ Decreased
✓ Stayed the Same

Negative Thoughts:

Fight with co-worker.

Did your pain increase, decrease, or remain the same when you thought about it?

✓ Increased
____ Decreased
____ Stayed the Same

1 DAILY
MOOD CHART

DAY _Monday_   DATE _Sept. 26, 2011_   WEIGHT _223_

Connect the points on your Mood Satisfaction Chart so your medical team can see when and why your mental state changed.

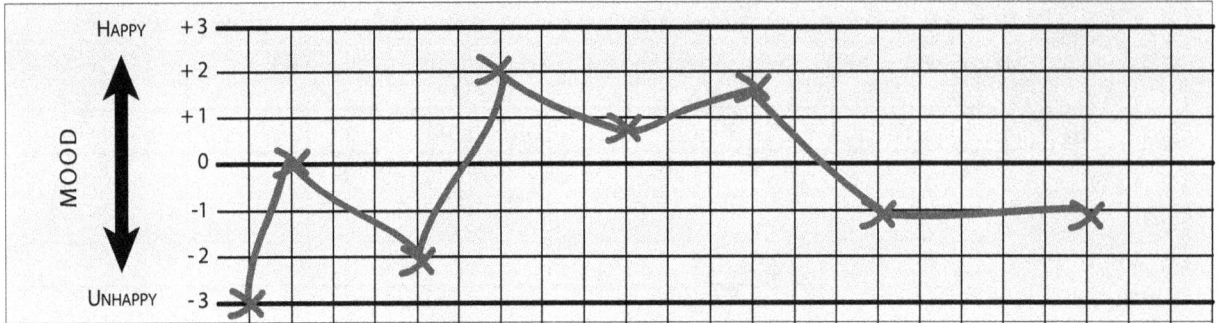

2 ACTIVITY LOG

Woke up · Shower · Exercise · Work → · Lunch · Work → · Dinner · Watch TV · Bed · Nightmare

3 MEDICATION LOG
NAME/DOSE

1 _Neurontin (600mg)_
2 _Tramadol (50mg)_
3 _Lisinopril (10mg)_
4
5
6
7
8

4 PHYSIOLOGY

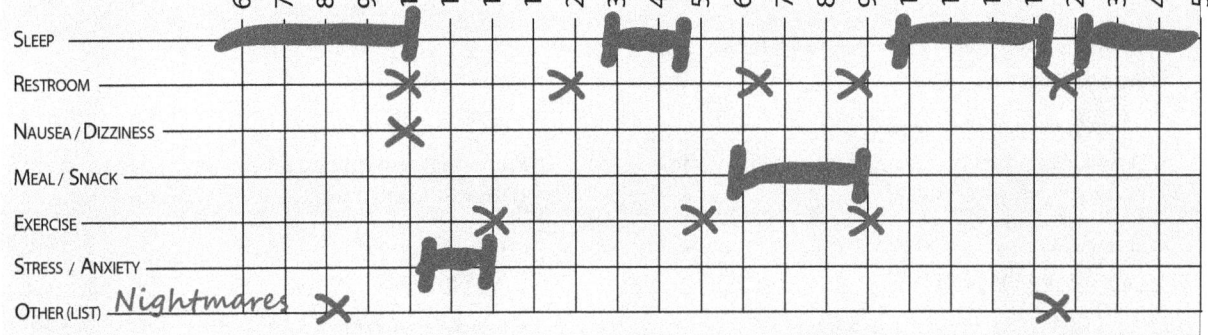

SLEEP
RESTROOM
NAUSEA / DIZZINESS
MEAL / SNACK
EXERCISE
STRESS / ANXIETY
OTHER (LIST) _Nightmares_

1 DAILY RESULTS
OF MEDICATIONS AND TREATMENTS

As you and your medical team develop new treatment plans, it will be especially helpful to record any side effects you experience as you add new treatments. This can help determine which types of treatments will work best for you.

Contact your care provider with any bad reactions or side effects to determine if you should discontinue the medication or treatment.

MEDICATION / TREATMENT	AMOUNT / TIME / COMMENTS
Gabapentin	Slightly more drowsy than usual
Tramadol	More painful throughout the day
Alprazolam	Try taking about 30 minutes before bed tomorrow
Stretching	Helped a little, but will be difficult to fit in daily

MEDICAL
HISTORY

1 PERSONAL
MEDICAL TEAM SUMMARY

NAME	PHONE	FAX	NOTES
ADDRESS			

NAME	PHONE	FAX	NOTES
ADDRESS			

NAME	PHONE	FAX	NOTES
ADDRESS			

NAME	PHONE	FAX	NOTES
ADDRESS			

NAME	PHONE	FAX	NOTES
ADDRESS			

1 PERSONAL
MEDICAL TEAM SUMMARY (CONTINUED)

NAME	PHONE	FAX	NOTES
ADDRESS			

NAME	PHONE	FAX	NOTES
ADDRESS			

NAME	PHONE	FAX	NOTES
ADDRESS			

NAME	PHONE	FAX	NOTES
ADDRESS			

NAME	PHONE	FAX	NOTES
ADDRESS			

2 CURRENT PERSCRIPTION MEDICATIONS

DRUG NAME	DOSAGE	FREQUENCY	TREATMENT FOR	SIDE EFFECTS

3 CURRENT OVER THE COUNTER MEDICATIONS (ASPIRIN, ETC.)

DRUG NAME	DOSAGE	FREQUENCY	TREATMENT FOR	SIDE EFFECTS

4 DRUG ALLERGY SUMMARY

DRUG NAME (include prescription and other medicines)	REACTION

5 PAIN SURVEY

	None	Mild	Moderate	Severe	Unable	
Place a check (✓) in the appropriate box. ACTIVITY						HELPFUL TREATMENTS / COMMENTS
Pain when performing the following?						
Bending						
Caring for Infirm Family						
Carrying Groceries						
Changing Position (Sit to Stand)						
Climbing Stairs						
Driving						
Extended Computer Use						
Feeding (Self)						
Household Chores						
Kneeling						
Lifting Children						
Lifting objects						
Pet Care						
Reading (Concentration)						
Self care - Bathing						
Self care - Dressing						
Self care - Shaving						
Sexual Activities						
Sleeping						
Sitting (Prolonged)						
Standing (Prolonged)						
Walking						
Yard Work						
Sports / Recreational Activities / Exercise						
List:						
List:						
List:						
List:						
List:						
List any other activities that cause pain:						

6 PERSONAL & FAMILY
HEALTH HISTORY (PAGE 1 OF 3)

						MATERNAL			PATERNAL			
Place a check (✓) in the corresponding box for each condition as it applies to you and you relatives. CONDITION	YOU	YOUR MOTHER	YOUR FATHER	BROTHER(S)	SISTER(S)	GRANDMOTHER	GRANDFATHER	AUNT(S) / UNCLE(S)	GRANDMOTHER	GRANDFATHER	AUNT(S) / UNCLE(S)	COMMENTS
Head (Ear, Nose, Throat / Eyes / Jaw):												
Migraine Headaches												
Severe / Frequent Headaches												
Jaw Pain / TMJ												
Dizziness or Faintness												
Epilepsy / Seizures or Convulsions												
Near or Farsighted (Glasses)												
Glaucoma												
Cataracts												
Blindness												
Recurrent Ear Infecitons												
Deafness / Reduced Hearing												
Hay Fever												
Recurrent Sinusitis												
Overactive Thyroid (Hyperthyroidism)												
Underactive Thyroid (Hypothyroidism)												
Goiter												
Other:_____												
Psychological:												
Smoking												
Alcoholism												
Chemical Dependency												
Anxiety												
Serious Depression												
Post Traumatic Stress Disorder (PTSD)												
Nervous Breakdown												
Suicide / Attempt												
Bipolar Disorder												
Personality Disorder:_____												
Neurological (Nerves):												
Insomnia												
Sleep Apnea												
Peripheral Neuropathy												
Paralysis												
Orthopedic (Bones, Muscles, etc.):												
Arthritis / Swollen Joints / Rheumatism												
Osteoporosis												
Varicose Veins												
Connective Tissue Disorder												
Gout												
Broken Bones												
Cortisone Treatments												
Artificial Joints												
Swollen Feet or Ankles												
Back Problems / Injury												

6 HEALTH HISTORY (CONTINUED - PAGE 2 OF 3)

Place a check (✓) in the corresponding box for each condition as it applies to you and you relatives.

Condition	You	Your Mother	Your Father	Brother(s)	Sister(s)	Maternal Grandmother	Maternal Grandfather	Maternal Aunt(s)/Uncle(s)	Paternal Grandmother	Paternal Grandfather	Paternal Aunt(s)/Uncle(s)	Comments
Digestive (Stomache, Intestines, etc.):												
Hiatal Hernia / Chronic Heartburn												
Stomach or Duodenal Ulcer												
Hepatitis												
Cirrhosis / Liver Disease												
Gall Stones												
Irritable Bowel Syndrome (IBS)												
Ulcerative Colitis												
Diverticulitis (-osis)												
Polyps (Colon)												
Dysentery or Serious Diarrhea												
Rectal Trouble												
Hemorrhoids												
Recurrent Urinary Tract Infections (UTI)												
Frequent, Painful, or Difficult Urination												
Incontinence												
Kidney Stones												
Other Kidney Disease:_____												
Cardiopulmonary (Heart, Lungs, Blood):												
Phlebitis or Blood Clots / Emboli												
Anemia												
Asthma, Bronchitis or Emphysema												
Angina												
Heart Attack / Surgery												
Heart Murmur												
Enlarged Heart												
Coronary Heart Disease												
Artificial Heart Valves												
Pacemaker												
High Blood Pressure												
Low Blood Pressure												
Stroke / TIA												
Shortness of Breath / Chest Pain												
Asthma												
Chronic Bronchitis												
Cough, persistent or bloody												
Emphysema												
Tuberculosis												
Systemic Disease / Disorders:												
Diabetes												
Psoriasis, Eczema, or Rosacea												
Gonorrhea, Syphilis or Venereal Disease												
AIDS / HIV Infection												
Hepatitis Type _____												
Herpes Infection												

6 HEALTH HISTORY (CONTINUED - PAGE 3 OF 3)

Place a check (✓) in the corresponding box for each condition as it applies to you and you relatives.

CONDITION	YOU	YOUR MOTHER	YOUR FATHER	BROTHER(S)	SISTER(S)	MATERNAL GRANDMOTHER	MATERNAL GRANDFATHER	MATERNAL AUNT(S) / UNCLE(S)	PATERNAL GRANDMOTHER	PATERNAL GRANDFATHER	PATERNAL AUNT(S) / UNCLE(S)	COMMENTS
Systemic Disease / Disorders:												
Chicken Pox												
Shingles												
Mumps or Measles												
Rheumatic or Scarlet Fever												
Cancer (Type:_____)												
Cancer (Type:_____)												
Cancer (Type:_____)												
Women:												
Severe Menstrual Cramping												
Pre Menstrual Dimorphic Disorder (PMDD)												
Abnormal PAP												
Ovarian Cyst(s)												
Fibroids(s)												
Endometriosis / Adhesions												
Breast Lump(s)												
Men:												
Enlarged Prostate												
Erectile Dysfunction												
Other Medical Condition:												
Other:												
Other:												
Other:												
Other:												

7 ANNUAL
PERSONAL MEDICAL SUMMARY

By completing this table, you and your medical team will be able to recognize trends and links from your past that will contribute to selecting the best treatment for you. Be brief, but include anything, especially unique or life-changing events and major illnesses or diagnoses, that could be informative.

YEAR	AGE	SCHOOL GRADE	MAIN ACTIVITIES / SPORTS	OCCUPATION	SIGNIFICANT EVENT	SIGNIFICANT DIAGNOSIS
	Born					

7 PERSONAL MEDICAL SUMMARY (CONTINUED)

By completing this table, you and your medical team will be able to recognize trends and links from your past that will contribute to selecting the best treatment for you. Be brief, but include anything, especially unique or life-changing events and major illnesses or diagnoses, that could be informative.

YEAR	AGE	GRADE	MAIN ACTIVITIES / SPORTS	OCCUPATION	SIGNIFICANT EVENT	SIGNIFICANT DIAGNOSIS

MONTHLY SUMMARIES

1 MONTHLY
PAIN OVERVIEW CHART

MONTH AT A GLANCE: Using the information documented on the daily pain graphing sheets, document the highest level of pain you experienced for each day. This will provide a means for recognizing patterns over a longer period of time.

MONTH	1	2	3	4	5	6	7	8	9	10	11	12	13	14	15	16	17	18	19	20	21	22	23	24	25	26	27	28	29	30	31	Number of Days with Pain	Drug Change (✓)
JAN																																	
FEB																																	
MAR																																	
APR																																	
MAY																																	
JUNE																																	
JULY																																	
AUG																																	
SEPT																																	
OCT																																	
NOV																																	
DEC																																	

YEAR _____

TYPE OF PAIN

WORST IMAGINABLE ▨

SEVERE Ⓢ

MODERATE Ⓜ

TOLERABLE ⊠

COMMENTS AND MORE INFORMATION: Make notes for and about visits with your healthcare provider, side effects from treatments you may be experiencing, any problems you are having, and more about some of your previous answers or questions.

2 EXERCISE RECORD CHART

MONTH AT A GLANCE: Document the type of exercise you practiced for each day. This will provide a means for recognizing patterns over a long period of time.

YEAR _____

MONTH	1	2	3	4	5	6	7	8	9	10	11	12	13	14	15	16	17	18	19	20	21	22	23	24	25	26	27	28	29	30	31	Number of Days Exercised	Weight at End of the Month
JAN																																	
FEB																																	
MAR																																	
APR																																	
MAY																																	
JUNE																																	
JULY																																	
AUG																																	
SEPT																																	
OCT																																	
NOV																																	
DEC																																	

TYPE OF EXERCISE

Cardio ⊠

Weights ⊡

Cardio and Weights ▨

Other ⊘

COMMENTS AND MORE INFORMATION: Make notes for and about visits with your healthcare provider, side effects from treatments you may be experiencing, any problems you are having, and more about some of your previous answers or questions.

_____

_____

_____

_____

_____

_____

3 MENSTRUAL RECORD CHART

MONTH AT A GLANCE: Document each day of your menstrual cycle and the type of flow for each including any spotting between periods. This will provide a means for recognizing patterns over a long period of time.

YEAR

MONTH	1	2	3	4	5	6	7	8	9	10	11	12	13	14	15	16	17	18	19	20	21	22	23	24	25	26	27	28	29	30	31	No. of days from start of period to beginning of next.	Breast Exam Done (✓)
JAN																																	
FEB																																	
MAR																																	
APR																																	
MAY																																	
JUNE																																	
JULY																																	
AUG																																	
SEPT																																	
OCT																																	
NOV																																	
DEC																																	

TYPE OF FLOW

NORMAL ⊠

EXCEPTIONALLY LIGHT ∅

EXCEPTIONALLY HEAVY ▦

SPOTTING ⑤

COMMENTS AND MORE INFORMATION: Make notes for and about visits with your healthcare provider, side effects from treatments you may be experiencing, any problems you are having, and more about some of your previous answers or questions.

4 MEDICATION SIDE EFFECTS

As you and your medical team develop new treatment plans, it will be especially helpful to record any side effects you experience as you add new treatments. This can help determine which types of treatments will work best for you.

Contact your care provider with any side effects.

MEDICATION NAME	DATE STARTED	DATE STOPPED	SIDE EFFECTS / COMMENTS

DAILY
SUMMARIES

1 DAILY
TREATMENT PLAN

As you and your medical team develop new treatment plans, record your plan for the day including new medications, increases or decreases to medications, exercises, physical therapy, or any other treatment efforts.

MEDICATION / TREATMENT	AMOUNT / TIME / COMMENTS

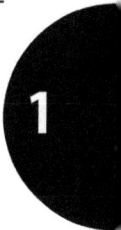

1 DAILY
PAIN CHART

DAY_____ DATE_____ WEIGHT_____

Connect the points on your Daily Pain and Satisfaction Charts so your medical team can see when your status changed.

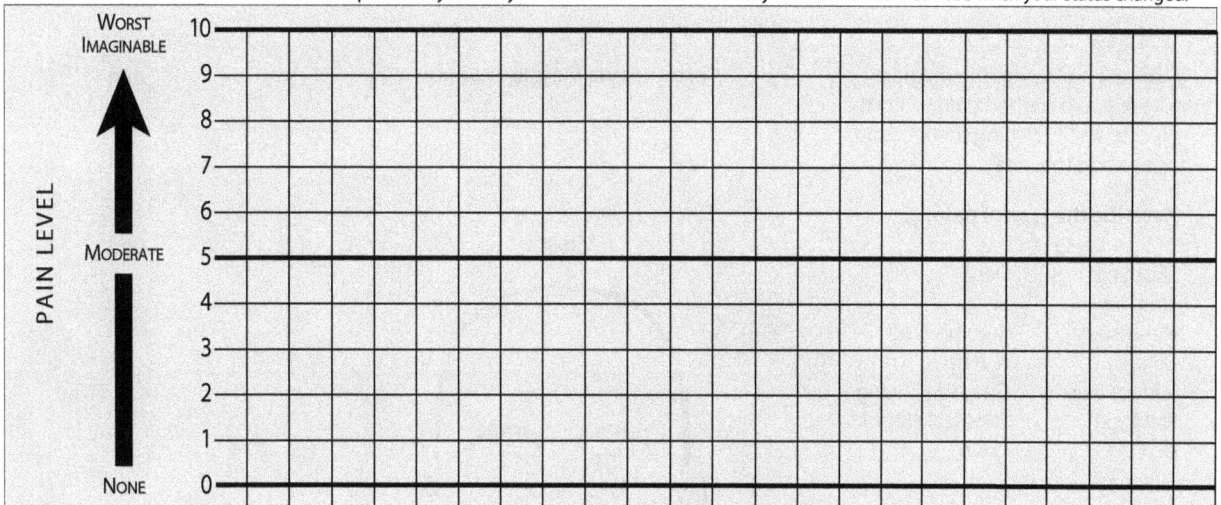

2 SATISFACTION

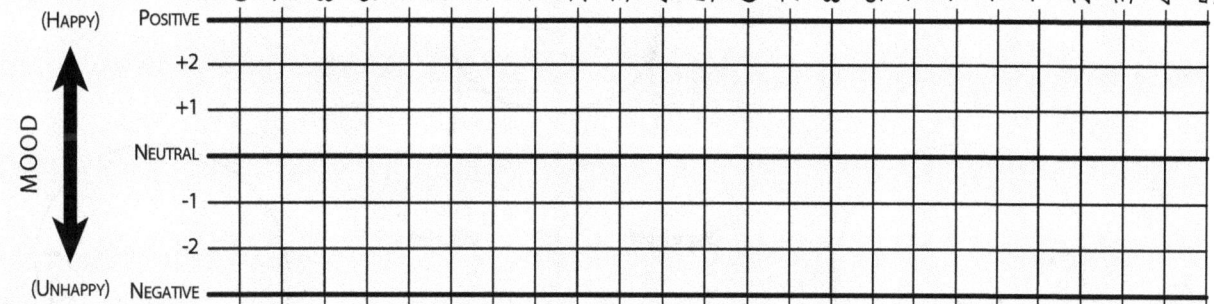

3 PHYSIOLOGY

SLEEP

RESTROOM

NAUSEA / DIZZINESS

MEAL / SNACK

EXERCISE

STRESS / ANXIETY

MEDICINE NAME / DOSE

1

2

3

BLOOD PRESSURE

PULSE

4 DAILY HEAD & FACE PAIN DIAGRAM

Mark each place on the diagram where you have had pain today by placing an 'X', circling the location, or shading the area .

Describe the type of pain:

Shooting	Deep
Tingling	Sharp
Numbness	Burning / Hot
Cold	Aching
Surface Pain	Gnawing / Biting
Stabbing	Electrical / Shocks
Dull	Other_____
Stinging	

COMMENTS AND MORE INFORMATION:

Front

Upper Right   **Upper Left**

Lower Right   **Lower Left**

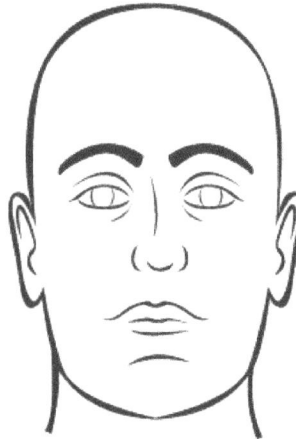

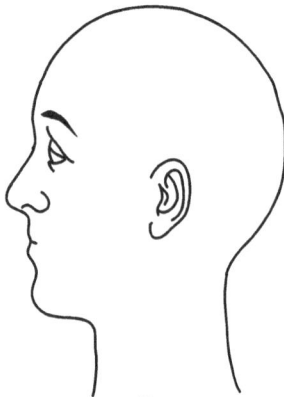

Your Right Side

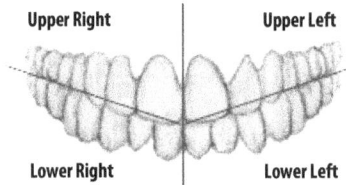

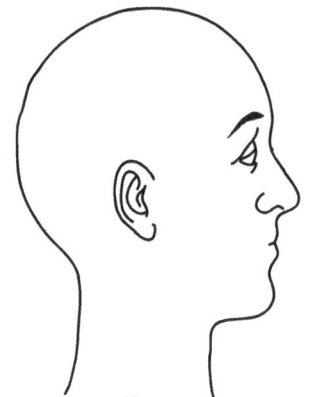

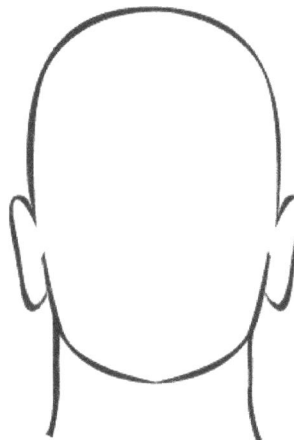

Your Right Side

Back

5 DAILY BODY PAIN DIAGRAM

Mark each place on the diagram where you have had pain today by placing an 'X', circling the location, or shading the area .

Describe the type of pain:

Shooting	Deep
Tingling	Sharp
Numbness	Burning / Hot
Cold	Aching
Surface Pain	Gnawing / Biting
Stabbing	Electrical / Shocks
Dull	Other_____
Stinging	

COMMENTS AND MORE INFORMATION:

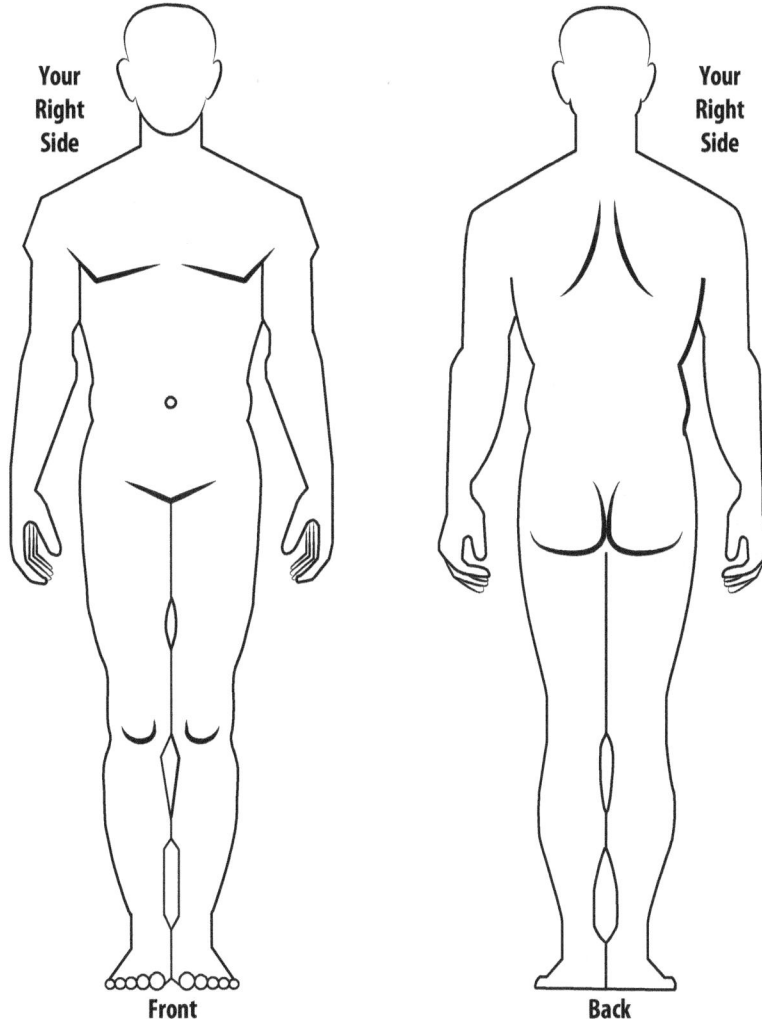

Your Right Side

Your Right Side

Front

Back

1

6 DAILY PAIN SUMMARY

Were there times during the day that you experienced unrelieved breakthrough pain? ____NO ____YES

How many times did this happen today?

1 2 3 4 5 6 7 8 9 10 more than 10

Did any specific activity start your breakthrough pain? ____NO ____YES: What activities?

_____

Put an "X" on the body diagram to show each place you've had *BREAKTHROUGH PAIN* today.

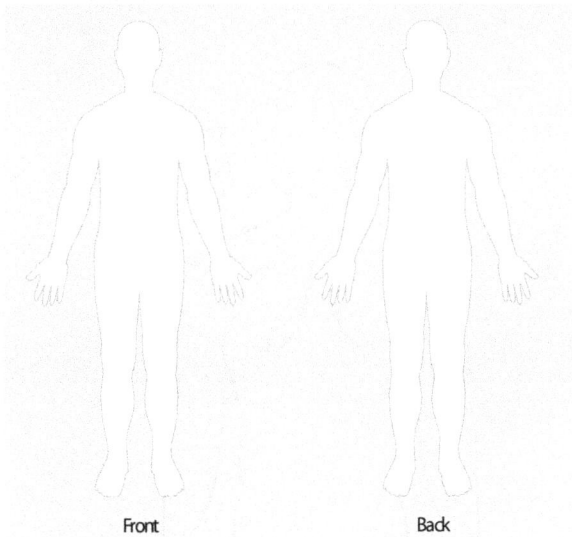

Front   Back

NON-DRUG THERAPIES
(other than prescription or other medicines)

_____

_____

ACTIVITIES/EXERCISE

_____

_____

What was your average level of pain today?

0 1 2 3 4 5 6 7 8 9 10

Other than prescription medicine, did you do anything else today to relieve the pain? ____NO ____YES: (Note any that you used.)
____ Non-prescription drugs (e.g., acetaminophen, ibuprofen)
____ Herbal remedies
____ Hot or cold packs
____ Exercise
____ Changing position (such as lying down or elevating your legs)
____ Physical therapy
____ Massage
____ Acupuncture
____ Rest
____ Psychological counseling
____ Talk to trusted friend, family, clergy
____ Prayer, meditation, guided imagery
____ Relaxation technique (hypnosis, biofeedback)
____ Creative technique (art or music therapy)
____ Other (e.g., specific chiropractic manipulation, osteopathic treatments):

_____

Check any of these common side effects that you've noticed after taking your pain medicine:
____ Drowsiness, sleepiness
____ Nausea, vomiting, upset stomach
____ Constipation
____ Lack of appetite
____ Other (describe):

_____

Did you sleep through the night? ____NO____YES

If not, how many times was your sleep disrupted? _____

How many hours did you sleep during the night? _____

COMMENTS AND MORE INFORMATION: Make notes for and about visits with your healthcare provider, side effects from treatments you may be experiencing, any problems you are having coping with your pain, and more about some of your previous answers or questions.

_____

_____

_____

1 DAILY DIARY

SATISFACTION CHART

Day_____ Date_____ Weight_____

Connect the points on your Daily Satisfaction Chart so your medical team can see when and why your mental state changed.

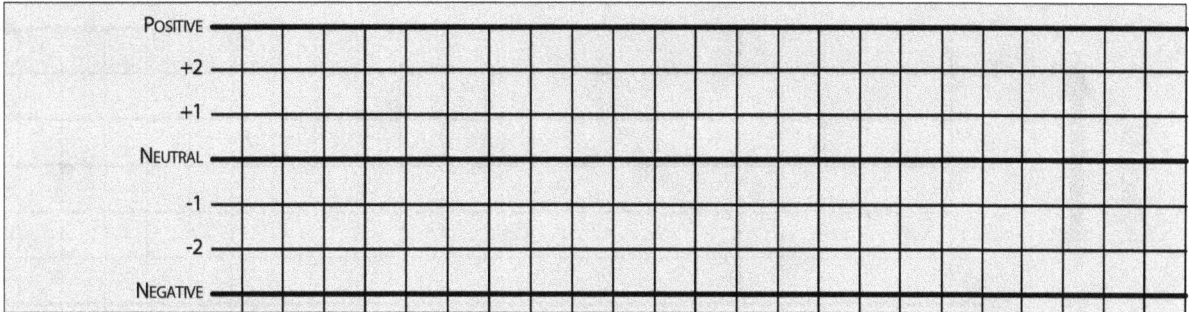

| POSITIVE |
| +2 |
| +1 |
| NEUTRAL |
| -1 |
| -2 |
| NEGATIVE |

2 ACTIVITY LOG

TRIGGERS AND SIGNIFICANT EVENTS

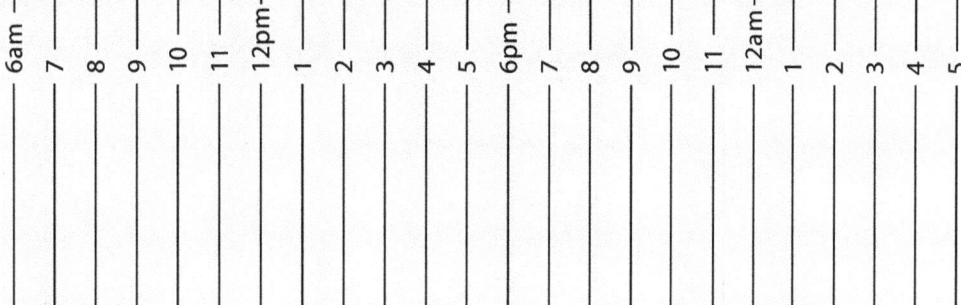

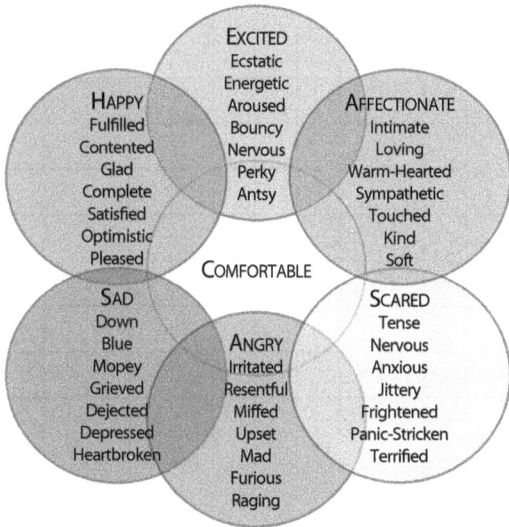

6am 7 8 9 10 11 12pm 1 2 3 4 5 6pm 7 8 9 10 11 12am 1 2 3 4 5

EXCITED
Ecstatic
Energetic
Aroused
Bouncy
Nervous
Perky
Antsy

HAPPY
Fulfilled
Contented
Glad
Complete
Satisfied
Optimistic
Pleased

AFFECTIONATE
Intimate
Loving
Warm-Hearted
Sympathetic
Touched
Kind
Soft

COMFORTABLE

SAD
Down
Blue
Mopey
Grieved
Dejected
Depressed
Heartbroken

ANGRY
Irritated
Resentful
Miffed
Upset
Mad
Furious
Raging

SCARED
Tense
Nervous
Anxious
Jittery
Frightened
Panic-Stricken
Terrified

Describe any changes in your pain today:

_____
_____
_____
_____

Did anything unusual happen today?

_____
_____
_____
_____

What did you spend the most time time thinking about today?

Positive Thoughts:

_____

Did your pain increase, decrease, or remain the same when you thought about it?
____ Increased
____ Decreased
____ Stayed the Same

Negative Thoughts:

_____

Did your pain increase, decrease, or remain the same when you thought about it?
____ Increased
____ Decreased
____ Stayed the Same

DAY_____ DATE_____ WEIGHT_____

1 DAILY
MOOD CHART

Connect the points on your Mood Satisfaction Chart so your medical team can see when and why your mental state changed.

HAPPY +3
       +2
       +1
MOOD   0
       -1
       -2
SAD   -3

2 ACTIVITY LOG

6am 7 8 9 10 11 12pm 1 2 3 4 5 6pm 7 8 9 10 11 12am 1 2 3 4 5

3 MEDICATION LOG
NAME/DOSE

1
2
3
4
5
6
7
8

4 PHYSIOLOGY

6am 7 8 9 10 11 12pm 1 2 3 4 5 6pm 7 8 9 10 11 12am 1 2 3 4 5

SLEEP
URINATION
DEFECATION
NAUSEA
EATING
EXERCISE
OTHER (LIST)

1 DAILY RESULTS
OF MEDICATIONS AND TREATMENTS

As you and your medical team develop new treatment plans, it will be especially helpful to record any side effects you experience as you add new treatments. This can help determine which types of treatments will work best for you.

Contact your care provider with any bad reactions or side effects to determine if you should discontinue the medication or treatment.

MEDICATION / TREATMENT	AMOUNT / TIME / COMMENTS

1 DAILY
TREATMENT PLAN

As you and your medical team develop new treatment plans, record your plan for the day including new medications, increases or decreases to medications, exercises, physical therapy, or any other treatment efforts.

2

MEDICATION / TREATMENT	AMOUNT / TIME / COMMENTS

1 DAILY
PAIN CHART

Day_____ Date_____ Weight_____

Connect the points on your Daily Pain and Satisfaction Charts so your medical team can see when your status changed.

WORST IMAGINABLE 10
9
8
7
6
MODERATE 5
4
3
2
1
NONE 0

PAIN LEVEL

2 SATISFACTION

6am 7 8 9 10 11 12pm 1 2 3 4 5 6pm 7 8 9 10 11 12am 1 2 3 4 5

(HAPPY) POSITIVE
+2
+1
NEUTRAL
-1
-2
(UNHAPPY) NEGATIVE

MOOD

3 PHYSIOLOGY

6am 7 8 9 10 11 12pm 1 2 3 4 5 6pm 7 8 9 10 11 12am 1 2 3 4 5

SLEEP
RESTROOM
NAUSEA / DIZZINESS
MEAL / SNACK
EXERCISE
STRESS / ANXIETY
MEDICINE NAME / DOSE
1
2
3
BLOOD PRESSURE
PULSE

4 DAILY HEAD & FACE PAIN DIAGRAM

2

Mark each place on the diagram where you have had pain today by placing an 'X', circling the location, or shading the area .

Describe the type of pain:

Shooting	Deep
Tingling	Sharp
Numbness	Burning / Hot
Cold	Aching
Surface Pain	Gnawing / Biting
Stabbing	Electrical / Shocks
Dull	Other_____
Stinging	

COMMENTS AND MORE INFORMATION:

Front

Upper Right   **Upper Left**

Lower Right   **Lower Left**

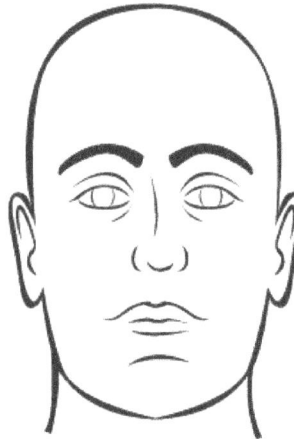

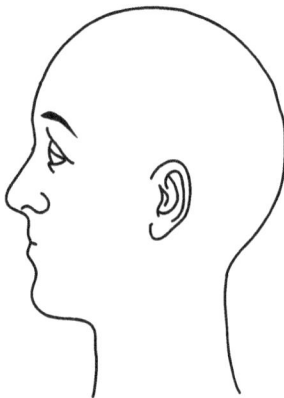

Your Right Side

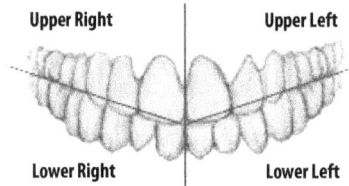

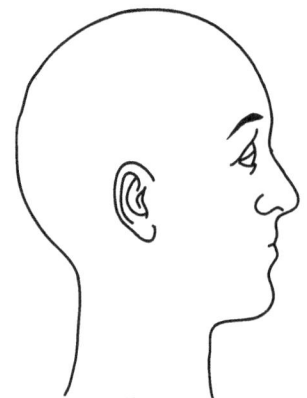

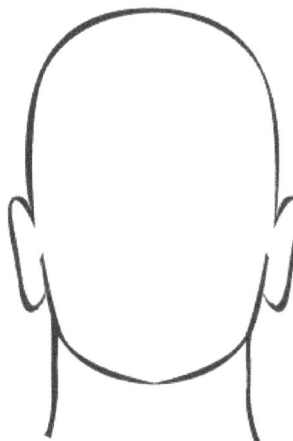

Your Right Side

Back

5 DAILY BODY PAIN DIAGRAM

Mark each place on the diagram where you have had pain today by placing an 'X', circling the location, or shading the area .

Describe the type of pain:

Shooting	Deep
Tingling	Sharp
Numbness	Burning / Hot
Cold	Aching
Surface Pain	Gnawing / Biting
Stabbing	Electrical / Shocks
Dull	Other_____
Stinging	

COMMENTS AND MORE INFORMATION:

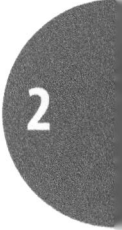

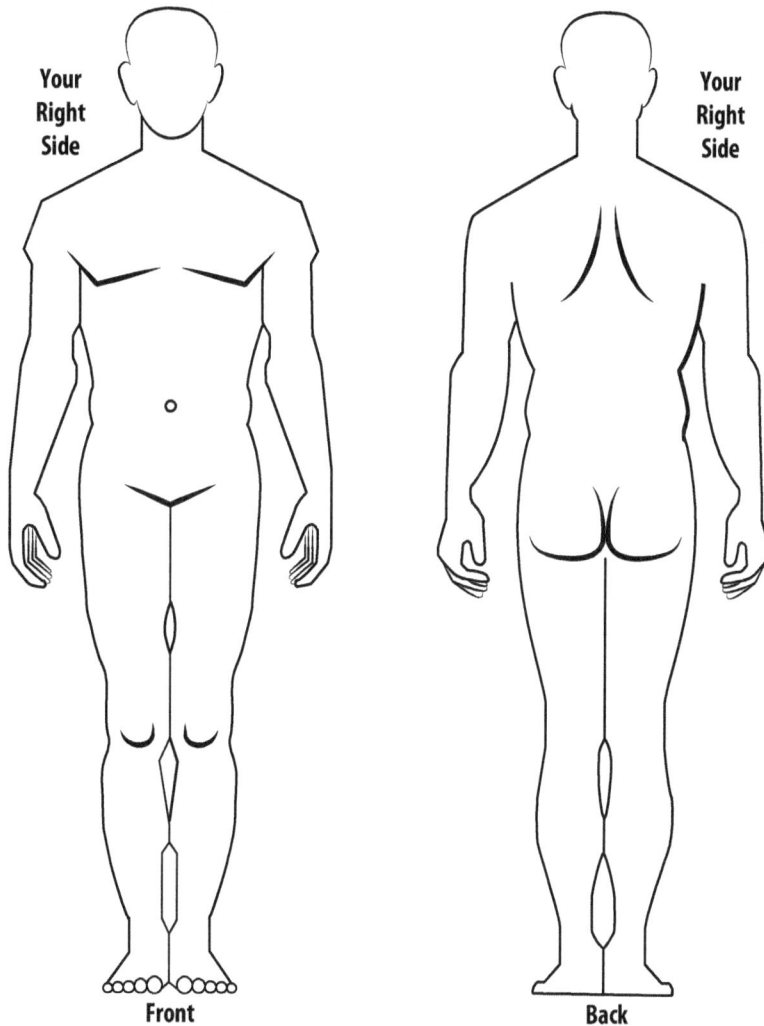

Your Right Side

Your Right Side

Front

Back

6 DAILY PAIN SUMMARY

Were there times during the day that you experienced unrelieved breakthrough pain? ____NO ____YES

How many times did this happen today?

1 2 3 4 5 6 7 8 9 10 more than 10

Did any specific activity start your breakthrough pain? ____NO ____YES: What activities?

_____

Put an "X" on the body diagram to show each place you've had **BREAKTHROUGH PAIN** today.

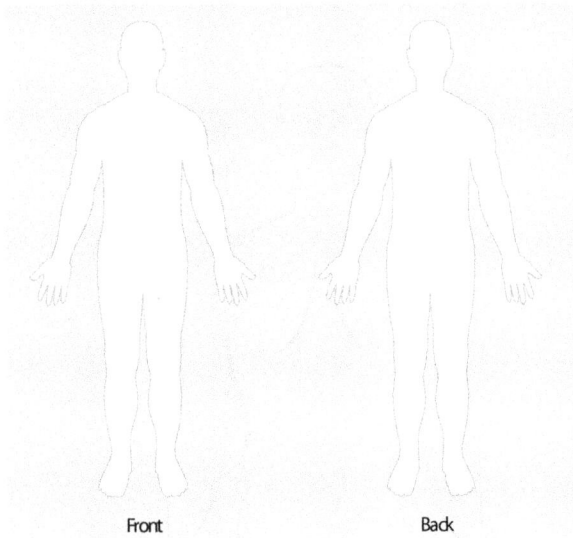

Front   Back

NON-DRUG THERAPIES
(other than prescription or other medicines)

_____

_____

ACTIVITIES/EXERCISE

_____

_____

What was your average level of pain today?

0 1 2 3 4 5 6 7 8 9 10

Other than prescription medicine, did you do anything else today to relieve the pain? ____NO ____YES:
(Note any that you used.)
____ Non-prescription drugs (e.g., acetaminophen, ibuprofen)
____ Herbal remedies
____ Hot or cold packs
____ Exercise
____ Changing position (such as lying down or elevating your legs)
____ Physical therapy
____ Massage
____ Acupuncture
____ Rest
____ Psychological counseling
____ Talk to trusted friend, family, clergy
____ Prayer, meditation, guided imagery
____ Relaxation technique (hypnosis, biofeedback)
____ Creative technique (art or music therapy)
____ Other (e.g., specific chiropractic manipulation, osteopathic treatments):

_____

Check any of these common side effects that you've noticed after taking your pain medicine:
____ Drowsiness, sleepiness
____ Nausea, vomiting, upset stomach
____ Constipation
____ Lack of appetite
____ Other (describe):

_____

Did you sleep through the night? ____NO____YES

If not, how many times was your sleep disrupted? _____

How many hours did you sleep during the night? _____

COMMENTS AND MORE INFORMATION: Make notes for and about visits with your healthcare provider, side effects from treatments you may be experiencing, any problems you are having coping with your pain, and more about some of your previous answers or questions.

_____

_____

_____

1 DAILY DIARY

DAY_____ DATE_____ WEIGHT_____

SATISFACTION CHART Connect the points on your Daily Satisfaction Chart so your medical team can see when and why your mental state changed.

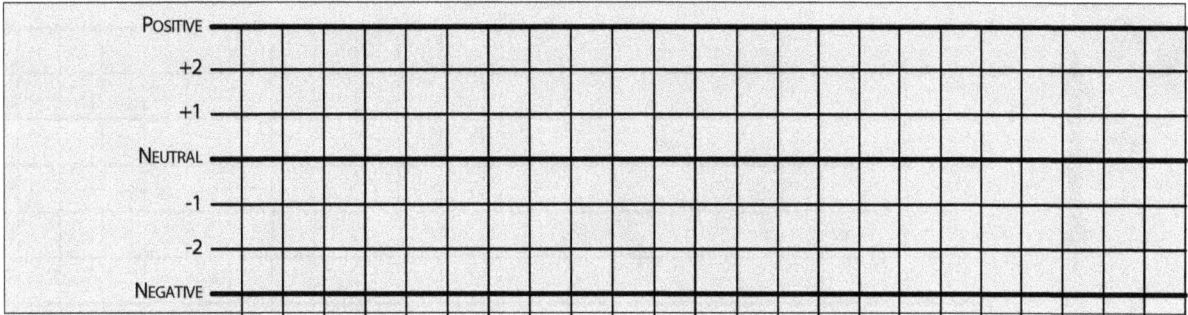

POSITIVE		
+2		
+1		
NEUTRAL		
-1		
-2		
NEGATIVE		

2 ACTIVITY LOG

TRIGGERS AND SIGNIFICANT EVENTS

6am 7 8 9 10 11 12pm 1 2 3 4 5 6pm 7 8 9 10 11 12am 1 2 3 4 5

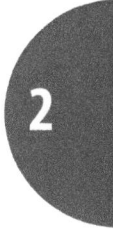

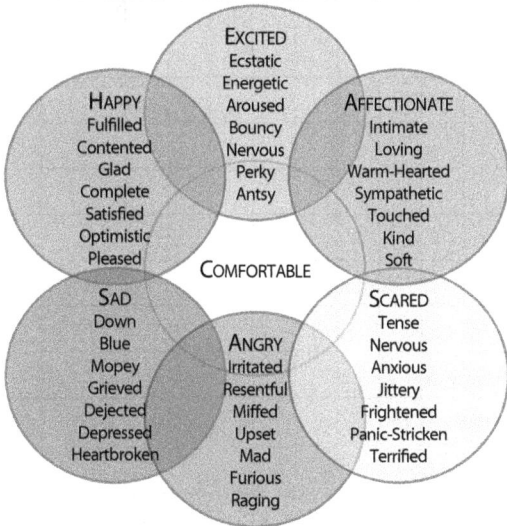

EXCITED
Ecstatic
Energetic
Aroused
Bouncy
Nervous
Perky
Antsy

HAPPY
Fulfilled
Contented
Glad
Complete
Satisfied
Optimistic
Pleased

AFFECTIONATE
Intimate
Loving
Warm-Hearted
Sympathetic
Touched
Kind
Soft

COMFORTABLE

SAD
Down
Blue
Mopey
Grieved
Dejected
Depressed
Heartbroken

ANGRY
Irritated
Resentful
Miffed
Upset
Mad
Furious
Raging

SCARED
Tense
Nervous
Anxious
Jittery
Frightened
Panic-Stricken
Terrified

Describe any changes in your pain today:

_____
_____
_____
_____

Did anything unusual happen today?

_____
_____
_____
_____

What did you spend the most time time thinking about today?

Positive Thoughts:

_____

Did your pain increase, decrease, or remain the same when you thought about it?
____ Increased
____ Decreased
____ Stayed the Same

Negative Thoughts:

_____

Did your pain increase, decrease, or remain the same when you thought about it?
____ Increased
____ Decreased
____ Stayed the Same

1 DAILY
MOOD CHART

Day_____ Date_____ Weight_____

Connect the points on your Mood Satisfaction Chart so your medical team can see when and why your mental state changed.

HAPPY

MOOD

SAD

	+3
	+2
	+1
	0
	-1
	-2
	-3

2 ACTIVITY LOG

6am 7 8 9 10 11 12pm 1 2 3 4 5 6pm 7 8 9 10 11 12am 1 2 3 4 5

3 MEDICATION LOG
NAME/DOSE

1————
2————
3————
4————
5————
6————
7————
8————

4 PHYSIOLOGY

6am 7 8 9 10 11 12pm 1 2 3 4 5 6pm 7 8 9 10 11 12am 1 2 3 4 5

SLEEP ———
URINATION ———
DEFECATION ———
NAUSEA ———
EATING ———
EXERCISE ———
OTHER (LIST) ———

1 DAILY RESULTS
OF MEDICATIONS AND TREATMENTS

As you and your medical team develop new treatment plans, it will be especially helpful to record any side effects you experience as you add new treatments. This can help determine which types of treatments will work best for you.

Contact your care provider with any bad reactions or side effects to determine if you should discontinue the medication or treatment.

2

MEDICATION / TREATMENT	AMOUNT / TIME / COMMENTS

1 DAILY
TREATMENT PLAN

As you and your medical team develop new treatment plans, record your plan for the day including new medications, increases or decreases to medications, exercises, physical therapy, or any other treatment efforts.

MEDICATION / TREATMENT	AMOUNT / TIME / COMMENTS

3

1 DAILY
PAIN CHART

DAY_____ DATE_____ WEIGHT_____

Connect the points on your Daily Pain and Satisfaction Charts so your medical team can see when your status changed.

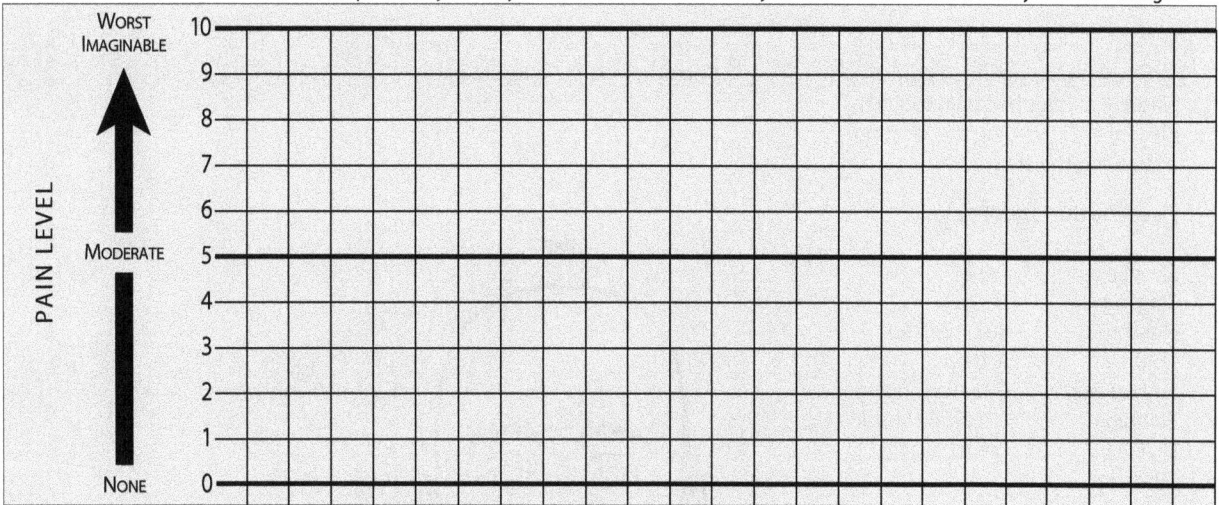

PAIN LEVEL

WORST IMAGINABLE — 10

9

8

7

6

MODERATE — 5

4

3

2

1

NONE — 0

2 SATISFACTION

MOOD

(HAPPY) POSITIVE

+2

+1

NEUTRAL

-1

-2

(UNHAPPY) NEGATIVE

6am 7 8 9 10 11 12pm 1 2 3 4 5 6pm 7 8 9 10 11 12am 1 2 3 4 5

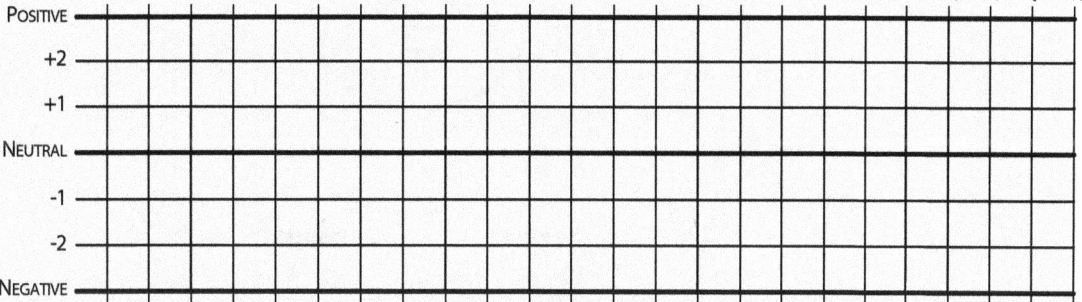

3 PHYSIOLOGY

6am 7 8 9 10 11 12pm 1 2 3 4 5 6pm 7 8 9 10 11 12am 1 2 3 4 5

SLEEP

RESTROOM

NAUSEA / DIZZINESS

MEAL / SNACK

EXERCISE

STRESS / ANXIETY

MEDICINE NAME / DOSE

1

2

3

BLOOD PRESSURE

PULSE

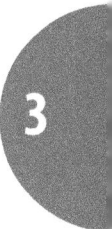

3

4 DAILY HEAD & FACE PAIN DIAGRAM

Mark each place on the diagram where you have had pain today by placing an 'X', circling the location, or shading the area .

Describe the type of pain:

Shooting	Deep
Tingling	Sharp
Numbness	Burning / Hot
Cold	Aching
Surface Pain	Gnawing / Biting
Stabbing	Electrical / Shocks
Dull	Other_____
Stinging	

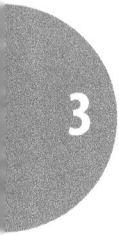

COMMENTS AND MORE INFORMATION:

Front

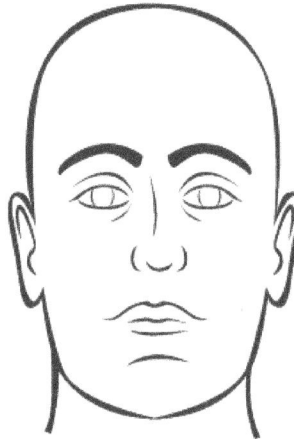

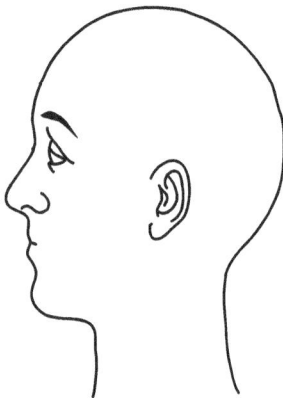

Your Right Side

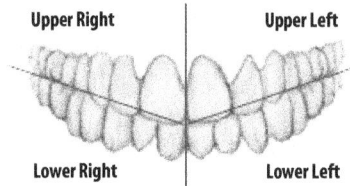

Upper Right   Upper Left

Lower Right   Lower Left

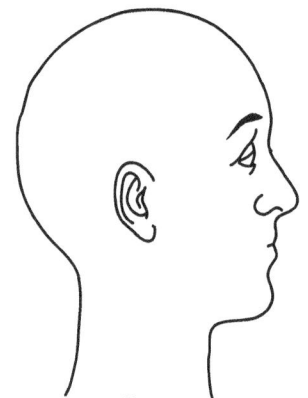

Your Right Side

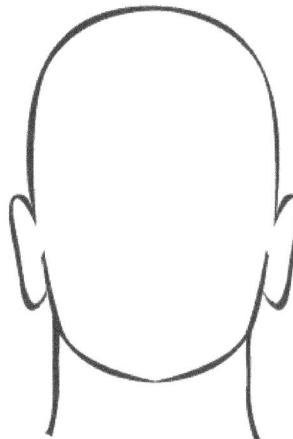

Back

5 DAILY BODY PAIN DIAGRAM

Mark each place on the diagram where you have had pain today by placing an 'X', circling the location, or shading the area .

Describe the type of pain:

Shooting	Deep
Tingling	Sharp
Numbness	Burning / Hot
Cold	Aching
Surface Pain	Gnawing / Biting
Stabbing	Electrical / Shocks
Dull	Other_____
Stinging	

COMMENTS AND MORE INFORMATION:

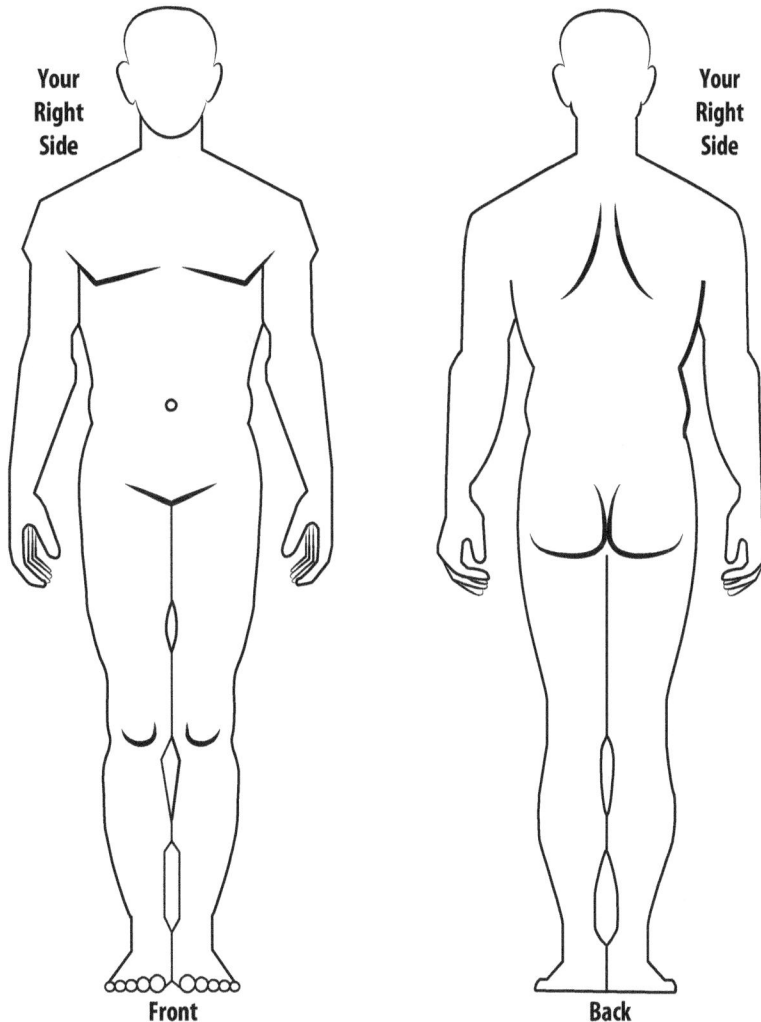

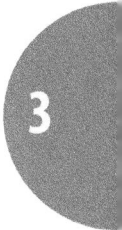

Your Right Side

Your Right Side

3

Front

Back

6 DAILY PAIN SUMMARY

Were there times during the day that you experienced unrelieved breakthrough pain? ____NO ____YES

How many times did this happen today?

1 2 3 4 5 6 7 8 9 10 more than 10

Did any specific activity start your breakthrough pain? ____NO ____YES: What activities?

_____

Put an "X" on the body diagram to show each place you've had *BREAKTHROUGH PAIN* today.

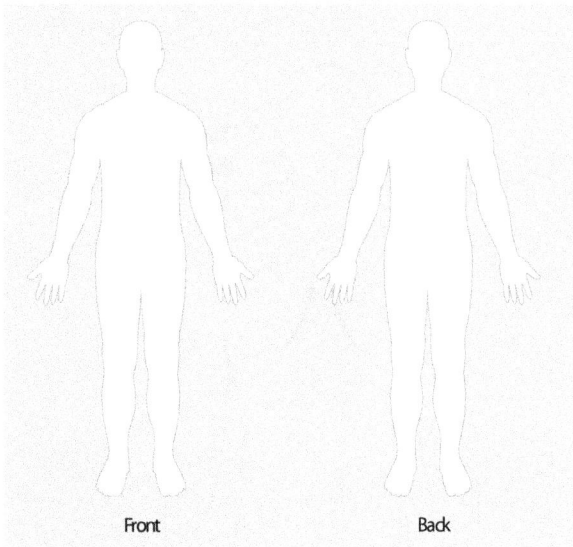

Front   Back

NON-DRUG THERAPIES
(other than prescription or other medicines)

_____

_____

ACTIVITIES/EXERCISE

_____

_____

What was your average level of pain today?

0 1 2 3 4 5 6 7 8 9 10

Other than prescription medicine, did you do anything else today to relieve the pain? ____NO ____YES: (Note any that you used.)
____ Non-prescription drugs (e.g., acetaminophen, ibuprofen)
____ Herbal remedies
____ Hot or cold packs
____ Exercise
____ Changing position (such as lying down or elevating your legs)
____ Physical therapy
____ Massage
____ Acupuncture
____ Rest
____ Psychological counseling
____ Talk to trusted friend, family, clergy
____ Prayer, meditation, guided imagery
____ Relaxation technique (hypnosis, biofeedback)
____ Creative technique (art or music therapy)
____ Other (e.g., specific chiropractic manipulation, osteopathic treatments):

_____

Check any of these common side effects that you've noticed after taking your pain medicine:
____ Drowsiness, sleepiness
____ Nausea, vomiting, upset stomach
____ Constipation
____ Lack of appetite
____ Other (describe):

_____

Did you sleep through the night? ____NO____YES

If not, how many times was your sleep disrupted? _____

How many hours did you sleep during the night? _____

COMMENTS AND MORE INFORMATION: Make notes for and about visits with your healthcare provider, side effects from treatments you may be experiencing, any problems you are having coping with your pain, and more about some of your previous answers or questions.

_____

_____

_____

1 DAILY DIARY

SATISFACTION CHART Connect the points on your Daily Satisfaction Chart so your medical team can see when and why your mental state changed.

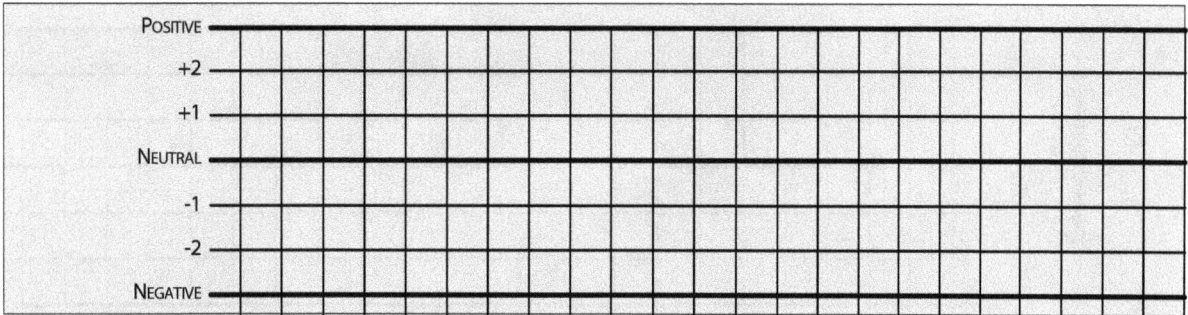

DAY_____ DATE_____ WEIGHT_____

POSITIVE
+2
+1
NEUTRAL
-1
-2
NEGATIVE

2 ACTIVITY LOG

6am 7 8 9 10 11 12pm 1 2 3 4 5 6pm 7 8 9 10 11 12am 1 2 3 4 5

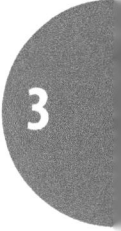

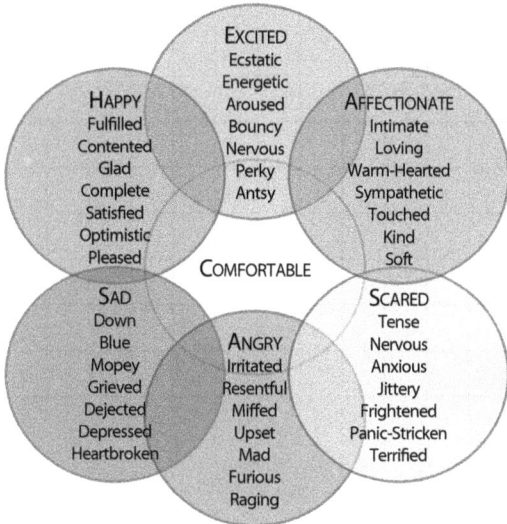

TRIGGERS AND SIGNIFICANT EVENTS

3

EXCITED
Ecstatic
Energetic
Aroused
Bouncy
Nervous
Perky
Antsy

HAPPY
Fulfilled
Contented
Glad
Complete
Satisfied
Optimistic
Pleased

AFFECTIONATE
Intimate
Loving
Warm-Hearted
Sympathetic
Touched
Kind
Soft

COMFORTABLE

SAD
Down
Blue
Mopey
Grieved
Dejected
Depressed
Heartbroken

ANGRY
Irritated
Resentful
Miffed
Upset
Mad
Furious
Raging

SCARED
Tense
Nervous
Anxious
Jittery
Frightened
Panic-Stricken
Terrified

Describe any changes in your pain today:
_____
_____
_____
_____
_____

Did anything unusual happen today?
_____
_____
_____
_____

What did you spend the most time time thinking about today?

Positive Thoughts:
_____
Did your pain increase, decrease, or remain the same when you thought about it?
____ Increased
____ Decreased
____ Stayed the Same

Negative Thoughts:
_____
Did your pain increase, decrease, or remain the same when you thought about it?
____ Increased
____ Decreased
____ Stayed the Same

1 DAILY
MOOD CHART

DAY_____ DATE_____ WEIGHT_____

Connect the points on your Mood Satisfaction Chart so your medical team can see when and why your mental state changed.

HAPPY   +3
         +2
         +1
MOOD   0
         -1
         -2
SAD   -3

2 ACTIVITY LOG

6am 7 8 9 10 11 12pm 1 2 3 4 5 6pm 7 8 9 10 11 12am 1 2 3 4 5

3 MEDICATION LOG
NAME/DOSE

1
2
3
4
5
6
7
8

4 PHYSIOLOGY

6am 7 8 9 10 11 12pm 1 2 3 4 5 6pm 7 8 9 10 11 12am 1 2 3 4 5

SLEEP
URINATION
DEFECATION
NAUSEA
EATING
EXERCISE
OTHER (LIST)

1 DAILY RESULTS
OF MEDICATIONS AND TREATMENTS

As you and your medical team develop new treatment plans, it will be especially helpful to record any side effects you experience as you add new treatments. This can help determine which types of treatments will work best for you.

Contact your care provider with any bad reactions or side effects to determine if you should discontinue the medication or treatment.

MEDICATION / TREATMENT	AMOUNT / TIME / COMMENTS

3

1 DAILY
TREATMENT PLAN

As you and your medical team develop new treatment plans, record your plan for the day including new medications, increases or decreases to medications, exercises, physical therapy, or any other treatment efforts.

Medication / Treatment	Amount / Time / Comments

4

1 DAILY
PAIN CHART

DAY_____ DATE_____ WEIGHT_____

Connect the points on your Daily Pain and Satisfaction Charts so your medical team can see when your status changed.

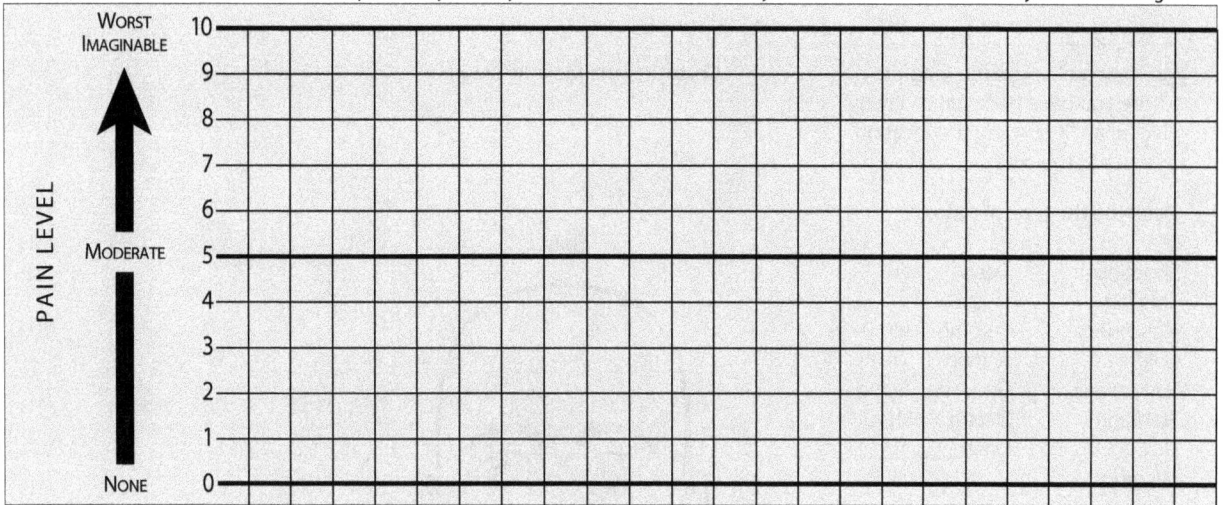

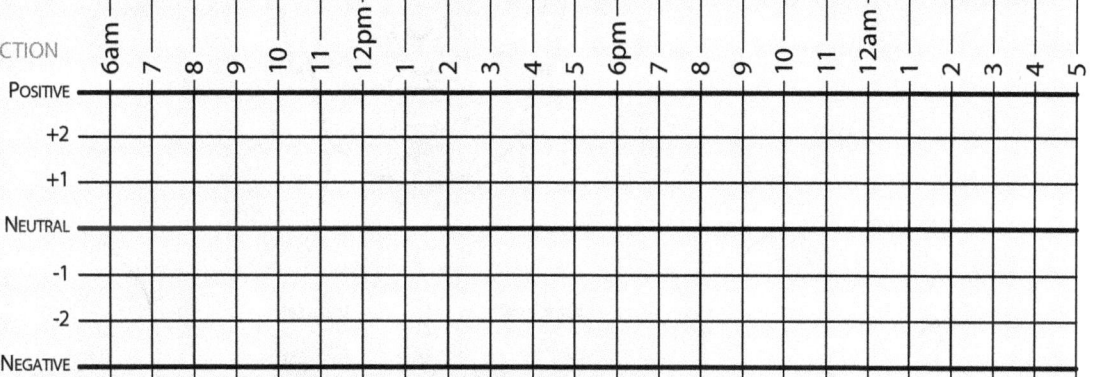

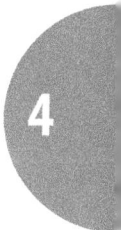

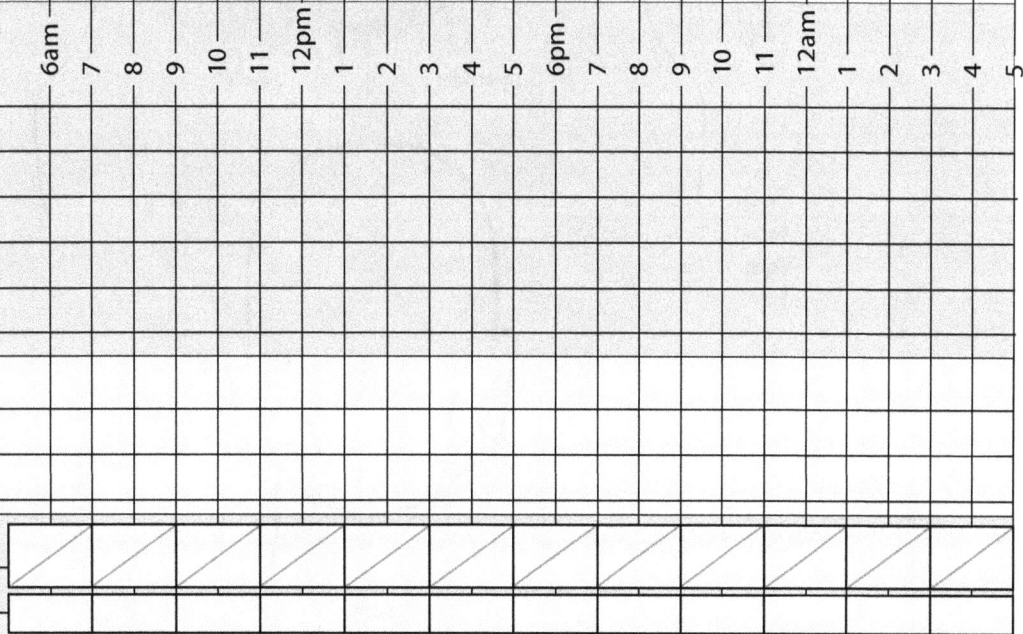

4 DAILY HEAD & FACE PAIN DIAGRAM

Mark each place on the diagram where you have had pain today by placing an 'X', circling the location, or shading the area .

Describe the type of pain:

Shooting	Deep
Tingling	Sharp
Numbness	Burning / Hot
Cold	Aching
Surface Pain	Gnawing / Biting
Stabbing	Electrical / Shocks
Dull	Other_____
Stinging	

COMMENTS AND MORE INFORMATION:

Front

Upper Right   **Upper Left**

Lower Right   **Lower Left**

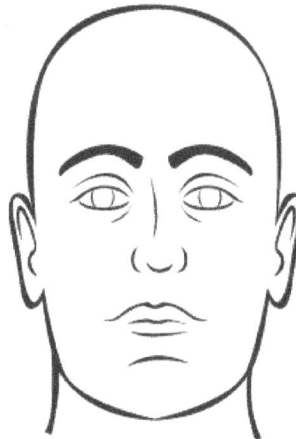

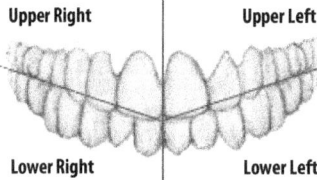

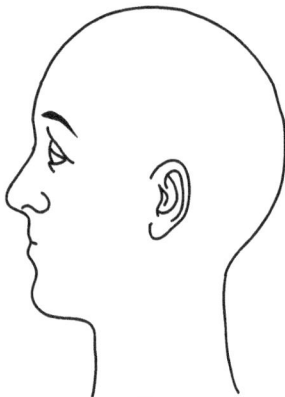

**Your
Right
Side**

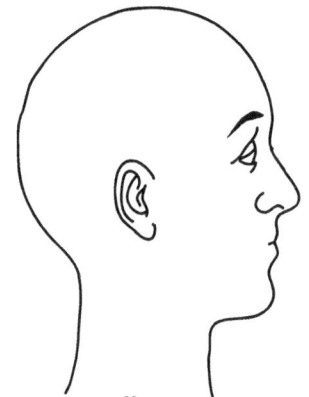

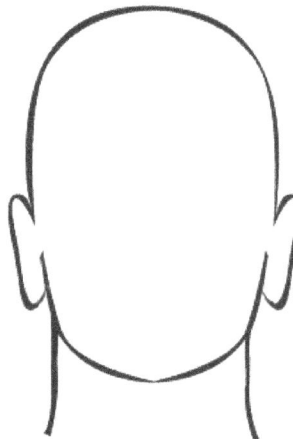

**Your
Right
Side**

Back

5 DAILY BODY PAIN DIAGRAM

Mark each place on the diagram where you have had pain today by placing an 'X', circling the location, or shading the area .

Describe the type of pain:

Shooting	Deep
Tingling	Sharp
Numbness	Burning / Hot
Cold	Aching
Surface Pain	Gnawing / Biting
Stabbing	Electrical / Shocks
Dull	Other_____
Stinging	

COMMENTS AND MORE INFORMATION:

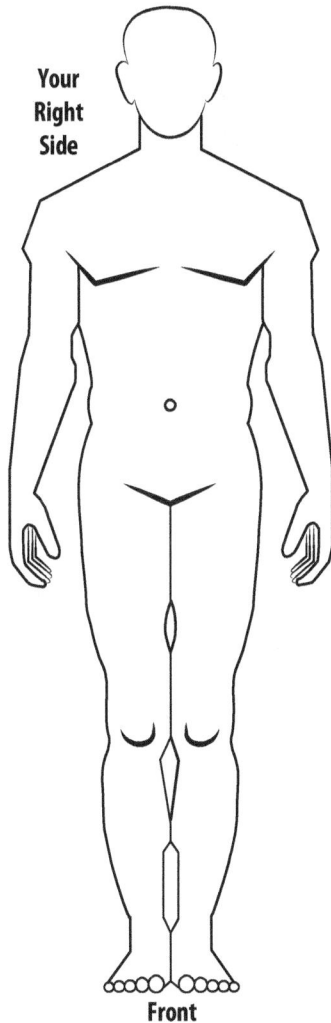

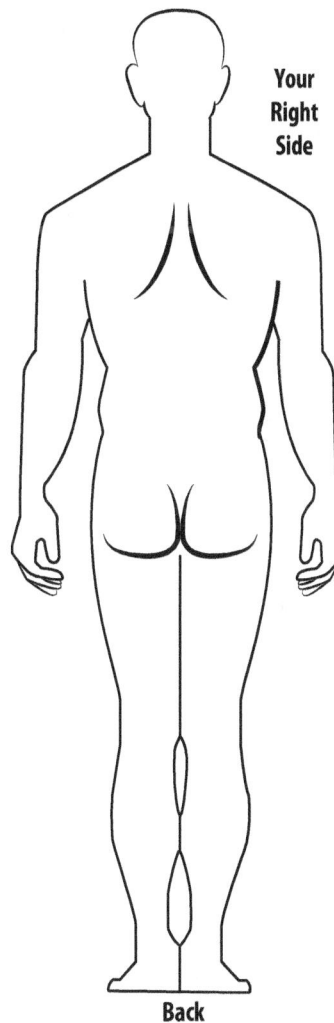

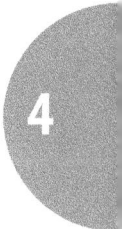

Your Right Side

Your Right Side

4

Front

Back

6 DAILY PAIN SUMMARY

Were there times during the day that you experienced unrelieved breakthrough pain? ____NO ____YES

How many times did this happen today?

1 2 3 4 5 6 7 8 9 10 more than 10

Did any specific activity start your breakthrough pain? ____NO ____YES: What activities?

_____

Put an "X" on the body diagram to show each place you've had *BREAKTHROUGH PAIN* today.

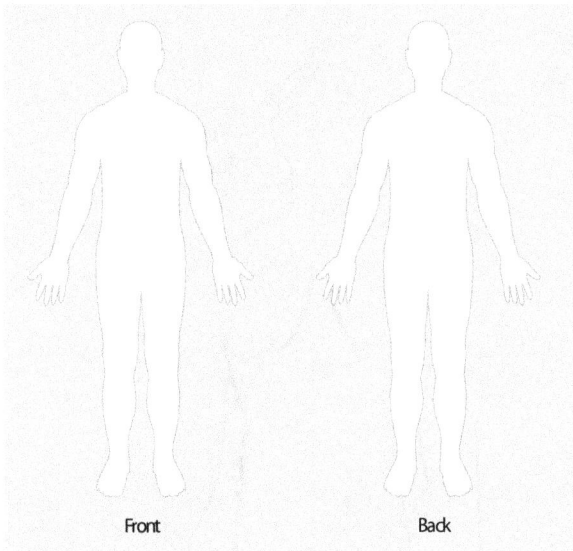

Front   Back

NON-DRUG THERAPIES
(other than prescription or other medicines)

_____

_____

ACTIVITIES/EXERCISE

_____

_____

What was your average level of pain today?

0 1 2 3 4 5 6 7 8 9 10

Other than prescription medicine, did you do anything else today to relieve the pain? ____NO ____YES: (Note any that you used.)
____ Non-prescription drugs (e.g., acetaminophen, ibuprofen)
____ Herbal remedies
____ Hot or cold packs
____ Exercise
____ Changing position (such as lying down or elevating your legs)
____ Physical therapy
____ Massage
____ Acupuncture
____ Rest
____ Psychological counseling
____ Talk to trusted friend, family, clergy
____ Prayer, meditation, guided imagery
____ Relaxation technique (hypnosis, biofeedback)
____ Creative technique (art or music therapy)
____ Other (e.g., specific chiropractic manipulation, osteopathic treatments):

_____

Check any of these common side effects that you've noticed after taking your pain medicine:
____ Drowsiness, sleepiness
____ Nausea, vomiting, upset stomach
____ Constipation
____ Lack of appetite
____ Other (describe):

_____

Did you sleep through the night? ____NO____YES

If not, how many times was your sleep disrupted? _____

How many hours did you sleep during the night? _____

COMMENTS AND MORE INFORMATION: Make notes for and about visits with your healthcare provider, side effects from treatments you may be experiencing, any problems you are having coping with your pain, and more about some of your previous answers or questions.

_____

_____

_____

1 DAILY DIARY

DAY_____ DATE_____ WEIGHT_____

SATISFACTION CHART Connect the points on your Daily Satisfaction Chart so your medical team can see when and why your mental state changed.

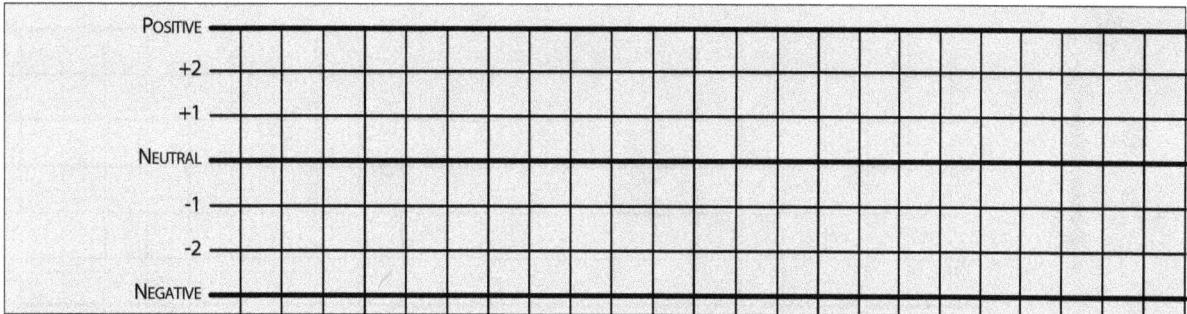

POSITIVE
+2
+1
NEUTRAL
-1
-2
NEGATIVE

2 ACTIVITY LOG

6am 7 8 9 10 11 12pm 1 2 3 4 5 6pm 7 8 9 10 11 12am 1 2 3 4 5

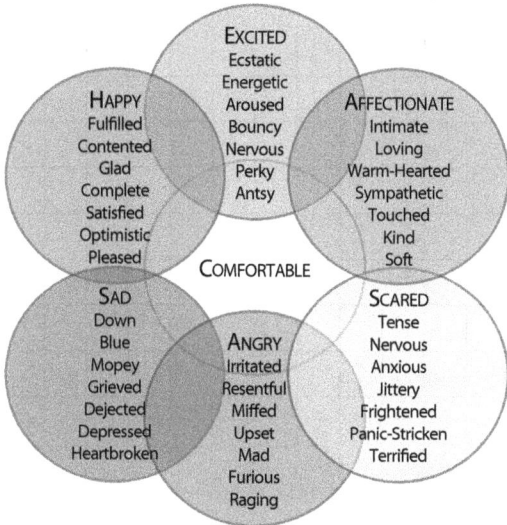

TRIGGERS AND SIGNIFICANT EVENTS

EXCITED
Ecstatic
Energetic
Aroused
Bouncy
Nervous
Perky
Antsy

HAPPY
Fulfilled
Contented
Glad
Complete
Satisfied
Optimistic
Pleased

AFFECTIONATE
Intimate
Loving
Warm-Hearted
Sympathetic
Touched
Kind
Soft

COMFORTABLE

SAD
Down
Blue
Mopey
Grieved
Dejected
Depressed
Heartbroken

ANGRY
Irritated
Resentful
Miffed
Upset
Mad
Furious
Raging

SCARED
Tense
Nervous
Anxious
Jittery
Frightened
Panic-Stricken
Terrified

Describe any changes in your pain today:

_____

_____

_____

_____

Did anything unusual happen today?

_____

_____

_____

_____

What did you spend the most time time thinking about today?

Positive Thoughts:

_____

Did your pain increase, decrease, or remain the same when you thought about it?
____ Increased
____ Decreased
____ Stayed the Same

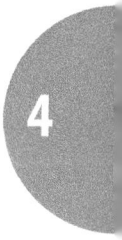

Negative Thoughts:

_____

Did your pain increase, decrease, or remain the same when you thought about it?
____ Increased
____ Decreased
____ Stayed the Same

4

DAY_____ DATE_____ WEIGHT_____

1 DAILY
MOOD CHART

Connect the points on your Mood Satisfaction Chart so your medical team can see when and why your mental state changed.

HAPPY +3
       +2
       +1
MOOD   0
       -1
       -2
SAD   -3

2 ACTIVITY LOG

6am 7 8 9 10 11 12pm 1 2 3 4 5 6pm 7 8 9 10 11 12am 1 2 3 4 5

3 MEDICATION LOG
NAME/DOSE

1————
2————
3————
4————
5————
6————
7————
8————

4 PHYSIOLOGY

6am 7 8 9 10 11 12pm 1 2 3 4 5 6pm 7 8 9 10 11 12am 1 2 3 4 5

SLEEP ————
URINATION ————
DEFECATION ————
NAUSEA ————
EATING ————
EXERCISE ————
OTHER (LIST) ————

1 DAILY RESULTS
OF MEDICATIONS AND TREATMENTS

As you and your medical team develop new treatment plans, it will be especially helpful to record any side effects you experience as you add new treatments. This can help determine which types of treatments will work best for you.

Contact your care provider with any bad reactions or side effects to determine if you should discontinue the medication or treatment.

MEDICATION / TREATMENT	AMOUNT / TIME / COMMENTS

4

1 DAILY
TREATMENT PLAN

As you and your medical team develop new treatment plans, record your plan for the day including new medications, increases or decreases to medications, exercises, physical therapy, or any other treatment efforts.

MEDICATION / TREATMENT	AMOUNT / TIME / COMMENTS

5

1 DAILY PAIN CHART

DAY_____ DATE_____ WEIGHT_____

Connect the points on your Daily Pain and Satisfaction Charts so your medical team can see when your status changed.

PAIN LEVEL

WORST IMAGINABLE — 10
9
8
7
6
MODERATE — 5
4
3
2
1
NONE — 0

2 SATISFACTION

6am 7 8 9 10 11 12pm 1 2 3 4 5 6pm 7 8 9 10 11 12am 1 2 3 4 5

MOOD

(HAPPY) POSITIVE
+2
+1
NEUTRAL
-1
-2
(UNHAPPY) NEGATIVE

3 PHYSIOLOGY

6am 7 8 9 10 11 12pm 1 2 3 4 5 6pm 7 8 9 10 11 12am 1 2 3 4 5

SLEEP
RESTROOM
NAUSEA / DIZZINESS
MEAL / SNACK
EXERCISE
STRESS / ANXIETY
MEDICINE NAME / DOSE
1
2
3
BLOOD PRESSURE
PULSE

4 DAILY HEAD & FACE PAIN DIAGRAM

Mark each place on the diagram where you have had pain today by placing an 'X', circling the location, or shading the area .

COMMENTS AND MORE INFORMATION:

Describe the type of pain:

Shooting	Deep
Tingling	Sharp
Numbness	Burning / Hot
Cold	Aching
Surface Pain	Gnawing / Biting
Stabbing	Electrical / Shocks
Dull	Other_____
Stinging	

Front

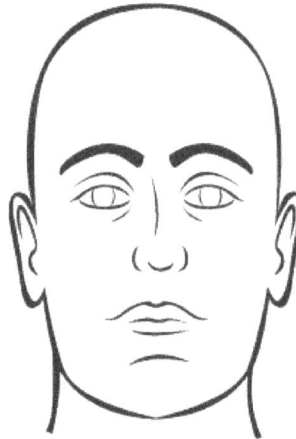

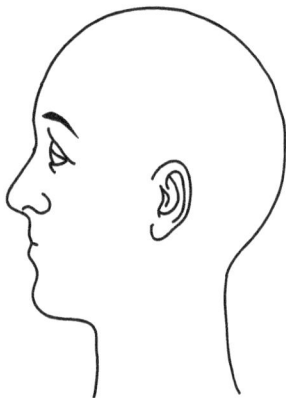

Your Right Side

Upper Right   Upper Left

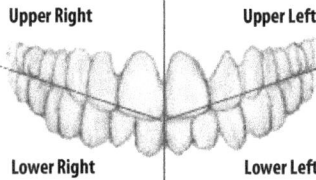

Lower Right   Lower Left

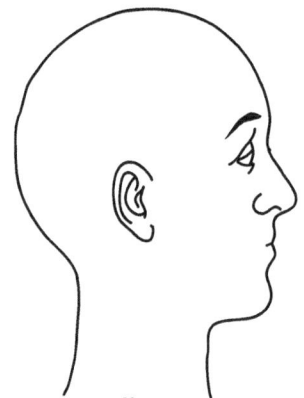

Your Right Side

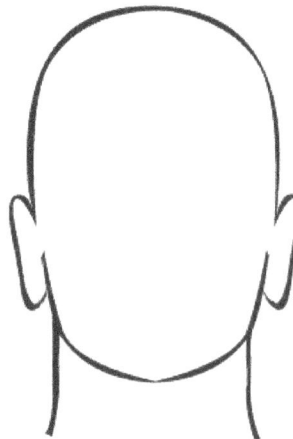

Back

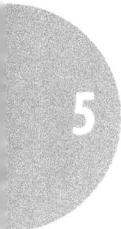

5 DAILY BODY PAIN DIAGRAM

Mark each place on the diagram where you have had pain today by placing an 'X', circling the location, or shading the area .

Describe the type of pain:

Shooting	Deep
Tingling	Sharp
Numbness	Burning / Hot
Cold	Aching
Surface Pain	Gnawing / Biting
Stabbing	Electrical / Shocks
Dull	Other_____
Stinging	

COMMENTS AND MORE INFORMATION:

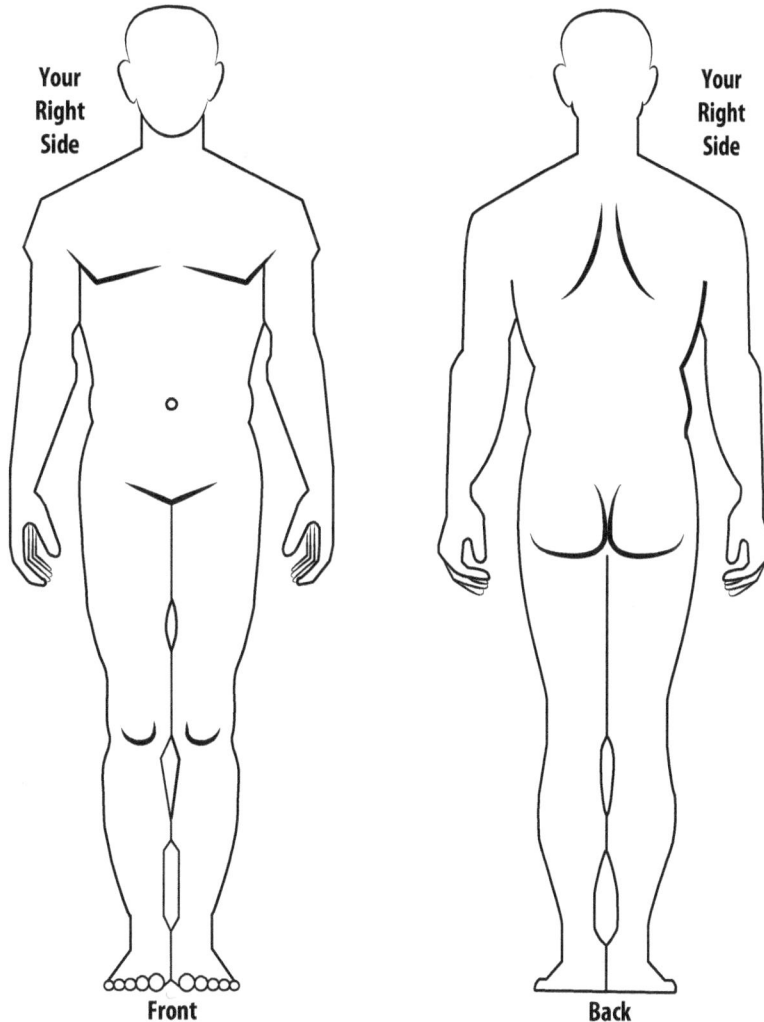

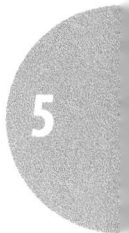

Your Right Side

Your Right Side

Front

Back

5

6 DAILY PAIN SUMMARY

Were there times during the day that you experienced unrelieved breakthrough pain? ____NO ____YES

How many times did this happen today?

1 2 3 4 5 6 7 8 9 10 more than 10

Did any specific activity start your breakthrough pain? ____NO ____YES: What activities?

_____

Put an "X" on the body diagram to show each place you've had *BREAKTHROUGH PAIN* today.

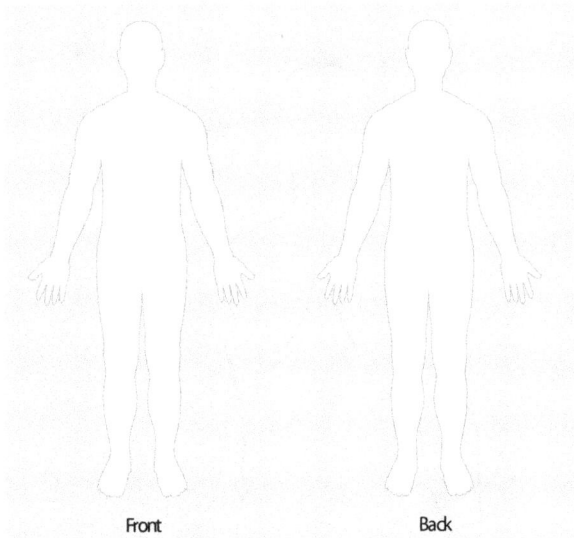

Front   Back

NON-DRUG THERAPIES
(other than prescription or other medicines)

_____

_____

ACTIVITIES/EXERCISE

_____

_____

What was your average level of pain today?

0   1   2   3   4   5   6   7   8   9   10

Other than prescription medicine, did you do anything else today to relieve the pain? ____NO ____YES: (Note any that you used.)
____ Non-prescription drugs (e.g., acetaminophen, ibuprofen)
____ Herbal remedies
____ Hot or cold packs
____ Exercise
____ Changing position (such as lying down or elevating your legs)
____ Physical therapy
____ Massage
____ Acupuncture
____ Rest
____ Psychological counseling
____ Talk to trusted friend, family, clergy
____ Prayer, meditation, guided imagery
____ Relaxation technique (hypnosis, biofeedback)
____ Creative technique (art or music therapy)
____ Other (e.g., specific chiropractic manipulation, osteopathic treatments):

_____

Check any of these common side effects that you've noticed after taking your pain medicine:
____ Drowsiness, sleepiness
____ Nausea, vomiting, upset stomach
____ Constipation
____ Lack of appetite
____ Other (describe):

_____

Did you sleep through the night? ____NO____YES

If not, how many times was your sleep disrupted? _____

How many hours did you sleep during the night? _____

COMMENTS AND MORE INFORMATION: Make notes for and about visits with your healthcare provider, side effects from treatments you may be experiencing, any problems you are having coping with your pain, and more about some of your previous answers or questions.

_____

_____

_____

1 DAILY DIARY

DAY_____ DATE_____ WEIGHT_____

SATISFACTION CHART Connect the points on your Daily Satisfaction Chart so your medical team can see when and why your mental state changed.

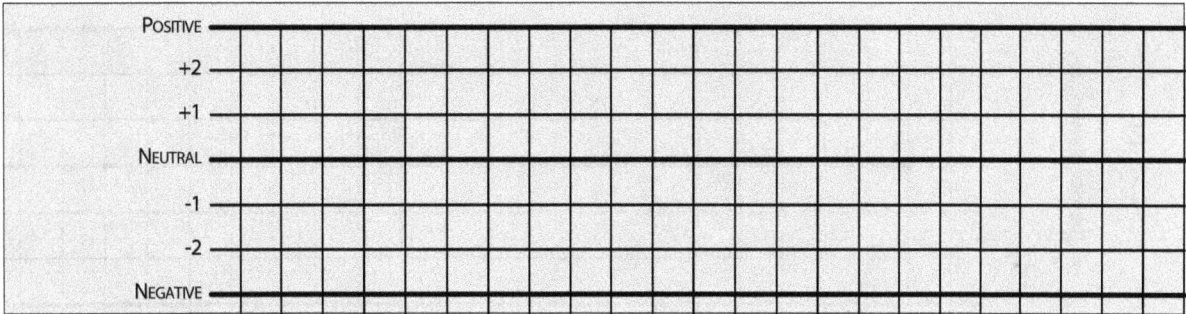

POSITIVE	
+2	
+1	
NEUTRAL	
-1	
-2	
NEGATIVE	

2 ACTIVITY LOG

TRIGGERS AND SIGNIFICANT EVENTS

6am 7 8 9 10 11 12pm 1 2 3 4 5 6pm 7 8 9 10 11 12am 1 2 3 4 5

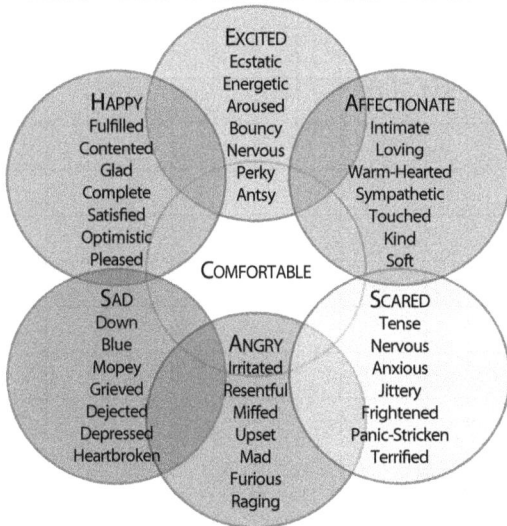

EXCITED
Ecstatic
Energetic
Aroused
Bouncy
Nervous
Perky
Antsy

HAPPY
Fulfilled
Contented
Glad
Complete
Satisfied
Optimistic
Pleased

AFFECTIONATE
Intimate
Loving
Warm-Hearted
Sympathetic
Touched
Kind
Soft

COMFORTABLE

SAD
Down
Blue
Mopey
Grieved
Dejected
Depressed
Heartbroken

ANGRY
Irritated
Resentful
Miffed
Upset
Mad
Furious
Raging

SCARED
Tense
Nervous
Anxious
Jittery
Frightened
Panic-Stricken
Terrified

Describe any changes in your pain today:

_____
_____
_____
_____

Did anything unusual happen today?

_____
_____
_____
_____

5

What did you spend the most time time thinking about today?

Positive Thoughts:	Negative Thoughts:
_____	_____
Did your pain increase, decrease, or remain the same when you thought about it?	Did your pain increase, decrease, or remain the same when you thought about it?
____ Increased	____ Increased
____ Decreased	____ Decreased
____ Stayed the Same	____ Stayed the Same

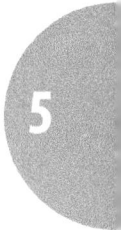

1 DAILY
MOOD CHART

DAY_____ DATE_____ WEIGHT_____

Connect the points on your Mood Satisfaction Chart so your medical team can see when and why your mental state changed.

HAPPY +3
+2
+1
MOOD 0
-1
-2
SAD -3

2 ACTIVITY LOG

6am 7 8 9 10 11 12pm 1 2 3 4 5 6pm 7 8 9 10 11 12am 1 2 3 4 5

3 MEDICATION LOG
NAME/DOSE

1
2
3
4
5
6
7
8

4 PHYSIOLOGY

6am 7 8 9 10 11 12pm 1 2 3 4 5 6pm 7 8 9 10 11 12am 1 2 3 4 5

SLEEP
URINATION
DEFECATION
NAUSEA
EATING
EXERCISE
OTHER (LIST)

1 DAILY RESULTS
OF MEDICATIONS AND TREATMENTS

As you and your medical team develop new treatment plans, it will be especially helpful to record any side effects you experience as you add new treatments. This can help determine which types of treatments will work best for you.

Contact your care provider with any bad reactions or side effects to determine if you should discontinue the medication or treatment.

MEDICATION / TREATMENT	AMOUNT / TIME / COMMENTS

5

1 DAILY
TREATMENT PLAN

As you and your medical team develop new treatment plans, record your plan for the day including new medications, increases or decreases to medications, exercises, physical therapy, or any other treatment efforts.

MEDICATION / TREATMENT	AMOUNT / TIME / COMMENTS

6

1 DAILY PAIN CHART

DAY_____ DATE_____ WEIGHT_____

Connect the points on your Daily Pain and Satisfaction Charts so your medical team can see when your status changed.

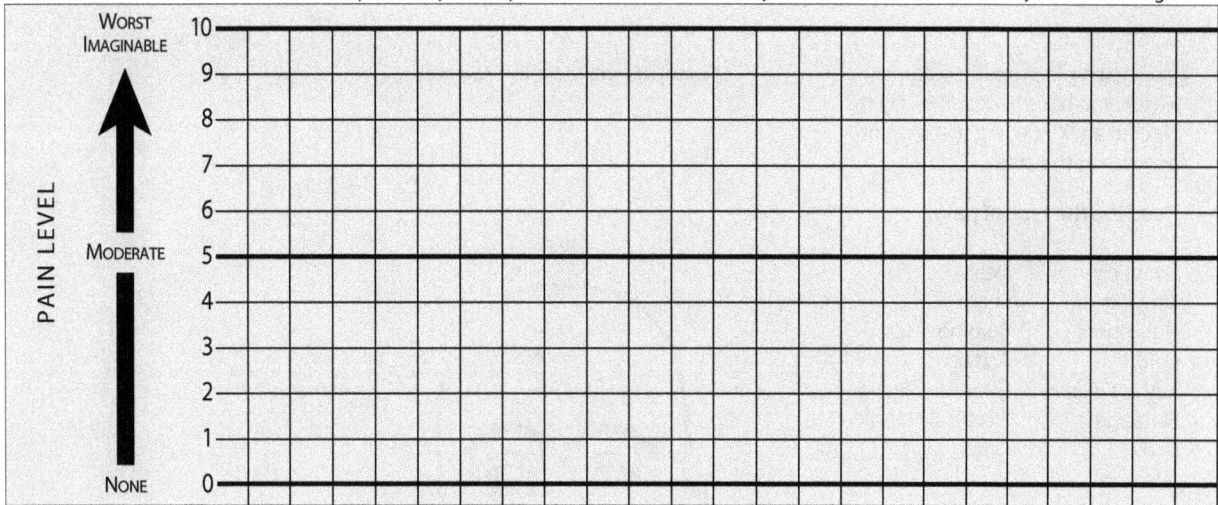

PAIN LEVEL

WORST IMAGINABLE — 10
9
8
7
6
MODERATE — 5
4
3
2
1
NONE — 0

6am 7 8 9 10 11 12pm 1 2 3 4 5 6pm 7 8 9 10 11 12am 1 2 3 4 5

2 SATISFACTION

MOOD

(HAPPY) POSITIVE
+2
+1
NEUTRAL
-1
-2
(UNHAPPY) NEGATIVE

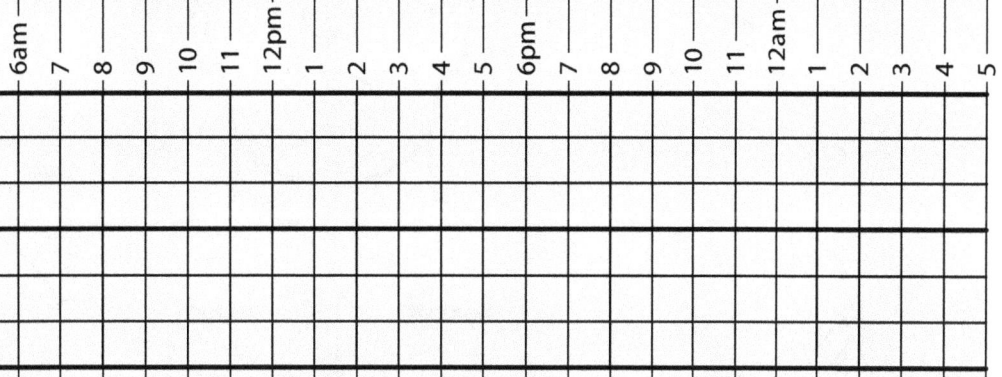

6am 7 8 9 10 11 12pm 1 2 3 4 5 6pm 7 8 9 10 11 12am 1 2 3 4 5

3 PHYSIOLOGY

6am 7 8 9 10 11 12pm 1 2 3 4 5 6pm 7 8 9 10 11 12am 1 2 3 4 5

SLEEP
RESTROOM
NAUSEA / DIZZINESS
MEAL / SNACK
EXERCISE
STRESS / ANXIETY
MEDICINE NAME / DOSE
1
2
3
BLOOD PRESSURE
PULSE

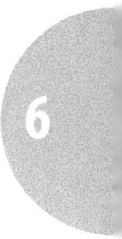

6

4 DAILY HEAD & FACE PAIN DIAGRAM

Mark each place on the diagram where you have had pain today by placing an 'X', circling the location, or shading the area .

Describe the type of pain:

Shooting	Deep
Tingling	Sharp
Numbness	Burning / Hot
Cold	Aching
Surface Pain	Gnawing / Biting
Stabbing	Electrical / Shocks
Dull	Other_____
Stinging	

COMMENTS AND MORE INFORMATION:

Front

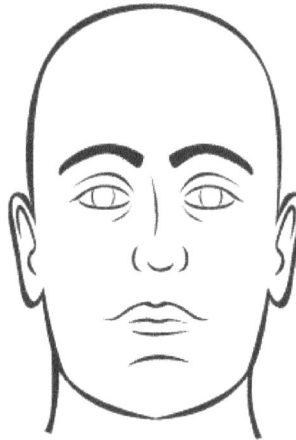

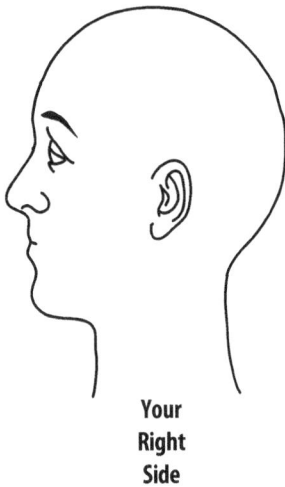

Your Right Side

Upper Right   Upper Left

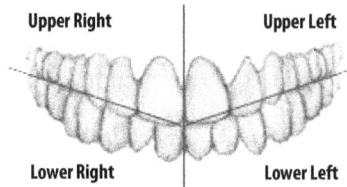

Lower Right   Lower Left

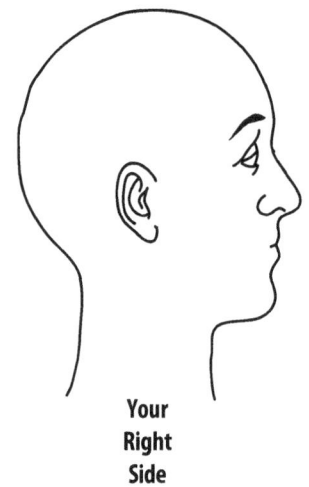

Your Right Side

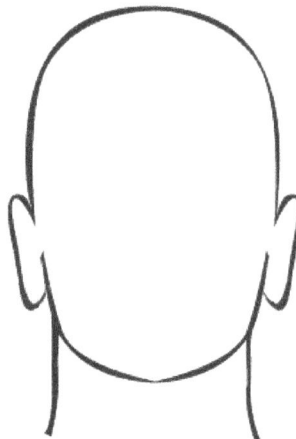

Back

6

5 DAILY BODY PAIN DIAGRAM

Mark each place on the diagram where you have had pain today by placing an 'X', circling the location, or shading the area .

Describe the type of pain:

Shooting	Deep
Tingling	Sharp
Numbness	Burning / Hot
Cold	Aching
Surface Pain	Gnawing / Biting
Stabbing	Electrical / Shocks
Dull	Other_____
Stinging	

COMMENTS AND MORE INFORMATION:

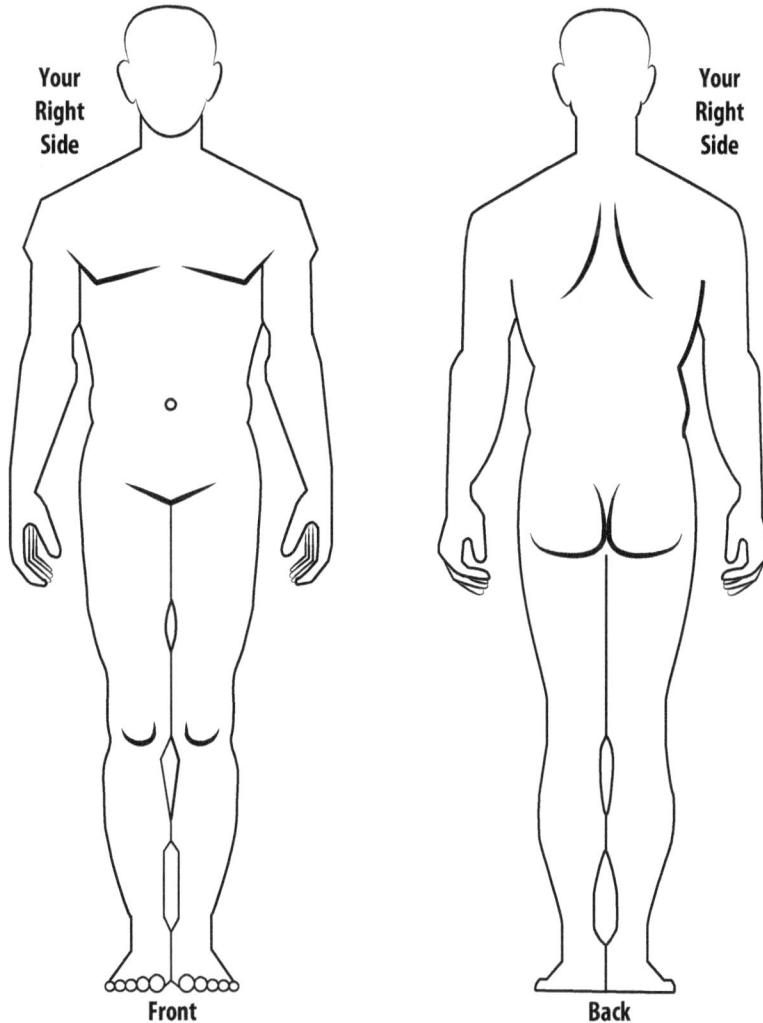

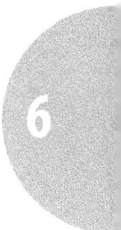

Your
Right
Side

Your
Right
Side

Front

Back

6

6 DAILY PAIN SUMMARY

Were there times during the day that you experienced unrelieved breakthrough pain? ____NO ____YES

How many times did this happen today?

1   2   3   4   5   6   7   8   9   10   more than 10

Did any specific activity start your breakthrough pain? ____NO ____YES: What activities?

_____

Put an "X" on the body diagram to show each place you've had *BREAKTHROUGH PAIN* today.

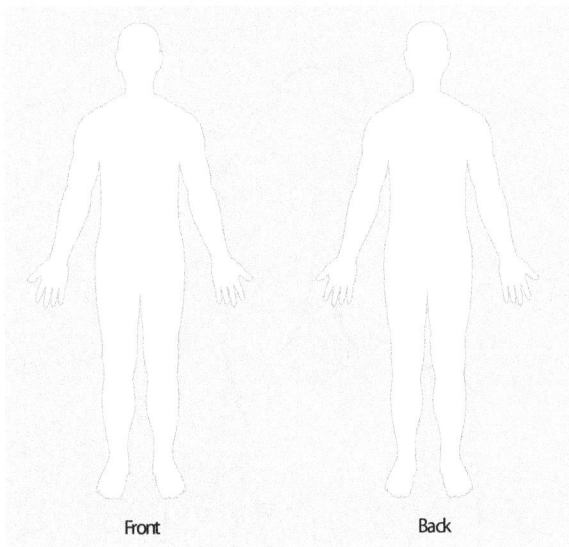

Front   Back

NON-DRUG THERAPIES
(other than prescription or other medicines)

_____

_____

ACTIVITIES/EXERCISE

_____

_____

What was your average level of pain today?

0   1   2   3   4   5   6   7   8   9   10

Other than prescription medicine, did you do anything else today to relieve the pain? ____NO ____YES:
(Note any that you used.)
____ Non-prescription drugs (e.g., acetaminophen, ibuprofen)
____ Herbal remedies
____ Hot or cold packs
____ Exercise
____ Changing position (such as lying down or elevating your legs)
____ Physical therapy
____ Massage
____ Acupuncture
____ Rest
____ Psychological counseling
____ Talk to trusted friend, family, clergy
____ Prayer, meditation, guided imagery
____ Relaxation technique (hypnosis, biofeedback)
____ Creative technique (art or music therapy)
____ Other (e.g., specific chiropractic manipulation, osteopathic treatments):

_____

Check any of these common side effects that you've noticed after taking your pain medicine:
____ Drowsiness, sleepiness
____ Nausea, vomiting, upset stomach
____ Constipation
____ Lack of appetite
____ Other (describe):

_____

Did you sleep through the night? ____NO____YES

If not, how many times was your sleep disrupted? _____

How many hours did you sleep during the night? _____

COMMENTS AND MORE INFORMATION: Make notes for and about visits with your healthcare provider, side effects from treatments you may be experiencing, any problems you are having coping with your pain, and more about some of your previous answers or questions.

_____

_____

_____

1 DAILY DIARY

SATISFACTION CHART

Day_____ Date_____ Weight_____

Connect the points on your Daily Satisfaction Chart so your medical team can see when and why your mental state changed.

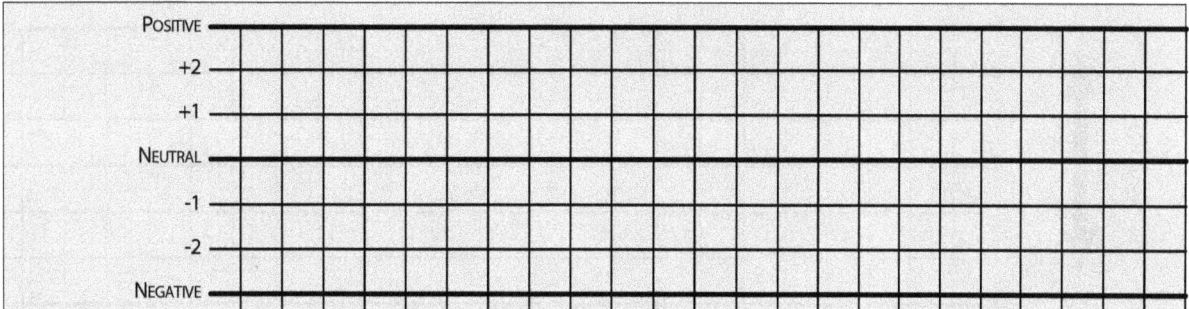

POSITIVE	
+2	
+1	
NEUTRAL	
-1	
-2	
NEGATIVE	

2 ACTIVITY LOG

6am 7 8 9 10 11 12pm 1 2 3 4 5 6pm 7 8 9 10 11 12am 1 2 3 4 5

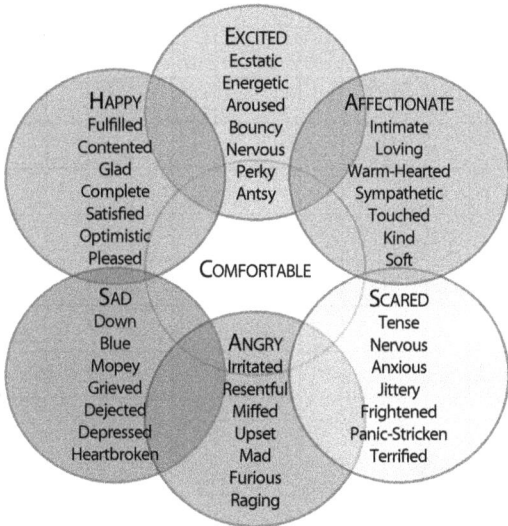

TRIGGERS AND SIGNIFICANT EVENTS

EXCITED
Ecstatic
Energetic
Aroused
Bouncy
Nervous
Perky
Antsy

HAPPY
Fulfilled
Contented
Glad
Complete
Satisfied
Optimistic
Pleased

AFFECTIONATE
Intimate
Loving
Warm-Hearted
Sympathetic
Touched
Kind
Soft

COMFORTABLE

SAD
Down
Blue
Mopey
Grieved
Dejected
Depressed
Heartbroken

ANGRY
Irritated
Resentful
Miffed
Upset
Mad
Furious
Raging

SCARED
Tense
Nervous
Anxious
Jittery
Frightened
Panic-Stricken
Terrified

Describe any changes in your pain today:

_____
_____
_____
_____

Did anything unusual happen today?

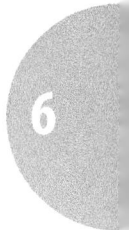

_____
_____
_____
_____

What did you spend the most time time thinking about today?

Positive Thoughts:

_____

Did your pain increase, decrease, or remain the same when you thought about it?
____ Increased
____ Decreased
____ Stayed the Same

Negative Thoughts:

_____

Did your pain increase, decrease, or remain the same when you thought about it?
____ Increased
____ Decreased
____ Stayed the Same

6

1 DAILY
MOOD CHART

DAY_____ DATE_____ WEIGHT_____

Connect the points on your Mood Satisfaction Chart so your medical team can see when and why your mental state changed.

MOOD

HAPPY	+3	
	+2	
	+1	
	0	
	-1	
	-2	
SAD	-3	

2 ACTIVITY LOG

6am 7 8 9 10 11 12pm 1 2 3 4 5 6pm 7 8 9 10 11 12am 1 2 3 4 5

3 MEDICATION LOG
NAME/DOSE

1
2
3
4
5
6
7
8

4 PHYSIOLOGY

6am 7 8 9 10 11 12pm 1 2 3 4 5 6pm 7 8 9 10 11 12am 1 2 3 4 5

SLEEP
URINATION
DEFECATION
NAUSEA
EATING
EXERCISE
OTHER (LIST)

6

1 DAILY RESULTS
OF MEDICATIONS AND TREATMENTS

As you and your medical team develop new treatment plans, it will be especially helpful to record any side effects you experience as you add new treatments. This can help determine which types of treatments will work best for you.

Contact your care provider with any bad reactions or side effects to determine if you should discontinue the medication or treatment.

MEDICATION / TREATMENT	AMOUNT / TIME / COMMENTS

6

1 DAILY
TREATMENT PLAN

As you and your medical team develop new treatment plans, record your plan for the day including new medications, increases or decreases to medications, exercises, physical therapy, or any other treatment efforts.

MEDICATION / TREATMENT	AMOUNT / TIME / COMMENTS

1 DAILY PAIN CHART

DAY_____ DATE_____ WEIGHT_____

Connect the points on your Daily Pain and Satisfaction Charts so your medical team can see when your status changed.

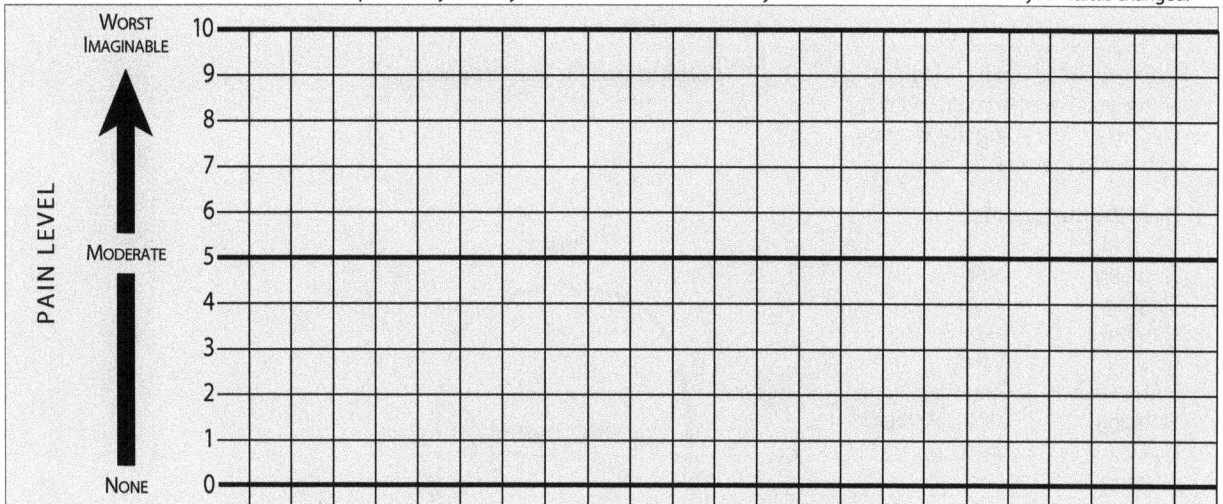

PAIN LEVEL

- WORST IMAGINABLE — 10
- 9
- 8
- 7
- 6
- MODERATE — 5
- 4
- 3
- 2
- 1
- NONE — 0

2 SATISFACTION

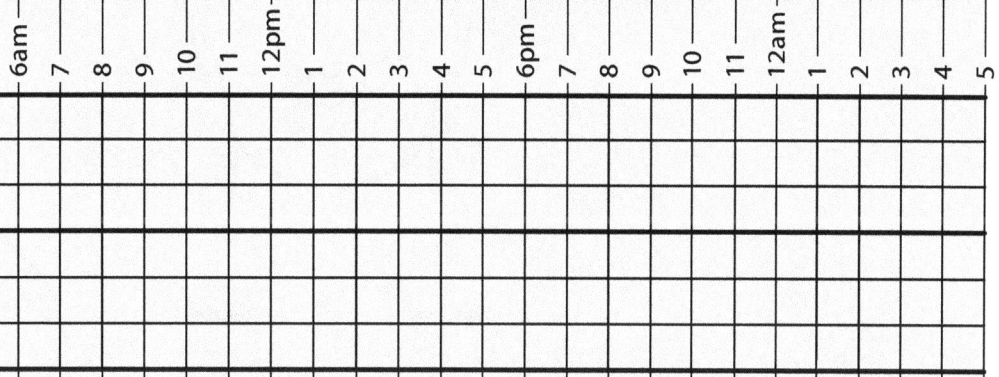

MOOD

- (HAPPY) POSITIVE
- +2
- +1
- NEUTRAL
- -1
- -2
- (UNHAPPY) NEGATIVE

Time axis: 6am, 7, 8, 9, 10, 11, 12pm, 1, 2, 3, 4, 5, 6pm, 7, 8, 9, 10, 11, 12am, 1, 2, 3, 4, 5

3 PHYSIOLOGY

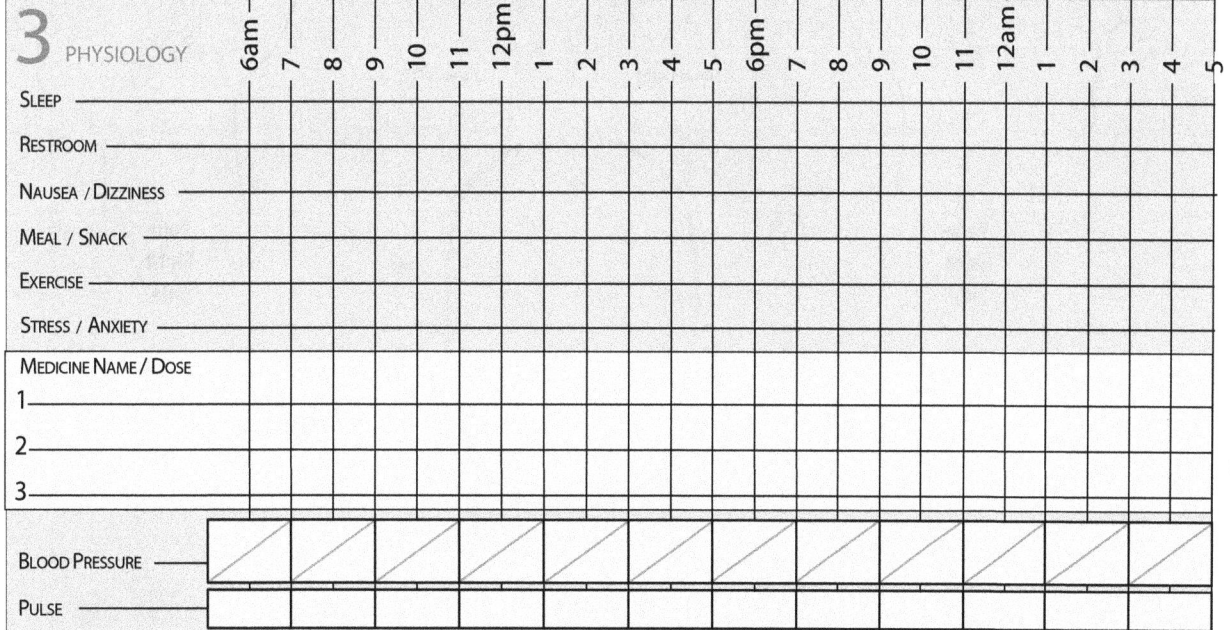

Time axis: 6am, 7, 8, 9, 10, 11, 12pm, 1, 2, 3, 4, 5, 6pm, 7, 8, 9, 10, 11, 12am, 1, 2, 3, 4, 5

- SLEEP
- RESTROOM
- NAUSEA / DIZZINESS
- MEAL / SNACK
- EXERCISE
- STRESS / ANXIETY
- MEDICINE NAME / DOSE
  1
  2
  3
- BLOOD PRESSURE
- PULSE

4 DAILY HEAD & FACE PAIN DIAGRAM

Mark each place on the diagram where you have had pain today by placing an 'X', circling the location, or shading the area.

Describe the type of pain:

Shooting	Deep
Tingling	Sharp
Numbness	Burning / Hot
Cold	Aching
Surface Pain	Gnawing / Biting
Stabbing	Electrical / Shocks
Dull	Other_____
Stinging	

COMMENTS AND MORE INFORMATION:

Front

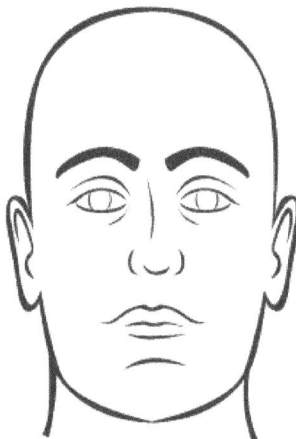

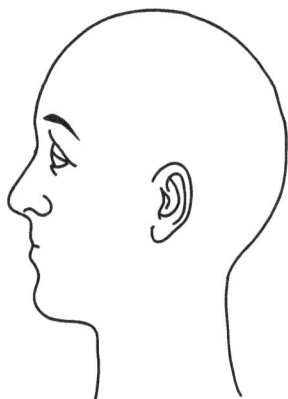

Your Right Side

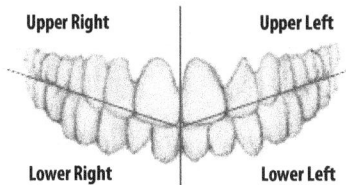

Upper Right   Upper Left

Lower Right   Lower Left

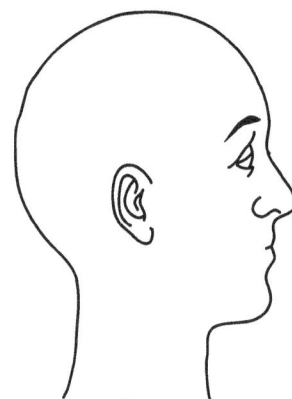

Your Right Side

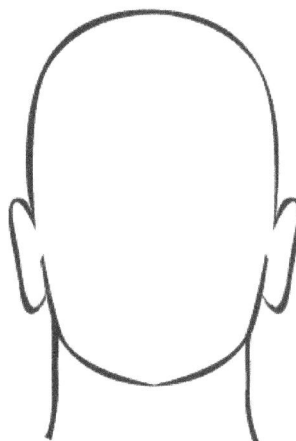

Back

5 DAILY BODY PAIN DIAGRAM

Mark each place on the diagram where you have had pain today by placing an 'X', circling the location, or shading the area .

Describe the type of pain:

Shooting	Deep
Tingling	Sharp
Numbness	Burning / Hot
Cold	Aching
Surface Pain	Gnawing / Biting
Stabbing	Electrical / Shocks
Dull	Other_____
Stinging	

COMMENTS AND MORE INFORMATION:

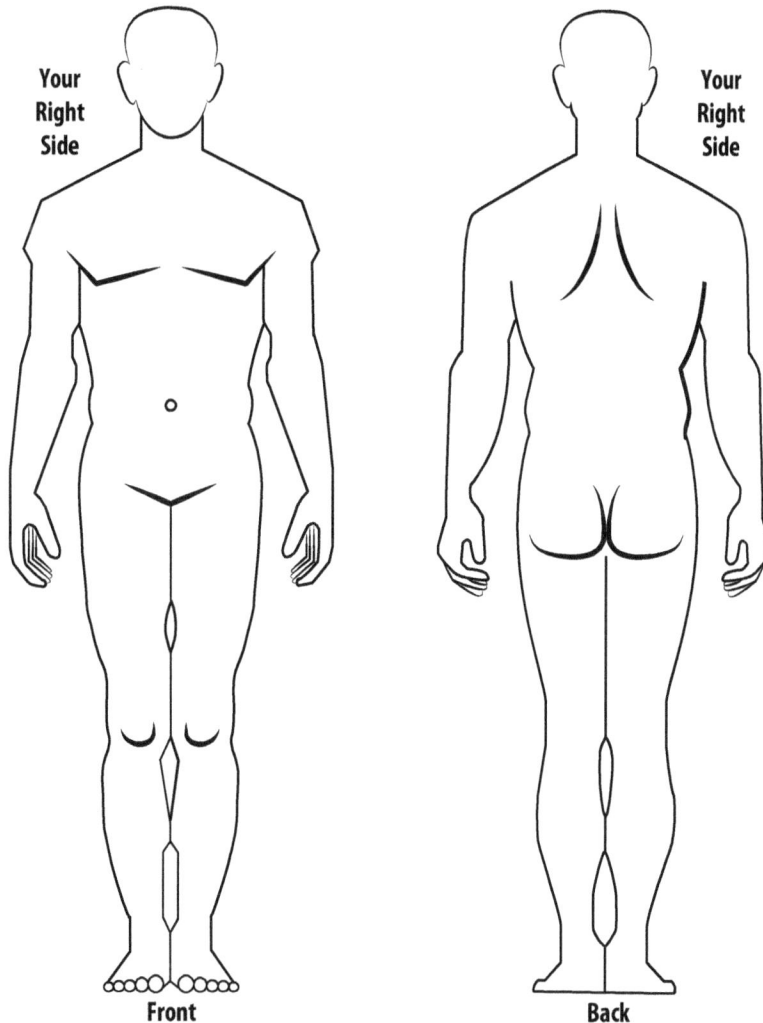

Your Right Side

Front

Your Right Side

Back

6 DAILY PAIN SUMMARY

Were there times during the day that you experienced unrelieved breakthrough pain? ____NO ____YES

How many times did this happen today?

1 2 3 4 5 6 7 8 9 10 more than 10

Did any specific activity start your breakthrough pain?
____NO ____YES: What activities?

_____

Put an "X" on the body diagram to show each place you've had **BREAKTHROUGH PAIN** today.

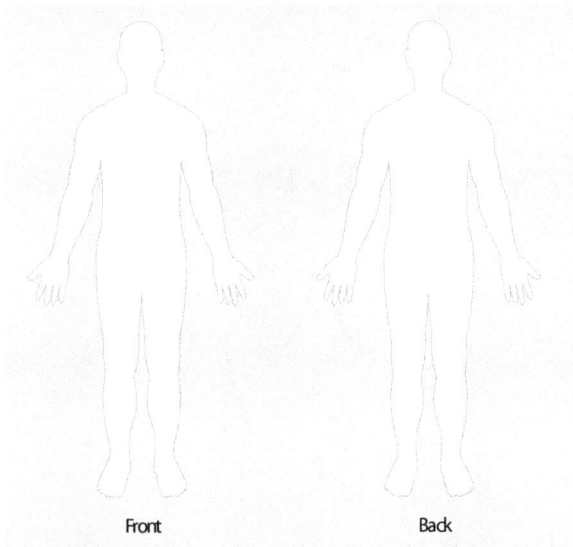

Front   Back

NON-DRUG THERAPIES
(other than prescription or other medicines)

_____

_____

ACTIVITIES/EXERCISE

_____

_____

What was your average level of pain today?

0 1 2 3 4 5 6 7 8 9 10

Other than prescription medicine, did you do anything else today to relieve the pain? ____NO ____YES:
(Note any that you used.)
____ Non-prescription drugs (e.g., acetaminophen, ibuprofen)
____ Herbal remedies
____ Hot or cold packs
____ Exercise
____ Changing position (such as lying down or elevating your legs)
____ Physical therapy
____ Massage
____ Acupuncture
____ Rest
____ Psychological counseling
____ Talk to trusted friend, family, clergy
____ Prayer, meditation, guided imagery
____ Relaxation technique (hypnosis, biofeedback)
____ Creative technique (art or music therapy)
____ Other (e.g., specific chiropractic manipulation, osteopathic treatments):

_____

Check any of these common side effects that you've noticed after taking your pain medicine:
____ Drowsiness, sleepiness
____ Nausea, vomiting, upset stomach
____ Constipation
____ Lack of appetite
____ Other (describe):

_____

Did you sleep through the night? ____NO____YES

If not, how many times was your sleep disrupted? _____

How many hours did you sleep during the night? _____

COMMENTS AND MORE INFORMATION: Make notes for and about visits with your healthcare provider, side effects from treatments you may be experiencing, any problems you are having coping with your pain, and more about some of your previous answers or questions.

_____

_____

_____

1 DAILY DIARY

SATISFACTION CHART   Connect the points on your Daily Satisfaction Chart so your medical team can see when and why your mental state changed.

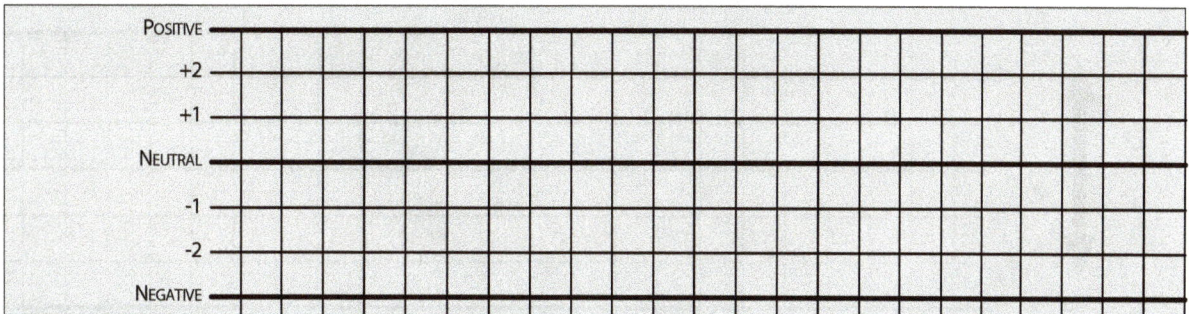

DAY_____ DATE_____ WEIGHT_____

POSITIVE
+2
+1
NEUTRAL
-1
-2
NEGATIVE

2 ACTIVITY LOG

6am 7 8 9 10 11 12pm 1 2 3 4 5 6pm 7 8 9 10 11 12am 1 2 3 4 5

TRIGGERS AND SIGNIFICANT EVENTS

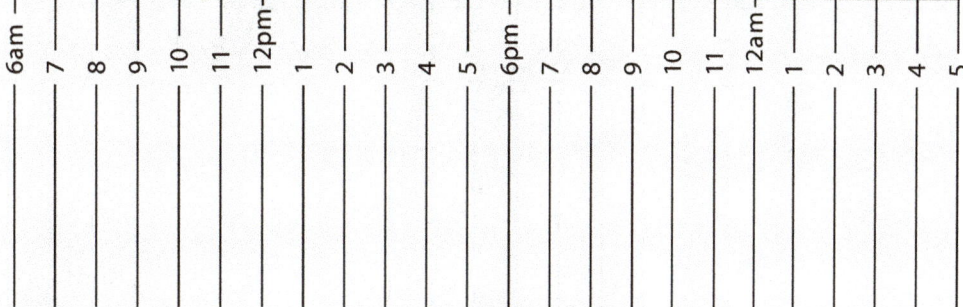

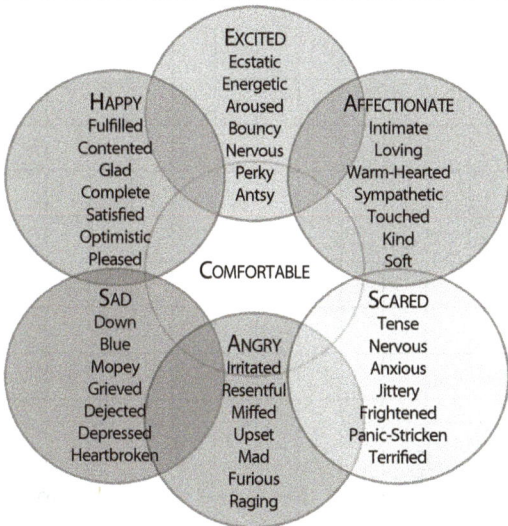

EXCITED
Ecstatic
Energetic
Aroused
Bouncy
Nervous
Perky
Antsy

HAPPY
Fulfilled
Contented
Glad
Complete
Satisfied
Optimistic
Pleased

AFFECTIONATE
Intimate
Loving
Warm-Hearted
Sympathetic
Touched
Kind
Soft

COMFORTABLE

SAD
Down
Blue
Mopey
Grieved
Dejected
Depressed
Heartbroken

ANGRY
Irritated
Resentful
Miffed
Upset
Mad
Furious
Raging

SCARED
Tense
Nervous
Anxious
Jittery
Frightened
Panic-Stricken
Terrified

Describe any changes in your pain today:

_____
_____
_____
_____

Did anything unusual happen today?

_____
_____
_____
_____

What did you spend the most time time thinking about today?

Positive Thoughts:

_____

Did your pain increase, decrease, or remain the same when you thought about it?
____ Increased
____ Decreased
____ Stayed the Same

Negative Thoughts:

_____

Did your pain increase, decrease, or remain the same when you thought about it?
____ Increased
____ Decreased
____ Stayed the Same

1 DAILY
MOOD CHART

DAY_____ DATE_____ WEIGHT_____

Connect the points on your Mood Satisfaction Chart so your medical team can see when and why your mental state changed.

	HAPPY	+3
		+2
		+1
MOOD		0
		-1
		-2
	SAD	-3

2 ACTIVITY LOG

6am 7 8 9 10 11 12pm 1 2 3 4 5 6pm 7 8 9 10 11 12am 1 2 3 4 5

3 MEDICATION LOG
NAME/DOSE

1————
2————
3————
4————
5————
6————
7————
8————

4 PHYSIOLOGY

6am 7 8 9 10 11 12pm 1 2 3 4 5 6pm 7 8 9 10 11 12am 1 2 3 4 5

SLEEP
URINATION
DEFECATION
NAUSEA
EATING
EXERCISE
OTHER (LIST)

1 DAILY RESULTS
OF MEDICATIONS AND TREATMENTS

As you and your medical team develop new treatment plans, it will be especially helpful to record any side effects you experience as you add new treatments. This can help determine which types of treatments will work best for you.

Contact your care provider with any bad reactions or side effects to determine if you should discontinue the medication or treatment.

MEDICATION / TREATMENT	AMOUNT / TIME / COMMENTS

8

1 DAILY
TREATMENT PLAN

As you and your medical team develop new treatment plans, record your plan for the day including new medications, increases or decreases to medications, exercises, physical therapy, or any other treatment efforts.

Medication / Treatment	Amount / Time / Comments

1 DAILY
PAIN CHART

DAY_____ DATE_____ WEIGHT_____

Connect the points on your Daily Pain and Satisfaction Charts so your medical team can see when your status changed.

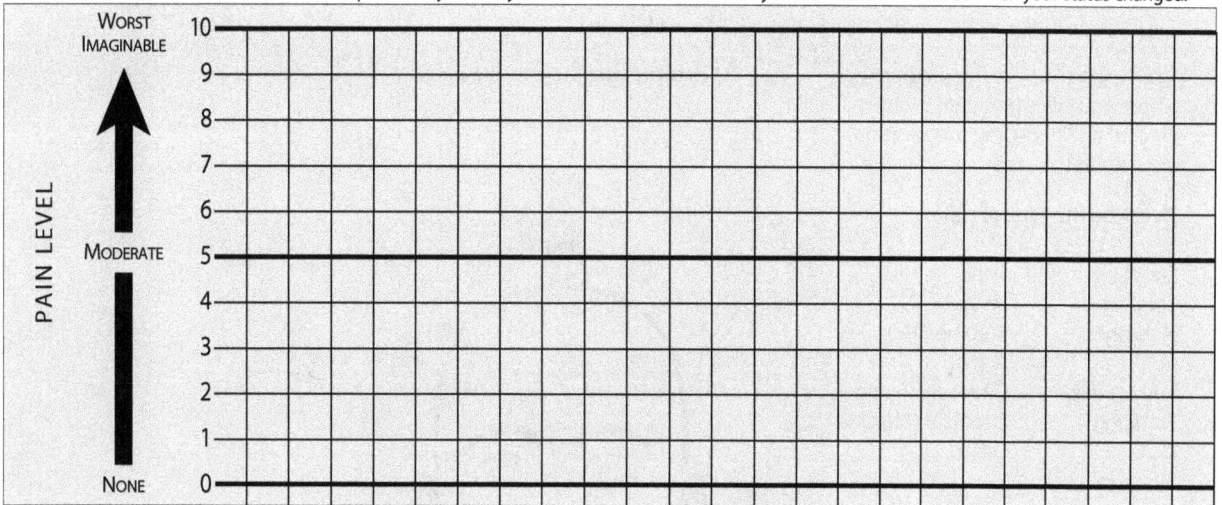

PAIN LEVEL

WORST IMAGINABLE — 10
9
8
7
6
MODERATE — 5
4
3
2
1
NONE — 0

2 SATISFACTION

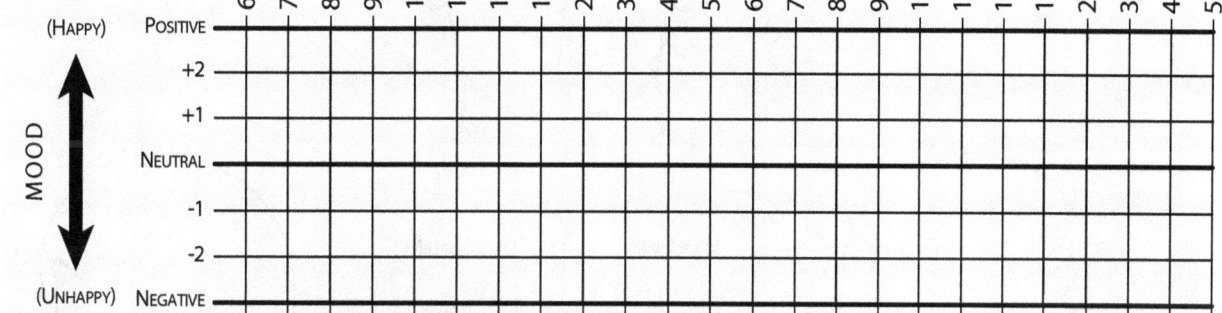

6am 7 8 9 10 11 12pm 1 2 3 4 5 6pm 7 8 9 10 11 12am 1 2 3 4 5

MOOD

(HAPPY) POSITIVE
+2
+1
NEUTRAL
-1
-2
(UNHAPPY) NEGATIVE

3 PHYSIOLOGY

6am 7 8 9 10 11 12pm 1 2 3 4 5 6pm 7 8 9 10 11 12am 1 2 3 4 5

SLEEP

RESTROOM

NAUSEA / DIZZINESS

MEAL / SNACK

EXERCISE

STRESS / ANXIETY

MEDICINE NAME / DOSE

1

2

3

BLOOD PRESSURE

PULSE

8

4 DAILY HEAD & FACE PAIN DIAGRAM

Mark each place on the diagram where you have had pain today by placing an 'X', circling the location, or shading the area .

Describe the type of pain:

Shooting	Deep
Tingling	Sharp
Numbness	Burning / Hot
Cold	Aching
Surface Pain	Gnawing / Biting
Stabbing	Electrical / Shocks
Dull	Other_____
Stinging	

COMMENTS AND MORE INFORMATION:

Front

Upper Right   Upper Left

Lower Right   Lower Left

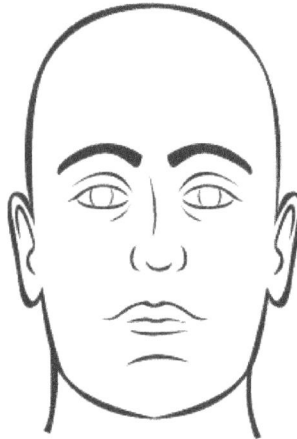

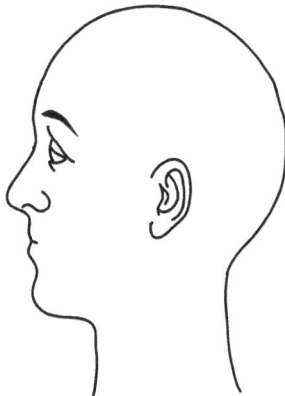

**Your
Right
Side**

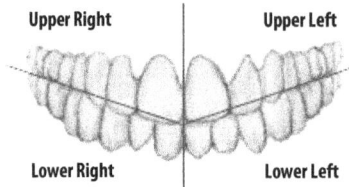

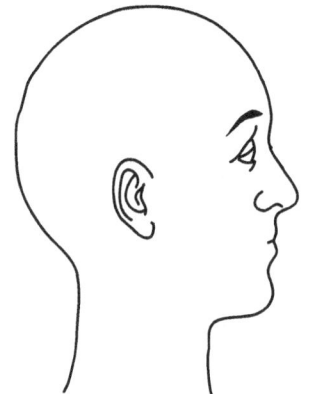

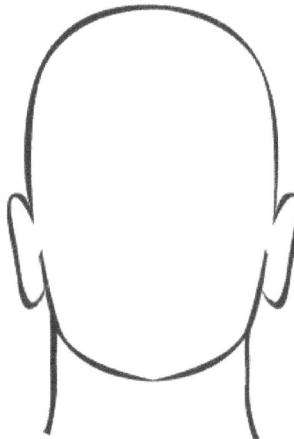

**Your
Right
Side**

Back

5 DAILY BODY PAIN DIAGRAM

8

Mark each place on the diagram where you have had pain today by placing an 'X', circling the location, or shading the area .

Describe the type of pain:

Shooting	Deep
Tingling	Sharp
Numbness	Burning / Hot
Cold	Aching
Surface Pain	Gnawing / Biting
Stabbing	Electrical / Shocks
Dull	Other_____
Stinging	

COMMENTS AND MORE INFORMATION:

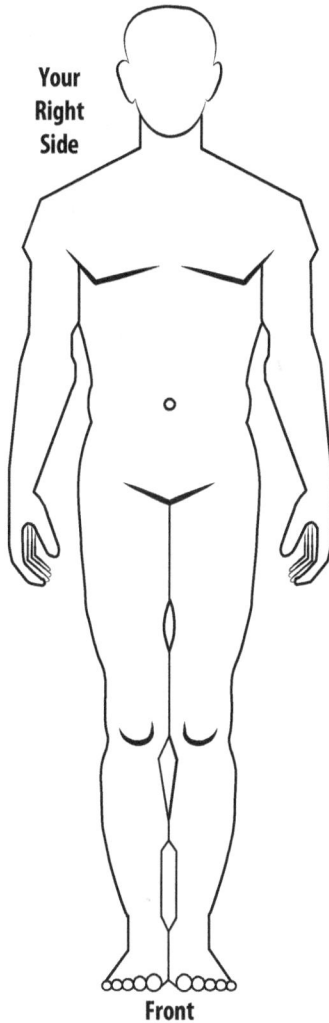

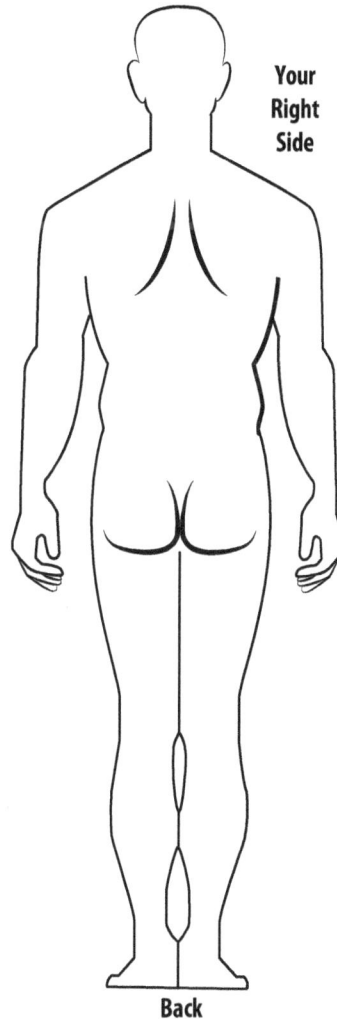

Your
Right
Side

Your
Right
Side

Front

Back

8

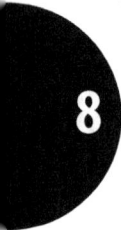

6 DAILY PAIN SUMMARY

Were there times during the day that you experienced unrelieved breakthrough pain? ____NO ____YES

How many times did this happen today?

1 2 3 4 5 6 7 8 9 10 more than 10

Did any specific activity start your breakthrough pain? ____NO ____YES: What activities?

_____

Put an "X" on the body diagram to show each place you've had *BREAKTHROUGH PAIN* today.

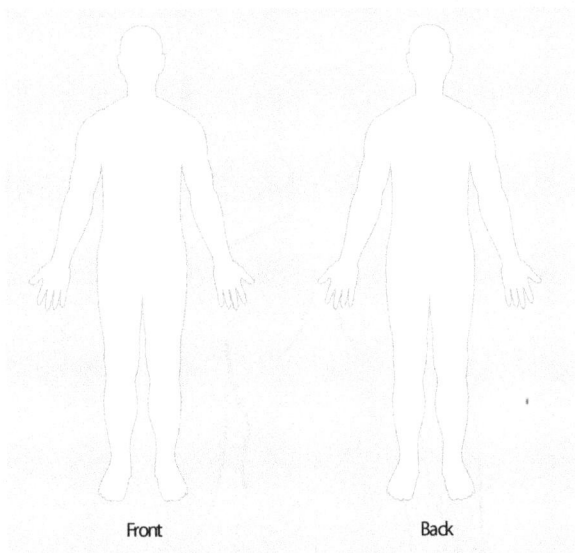

Front   Back

NON-DRUG THERAPIES
(other than prescription or other medicines)

_____

_____

ACTIVITIES/EXERCISE

_____

_____

What was your average level of pain today?

0   1   2   3   4   5   6   7   8   9   10

Other than prescription medicine, did you do anything else today to relieve the pain? ____NO ____YES: (Note any that you used.)

____ Non-prescription drugs (e.g., acetaminophen, ibuprofen)
____ Herbal remedies
____ Hot or cold packs
____ Exercise
____ Changing position (such as lying down or elevating your legs)
____ Physical therapy
____ Massage
____ Acupuncture
____ Rest
____ Psychological counseling
____ Talk to trusted friend, family, clergy
____ Prayer, meditation, guided imagery
____ Relaxation technique (hypnosis, biofeedback)
____ Creative technique (art or music therapy)
____ Other (e.g., specific chiropractic manipulation, osteopathic treatments):

_____

Check any of these common side effects that you've noticed after taking your pain medicine:
____ Drowsiness, sleepiness
____ Nausea, vomiting, upset stomach
____ Constipation
____ Lack of appetite
____ Other (describe):

_____

Did you sleep through the night? ____NO____YES

If not, how many times was your sleep disrupted? _____

How many hours did you sleep during the night? _____

COMMENTS AND MORE INFORMATION: Make notes for and about visits with your healthcare provider, side effects from treatments you may be experiencing, any problems you are having coping with your pain, and more about some of your previous answers or questions.

_____

_____

_____

1 DAILY DIARY

DAY_____ DATE_____ WEIGHT_____

SATISFACTION CHART Connect the points on your Daily Satisfaction Chart so your medical team can see when and why your mental state changed.

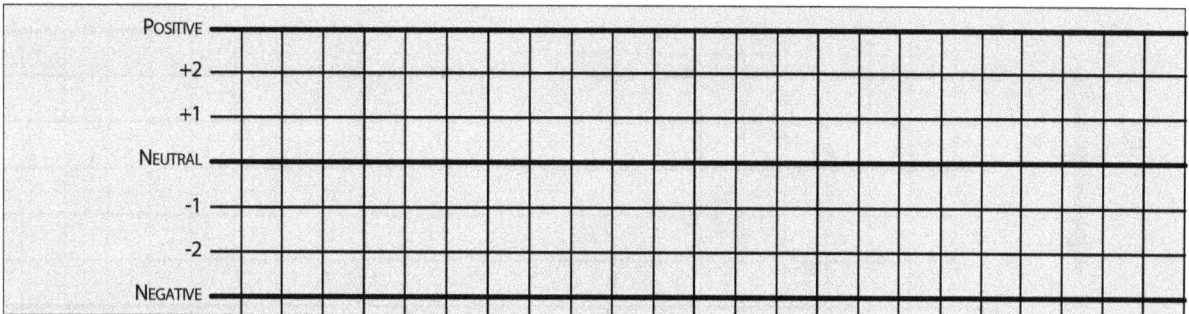

POSITIVE

+2

+1

NEUTRAL

-1

-2

NEGATIVE

2 ACTIVITY LOG

6am 7 8 9 10 11 12pm 1 2 3 4 5 6pm 7 8 9 10 11 12am 1 2 3 4 5

TRIGGERS AND SIGNIFICANT EVENTS

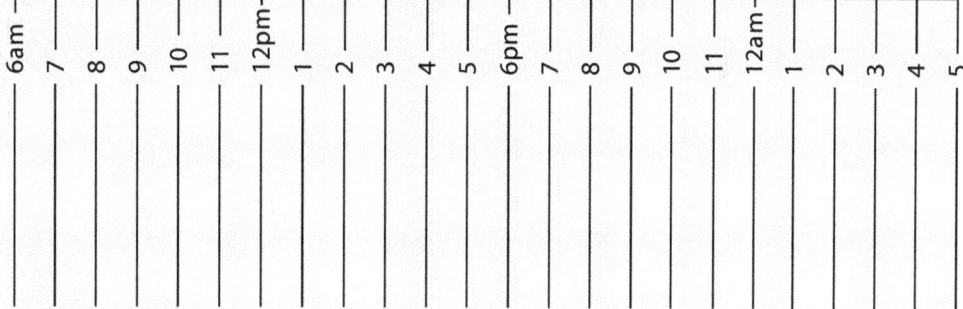

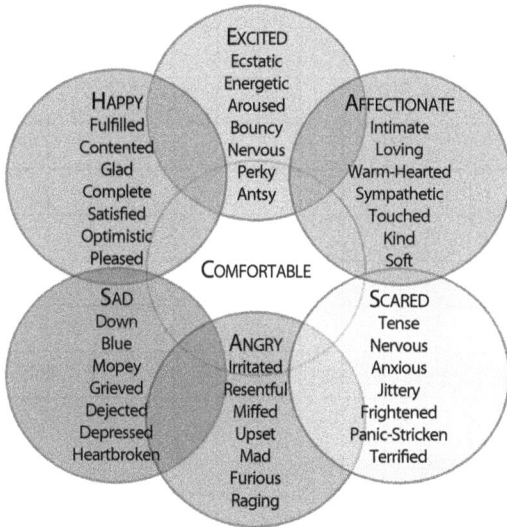

EXCITED
Ecstatic
Energetic
Aroused
Bouncy
Nervous
Perky
Antsy

HAPPY
Fulfilled
Contented
Glad
Complete
Satisfied
Optimistic
Pleased

AFFECTIONATE
Intimate
Loving
Warm-Hearted
Sympathetic
Touched
Kind
Soft

COMFORTABLE

SAD
Down
Blue
Mopey
Grieved
Dejected
Depressed
Heartbroken

ANGRY
Irritated
Resentful
Miffed
Upset
Mad
Furious
Raging

SCARED
Tense
Nervous
Anxious
Jittery
Frightened
Panic-Stricken
Terrified

Describe any changes in your pain today:

_____
_____
_____
_____

Did anything unusual happen today?

_____
_____
_____
_____

What did you spend the most time time thinking about today?

Positive Thoughts:

_____

Did your pain increase, decrease, or remain the same when you thought about it?
_____ Increased
_____ Decreased
_____ Stayed the Same

Negative Thoughts:

_____

Did your pain increase, decrease, or remain the same when you thought about it?
_____ Increased
_____ Decreased
_____ Stayed the Same

8

1 DAILY
MOOD CHART

DAY_____ DATE_____ WEIGHT_____

Connect the points on your Mood Satisfaction Chart so your medical team can see when and why your mental state changed.

HAPPY +3

+2

+1

MOOD 0

-1

-2

SAD -3

2 ACTIVITY LOG

6am 7 8 9 10 11 12pm 1 2 3 4 5 6pm 7 8 9 10 11 12am 1 2 3 4 5

3 MEDICATION LOG
NAME/DOSE

1———
2———
3———
4———
5———
6———
7———
8———

4 PHYSIOLOGY

6am 7 8 9 10 11 12pm 1 2 3 4 5 6pm 7 8 9 10 11 12am 1 2 3 4 5

SLEEP

URINATION

DEFECATION

NAUSEA

EATING

EXERCISE

OTHER (LIST)

1 DAILY RESULTS
OF MEDICATIONS AND TREATMENTS

As you and your medical team develop new treatment plans, it will be especially helpful to record any side effects you experience as you add new treatments. This can help determine which types of treatments will work best for you.

Contact your care provider with any bad reactions or side effects to determine if you should discontinue the medication or treatment.

MEDICATION / TREATMENT	AMOUNT / TIME / COMMENTS

1 DAILY
TREATMENT PLAN

As you and your medical team develop new treatment plans, record your plan for the day including new medications, increases or decreases to medications, exercises, physical therapy, or any other treatment efforts.

9

MEDICATION / TREATMENT	AMOUNT / TIME / COMMENTS

1 DAILY
PAIN CHART

DAY_____ DATE_____ WEIGHT_____

Connect the points on your Daily Pain and Satisfaction Charts so your medical team can see when your status changed.

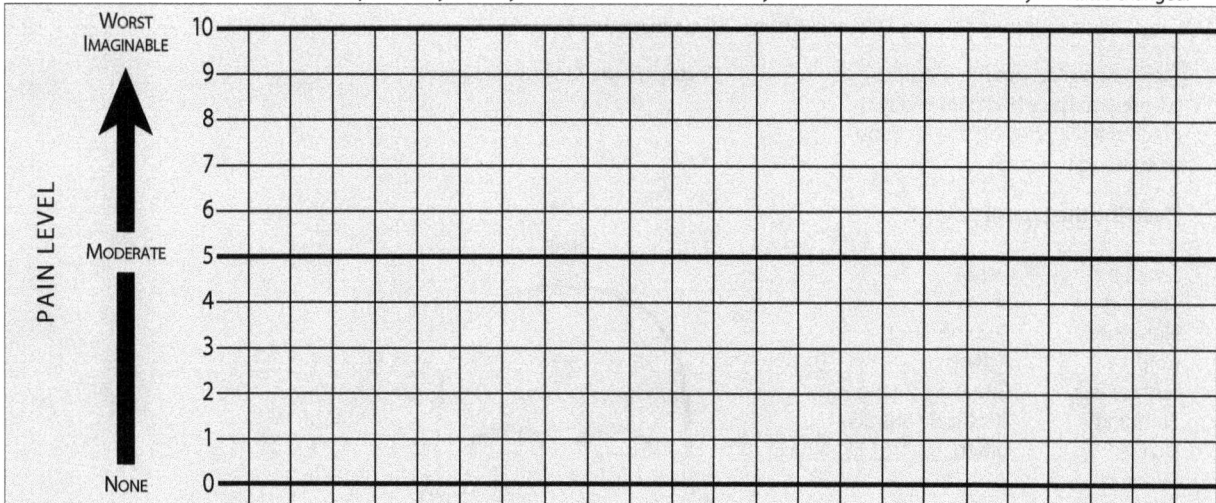

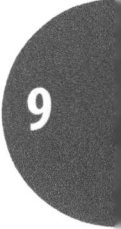

2 SATISFACTION

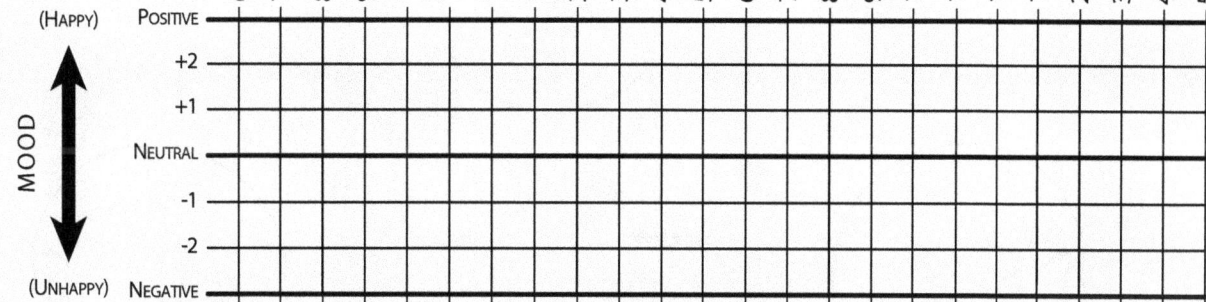

3 PHYSIOLOGY

	6am	7	8	9	10	11	12pm	1	2	3	4	5	6pm	7	8	9	10	11	12am	1	2	3	4	5
SLEEP																								
RESTROOM																								
NAUSEA / DIZZINESS																								
MEAL / SNACK																								
EXERCISE																								
STRESS / ANXIETY																								

MEDICINE NAME / DOSE

1_____

2_____

3_____

BLOOD PRESSURE ——

PULSE ——

4 DAILY HEAD & FACE PAIN DIAGRAM

9

Mark each place on the diagram where you have had pain today by placing an 'X', circling the location, or shading the area .

Describe the type of pain:

Shooting	Deep
Tingling	Sharp
Numbness	Burning / Hot
Cold	Aching
Surface Pain	Gnawing / Biting
Stabbing	Electrical / Shocks
Dull	Other_____
Stinging	

COMMENTS AND MORE INFORMATION:

Front

Upper Right   **Upper Left**

Lower Right   **Lower Left**

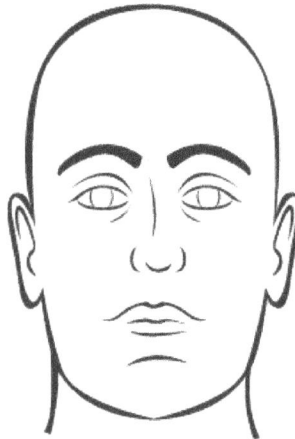

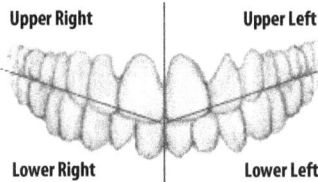

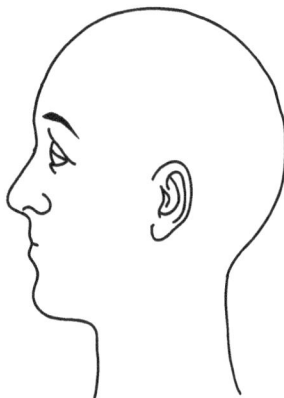

**Your
Right
Side**

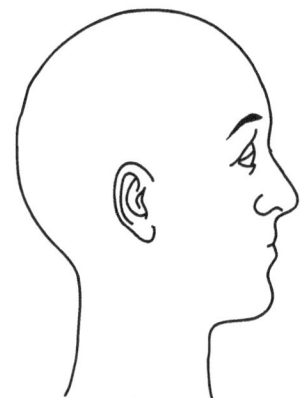

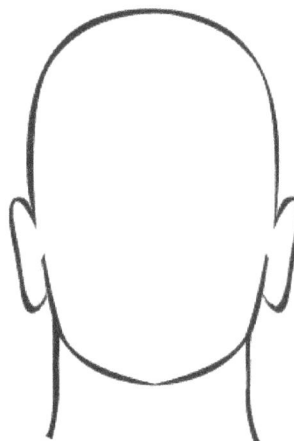

**Your
Right
Side**

Back

5 DAILY BODY PAIN DIAGRAM

Mark each place on the diagram where you have had pain today by placing an 'X', circling the location, or shading the area .

Describe the type of pain:

Shooting	Deep
Tingling	Sharp
Numbness	Burning / Hot
Cold	Aching
Surface Pain	Gnawing / Biting
Stabbing	Electrical / Shocks
Dull	Other_____
Stinging	

COMMENTS AND MORE INFORMATION:

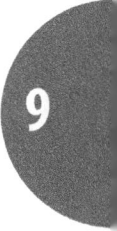

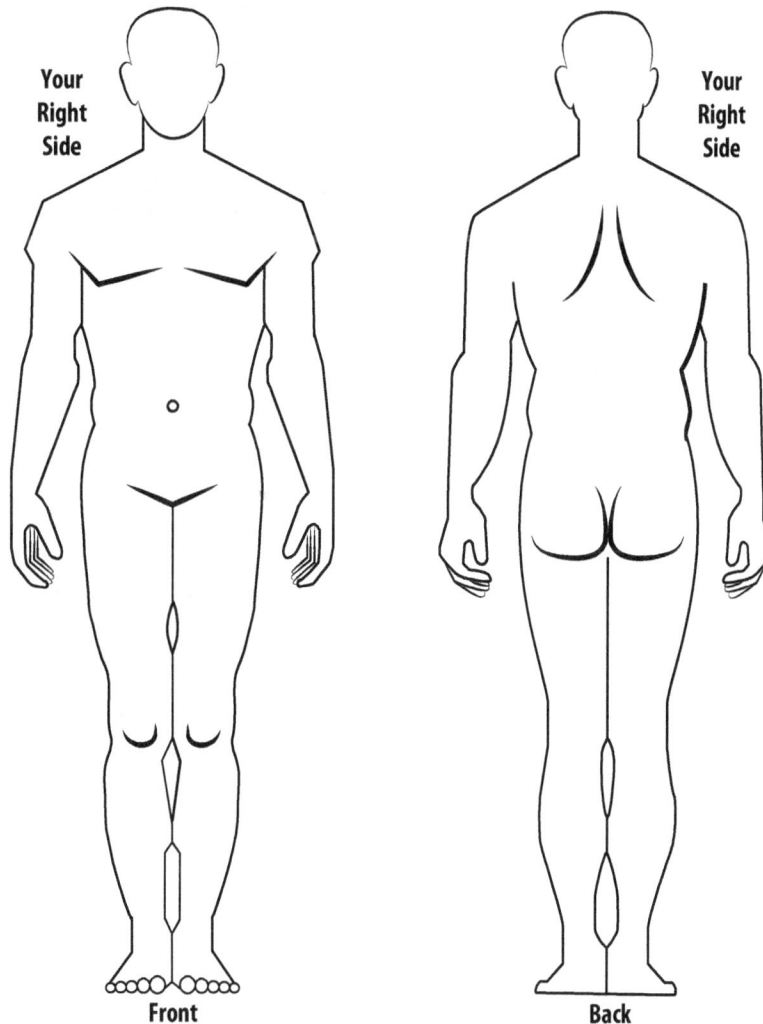

9

Your Right Side

Your Right Side

Front

Back

6 DAILY PAIN SUMMARY

Were there times during the day that you experienced unrelieved breakthrough pain? _____NO _____YES

How many times did this happen today?

1 2 3 4 5 6 7 8 9 10   more than 10

Did any specific activity start your breakthrough pain? _____NO _____YES: What activities?

_____

Put an "X" on the body diagram to show each place you've had *BREAKTHROUGH PAIN* today.

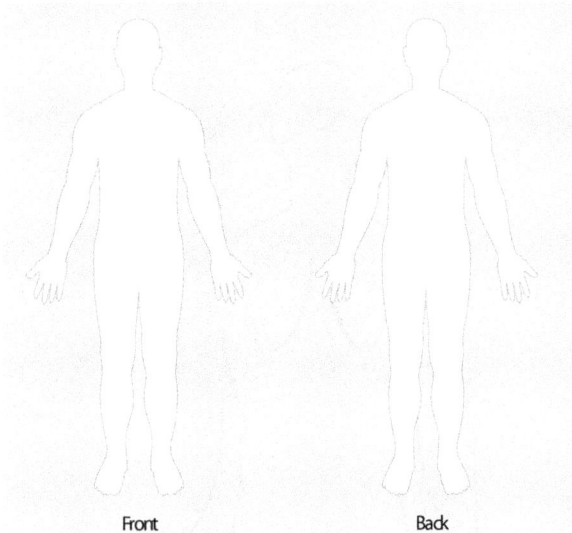

Front   Back

NON-DRUG THERAPIES
(other than prescription or other medicines)

_____

_____

ACTIVITIES/EXERCISE

_____

What was your average level of pain today?

0   1   2   3   4   5   6   7   8   9   10

Other than prescription medicine, did you do anything else today to relieve the pain? _____NO _____YES: (Note any that you used.)
_____ Non-prescription drugs (e.g., acetaminophen, ibuprofen)
_____ Herbal remedies
_____ Hot or cold packs
_____ Exercise
_____ Changing position (such as lying down or elevating your legs)
_____ Physical therapy
_____ Massage
_____ Acupuncture
_____ Rest
_____ Psychological counseling
_____ Talk to trusted friend, family, clergy
_____ Prayer, meditation, guided imagery
_____ Relaxation technique (hypnosis, biofeedback)
_____ Creative technique (art or music therapy)
_____ Other (e.g., specific chiropractic manipulation, osteopathic treatments):

_____

Check any of these common side effects that you've noticed after taking your pain medicine:
_____ Drowsiness, sleepiness
_____ Nausea, vomiting, upset stomach
_____ Constipation
_____ Lack of appetite
_____ Other (describe):

_____

Did you sleep through the night? _____NO_____YES

If not, how many times was your sleep disrupted? _____

How many hours did you sleep during the night? _____

COMMENTS AND MORE INFORMATION: Make notes for and about visits with your healthcare provider, side effects from treatments you may be experiencing, any problems you are having coping with your pain, and more about some of your previous answers or questions.

_____

_____

_____

1 DAILY DIARY

SATISFACTION CHART Connect the points on your Daily Satisfaction Chart so your medical team can see when and why your mental state changed.

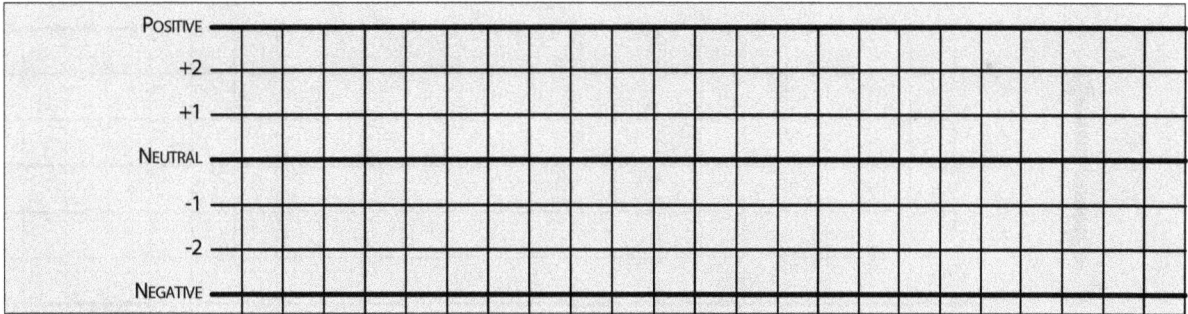

DAY_____ DATE_____ WEIGHT_____

9

POSITIVE
+2
+1
NEUTRAL
-1
-2
NEGATIVE

2 ACTIVITY LOG

6am 7 8 9 10 11 12pm 1 2 3 4 5 6pm 7 8 9 10 11 12am 1 2 3 4 5

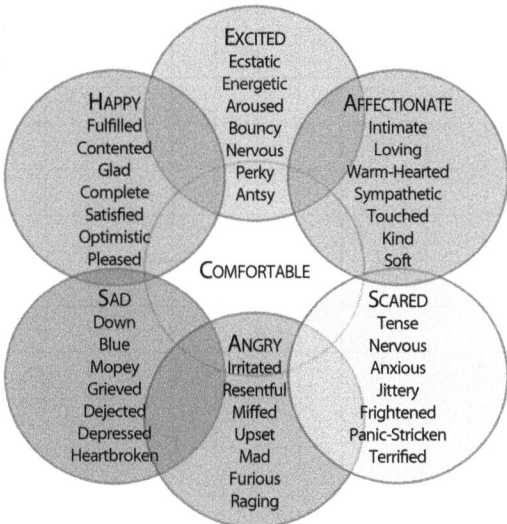

TRIGGERS AND SIGNIFICANT EVENTS

EXCITED
Ecstatic
Energetic
Aroused
Bouncy
Nervous
Perky
Antsy

HAPPY
Fulfilled
Contented
Glad
Complete
Satisfied
Optimistic
Pleased

AFFECTIONATE
Intimate
Loving
Warm-Hearted
Sympathetic
Touched
Kind
Soft

COMFORTABLE

SAD
Down
Blue
Mopey
Grieved
Dejected
Depressed
Heartbroken

ANGRY
Irritated
Resentful
Miffed
Upset
Mad
Furious
Raging

SCARED
Tense
Nervous
Anxious
Jittery
Frightened
Panic-Stricken
Terrified

Describe any changes in your pain today:
_____
_____
_____
_____

Did anything unusual happen today?
_____
_____
_____
_____

What did you spend the most time time thinking about today?

Positive Thoughts:
_____

Did your pain increase, decrease, or remain the same when you thought about it?
____ Increased
____ Decreased
____ Stayed the Same

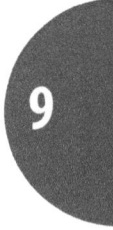

Negative Thoughts:
_____

Did your pain increase, decrease, or remain the same when you thought about it?
____ Increased
____ Decreased
____ Stayed the Same

9

1 DAILY
MOOD CHART

DAY_____ DATE_____ WEIGHT_____

Connect the points on your Mood Satisfaction Chart so your medical team can see when and why your mental state changed.

HAPPY   +3
             +2
             +1
MOOD   0
             -1
             -2
SAD   -3

2 ACTIVITY LOG

6am 7 8 9 10 11 12pm 1 2 3 4 5 6pm 7 8 9 10 11 12am 1 2 3 4 5

3 MEDICATION LOG
NAME/DOSE

1————
2————
3————
4————
5————
6————
7————
8————

4 PHYSIOLOGY

6am 7 8 9 10 11 12pm 1 2 3 4 5 6pm 7 8 9 10 11 12am 1 2 3 4 5

SLEEP ———
URINATION ———
DEFECATION ———
NAUSEA ———
EATING ———
EXERCISE ———
OTHER (LIST) ———

1 DAILY RESULTS
OF MEDICATIONS AND TREATMENTS

As you and your medical team develop new treatment plans, it will be especially helpful to record any side effects you experience as you add new treatments. This can help determine which types of treatments will work best for you.

Contact your care provider with any bad reactions or side effects to determine if you should discontinue the medication or treatment.

MEDICATION / TREATMENT	AMOUNT / TIME / COMMENTS

9

1 DAILY
TREATMENT PLAN

As you and your medical team develop new treatment plans, record your plan for the day including new medications, increases or decreases to medications, exercises, physical therapy, or any other treatment efforts.

MEDICATION / TREATMENT	AMOUNT / TIME / COMMENTS

10

1 DAILY
PAIN CHART

DAY_____ DATE_____ WEIGHT_____

Connect the points on your Daily Pain and Satisfaction Charts so your medical team can see when your status changed.

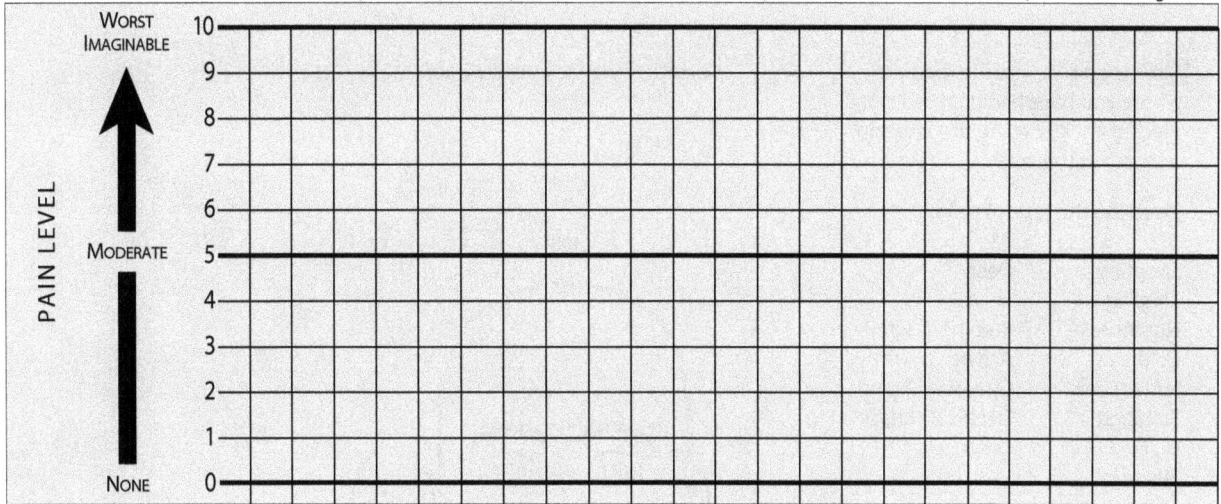

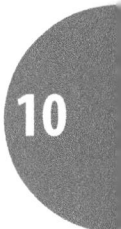

2 SATISFACTION

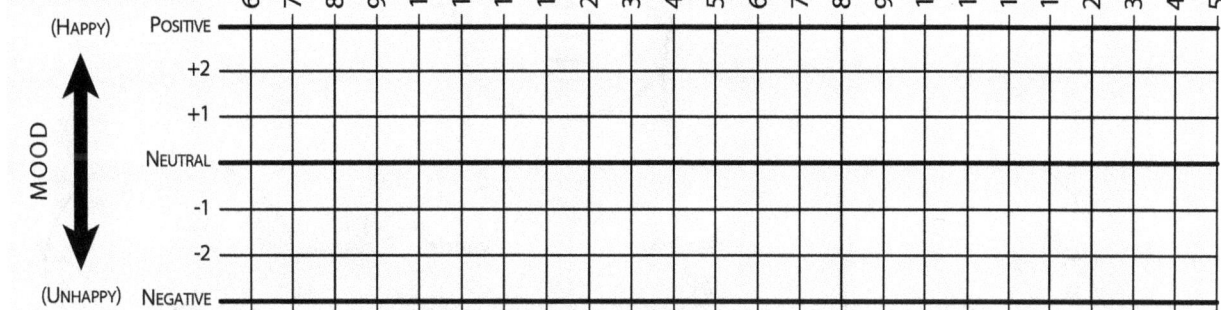

3 PHYSIOLOGY

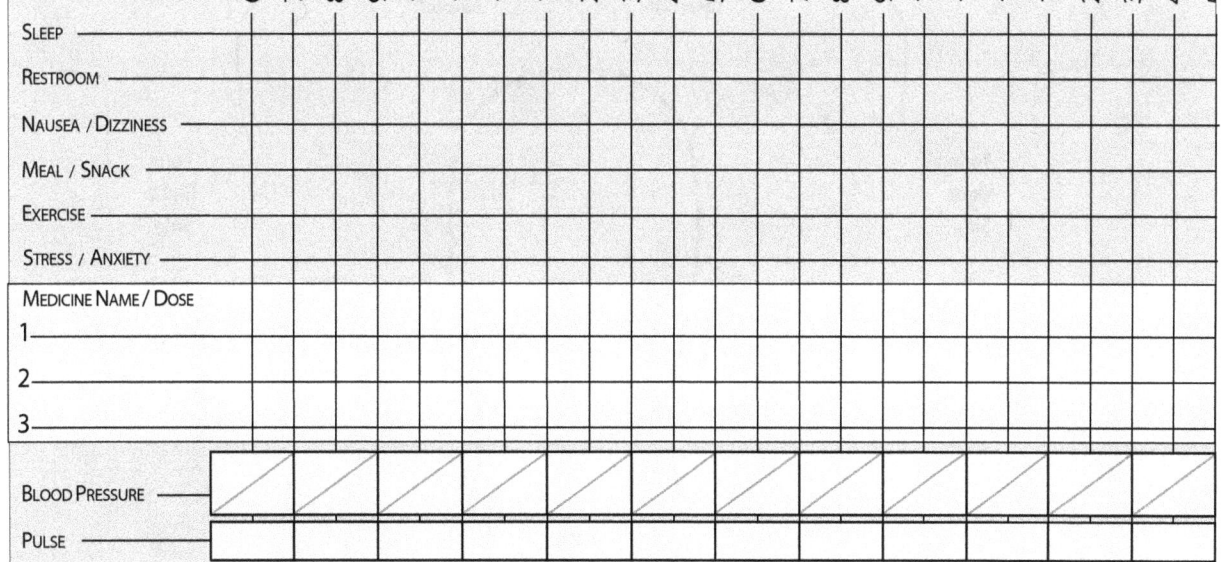

4 DAILY HEAD & FACE PAIN DIAGRAM

Mark each place on the diagram where you have had pain today by placing an 'X', circling the location, or shading the area .

COMMENTS AND MORE INFORMATION:

Describe the type of pain:

Shooting   Deep
Tingling   Sharp
Numbness   Burning / Hot
Cold   Aching
Surface Pain   Gnawing / Biting
Stabbing   Electrical / Shocks
Dull   Other_____
Stinging

10

Front

Upper Right   Upper Left

Lower Right   Lower Left

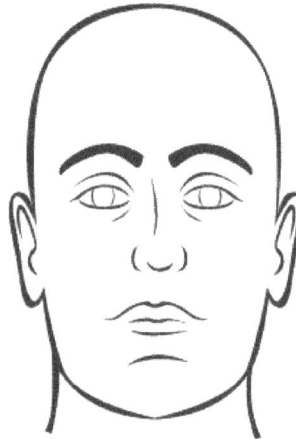

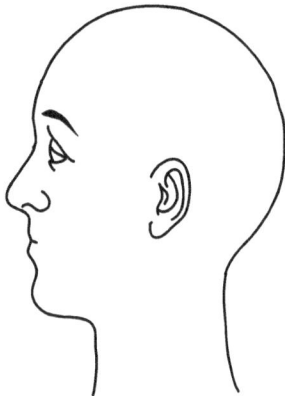

Your Right Side

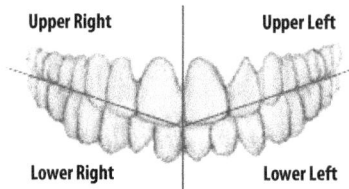

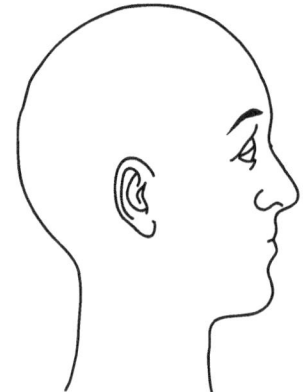

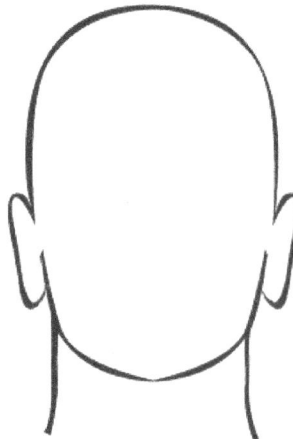

Your Right Side

Back

5 DAILY BODY PAIN DIAGRAM

Mark each place on the diagram where you have had pain today by placing an 'X', circling the location, or shading the area .

Describe the type of pain:

Shooting   Deep
Tingling   Sharp
Numbness   Burning / Hot
Cold   Aching
Surface Pain   Gnawing / Biting
Stabbing   Electrical / Shocks
Dull   Other_____
Stinging

COMMENTS AND MORE INFORMATION:

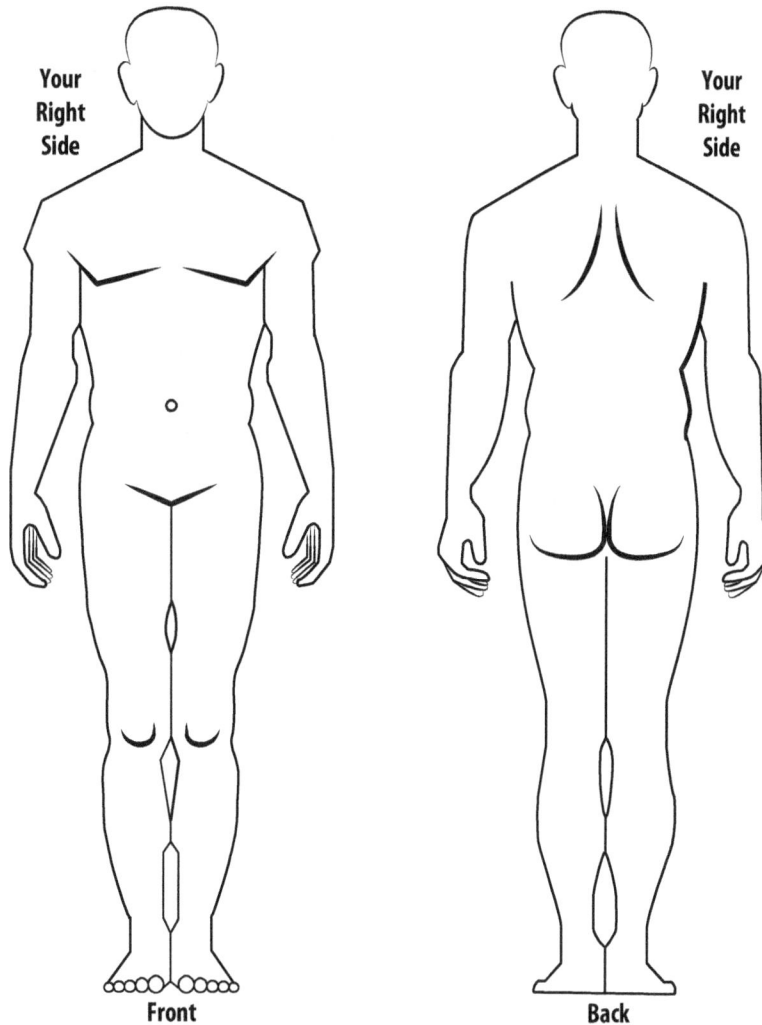

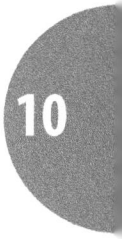

10

Your
Right
Side

Your
Right
Side

Front

Back

6 DAILY PAIN SUMMARY

Were there times during the day that you experienced unrelieved breakthrough pain? ____NO ____YES

How many times did this happen today?

1 2 3 4 5 6 7 8 9 10 more than 10

Did any specific activity start your breakthrough pain? ____NO ____YES: What activities?

_____

Put an "X" on the body diagram to show each place you've had **BREAKTHROUGH PAIN** today.

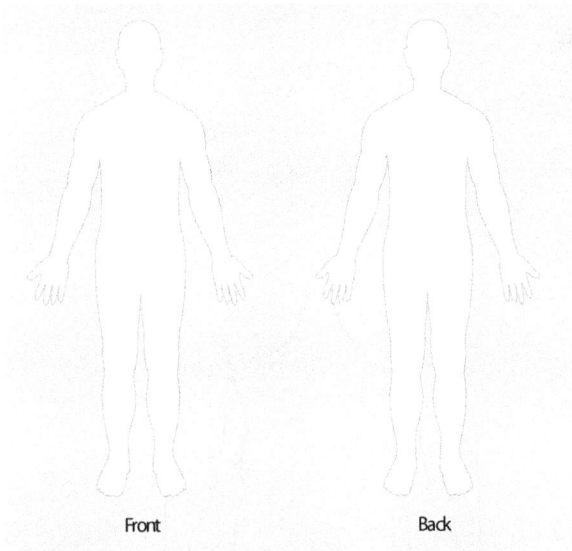

Front   Back

NON-DRUG THERAPIES
(other than prescription or other medicines)

_____

_____

ACTIVITIES/EXERCISE

_____

What was your average level of pain today?

0 1 2 3 4 5 6 7 8 9 10

Other than prescription medicine, did you do anything else today to relieve the pain? ____NO ____YES: (Note any that you used.)
____ Non-prescription drugs (e.g., acetaminophen, ibuprofen)
____ Herbal remedies
____ Hot or cold packs
____ Exercise
____ Changing position (such as lying down or elevating your legs)
____ Physical therapy
____ Massage
____ Acupuncture
____ Rest
____ Psychological counseling
____ Talk to trusted friend, family, clergy
____ Prayer, meditation, guided imagery
____ Relaxation technique (hypnosis, biofeedback)
____ Creative technique (art or music therapy)
____ Other (e.g., specific chiropractic manipulation, osteopathic treatments):

_____

Check any of these common side effects that you've noticed after taking your pain medicine:
____ Drowsiness; sleepiness
____ Nausea, vomiting, upset stomach
____ Constipation
____ Lack of appetite
____ Other (describe):

_____

Did you sleep through the night? ____NO____YES

If not, how many times was your sleep disrupted? _____

How many hours did you sleep during the night? _____

COMMENTS AND MORE INFORMATION: Make notes for and about visits with your healthcare provider, side effects from treatments you may be experiencing, any problems you are having coping with your pain, and more about some of your previous answers or questions.

_____

_____

_____

10

1 DAILY DIARY

SATISFACTION CHART

DAY_____ DATE_____ WEIGHT_____

Connect the points on your Daily Satisfaction Chart so your medical team can see when and why your mental state changed.

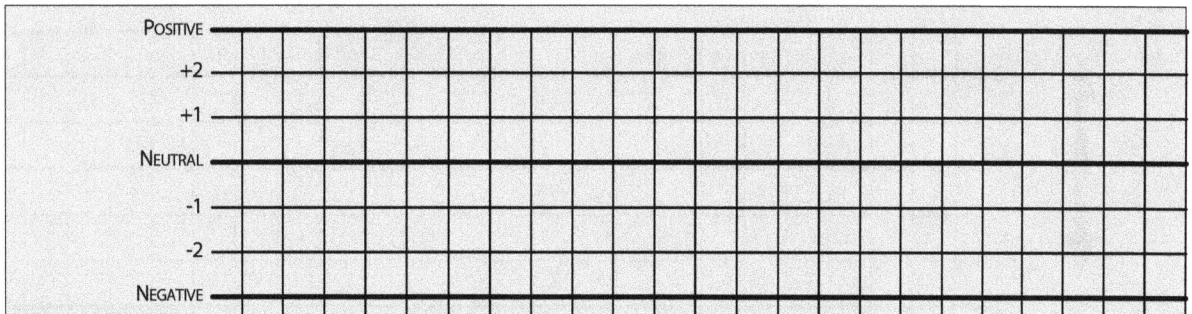

POSITIVE

+2

+1

NEUTRAL

-1

-2

NEGATIVE

2 ACTIVITY LOG

TRIGGERS AND SIGNIFICANT EVENTS

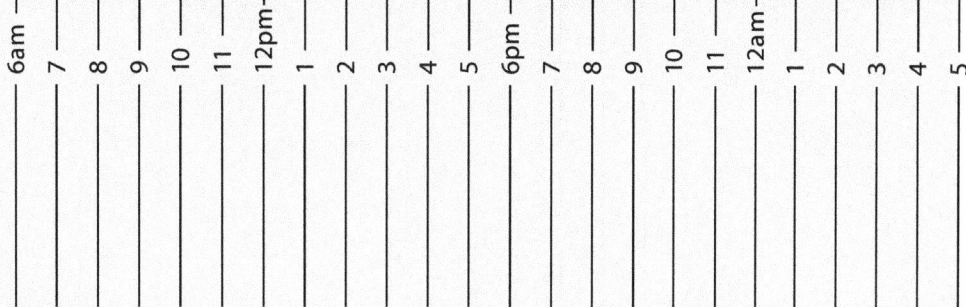

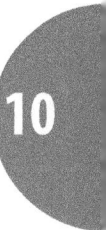

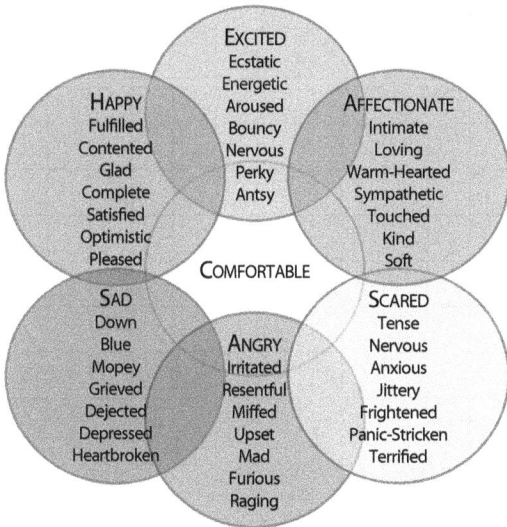

6am 7 8 9 10 11 12pm 1 2 3 4 5 6pm 7 8 9 10 11 12am 1 2 3 4 5

10

EXCITED
Ecstatic
Energetic
Aroused
Bouncy
Nervous
Perky
Antsy

HAPPY
Fulfilled
Contented
Glad
Complete
Satisfied
Optimistic
Pleased

AFFECTIONATE
Intimate
Loving
Warm-Hearted
Sympathetic
Touched
Kind
Soft

COMFORTABLE

SAD
Down
Blue
Mopey
Grieved
Dejected
Depressed
Heartbroken

ANGRY
Irritated
Resentful
Miffed
Upset
Mad
Furious
Raging

SCARED
Tense
Nervous
Anxious
Jittery
Frightened
Panic-Stricken
Terrified

Describe any changes in your pain today:

_____
_____
_____
_____
_____

Did anything unusual happen today?

_____
_____
_____
_____

What did you spend the most time time thinking about today?

Positive Thoughts:

_____

Did your pain increase, decrease, or remain the same when you thought about it?
____ Increased
____ Decreased
____ Stayed the Same

Negative Thoughts:

_____

Did your pain increase, decrease, or remain the same when you thought about it?
____ Increased
____ Decreased
____ Stayed the Same

1 DAILY
MOOD CHART

Day_____ Date_____ Weight_____

Connect the points on your Mood Satisfaction Chart so your medical team can see when and why your mental state changed.

MOOD		
HAPPY	+3	
	+2	
	+1	
	0	
	-1	
	-2	
SAD	-3	

2 ACTIVITY LOG

6am 7 8 9 10 11 12pm 1 2 3 4 5 6pm 7 8 9 10 11 12am 1 2 3 4 5

3 MEDICATION LOG
NAME/DOSE

1
2
3
4
5
6
7
8

4 PHYSIOLOGY

6am 7 8 9 10 11 12pm 1 2 3 4 5 6pm 7 8 9 10 11 12am 1 2 3 4 5

SLEEP
URINATION
DEFECATION
NAUSEA
EATING
EXERCISE
OTHER (LIST)

10

1 DAILY RESULTS
OF MEDICATIONS AND TREATMENTS

As you and your medical team develop new treatment plans, it will be especially helpful to record any side effects you experience as you add new treatments. This can help determine which types of treatments will work best for you.

Contact your care provider with any bad reactions or side effects to determine if you should discontinue the medication or treatment.

MEDICATION / TREATMENT	AMOUNT / TIME / COMMENTS

10

1 DAILY
TREATMENT PLAN

As you and your medical team develop new treatment plans, record your plan for the day including new medications, increases or decreases to medications, exercises, physical therapy, or any other treatment efforts.

MEDICATION / TREATMENT	AMOUNT / TIME / COMMENTS

11

1 DAILY
PAIN CHART

DAY_____ DATE_____ WEIGHT_____

Connect the points on your Daily Pain and Satisfaction Charts so your medical team can see when your status changed.

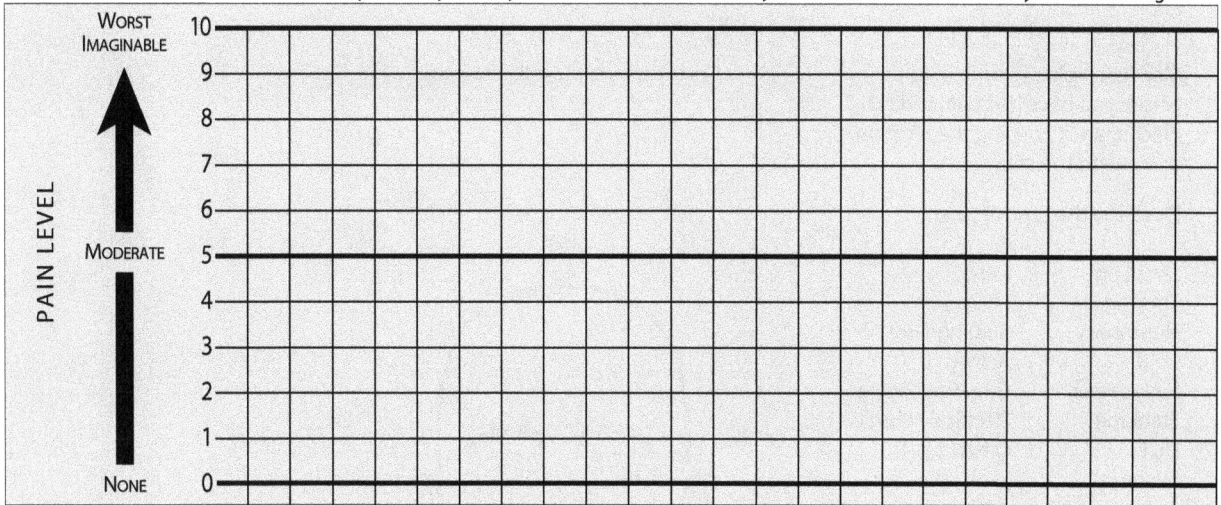

PAIN LEVEL

- WORST IMAGINABLE — 10
- 9
- 8
- 7
- 6
- MODERATE — 5
- 4
- 3
- 2
- 1
- NONE — 0

Times: 6am, 7, 8, 9, 10, 11, 12pm, 1, 2, 3, 4, 5, 6pm, 7, 8, 9, 10, 11, 12am, 1, 2, 3, 4, 5

2 SATISFACTION

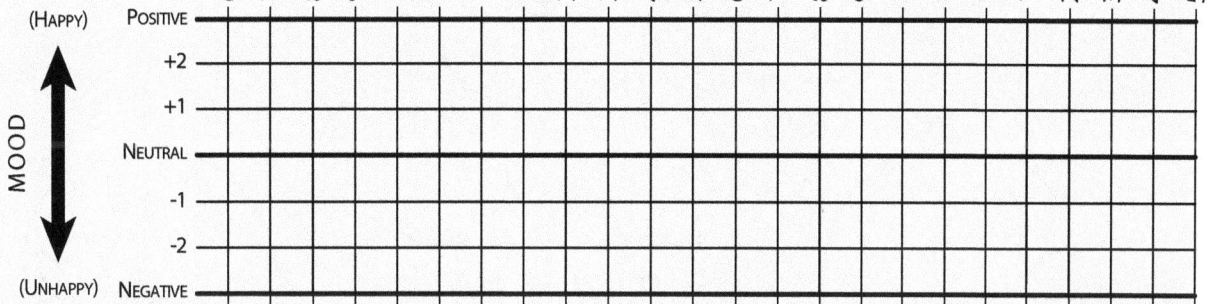

MOOD

- (HAPPY) POSITIVE
- +2
- +1
- NEUTRAL
- -1
- -2
- (UNHAPPY) NEGATIVE

Times: 6am, 7, 8, 9, 10, 11, 12pm, 1, 2, 3, 4, 5, 6pm, 7, 8, 9, 10, 11, 12am, 1, 2, 3, 4, 5

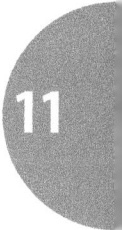

11

3 PHYSIOLOGY

Times: 6am, 7, 8, 9, 10, 11, 12pm, 1, 2, 3, 4, 5, 6pm, 7, 8, 9, 10, 11, 12am, 1, 2, 3, 4, 5

- SLEEP
- RESTROOM
- NAUSEA / DIZZINESS
- MEAL / SNACK
- EXERCISE
- STRESS / ANXIETY

MEDICINE NAME / DOSE

1
2
3

BLOOD PRESSURE

PULSE

4 DAILY HEAD & FACE PAIN DIAGRAM

Mark each place on the diagram where you have had pain today by placing an 'X', circling the location, or shading the area .

Describe the type of pain:

Shooting	Deep
Tingling	Sharp
Numbness	Burning / Hot
Cold	Aching
Surface Pain	Gnawing / Biting
Stabbing	Electrical / Shocks
Dull	Other_____
Stinging	

COMMENTS AND MORE INFORMATION:

Front

Upper Right   Upper Left

Lower Right   Lower Left

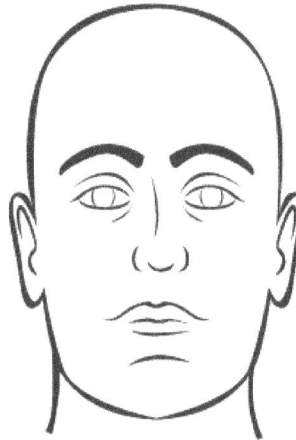

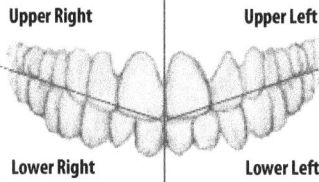

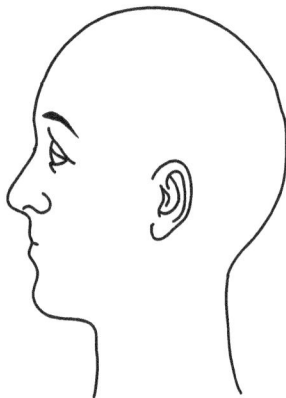

Your Right Side

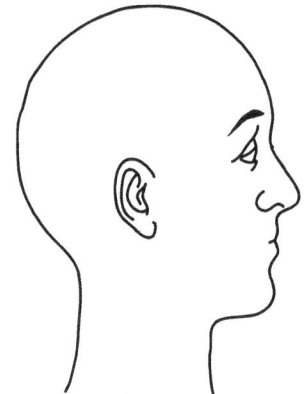

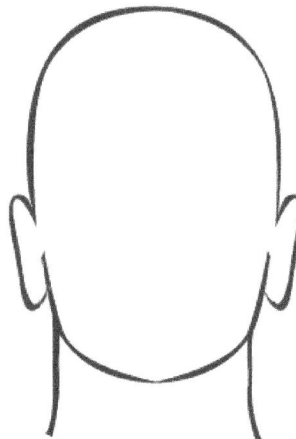

Your Right Side

Back

5 DAILY BODY PAIN DIAGRAM

Mark each place on the diagram where you have had pain today by placing an 'X', circling the location, or shading the area .

Describe the type of pain:

Shooting   Deep
Tingling   Sharp
Numbness   Burning / Hot
Cold   Aching
Surface Pain   Gnawing / Biting
Stabbing   Electrical / Shocks
Dull   Other_____
Stinging

COMMENTS AND MORE INFORMATION:

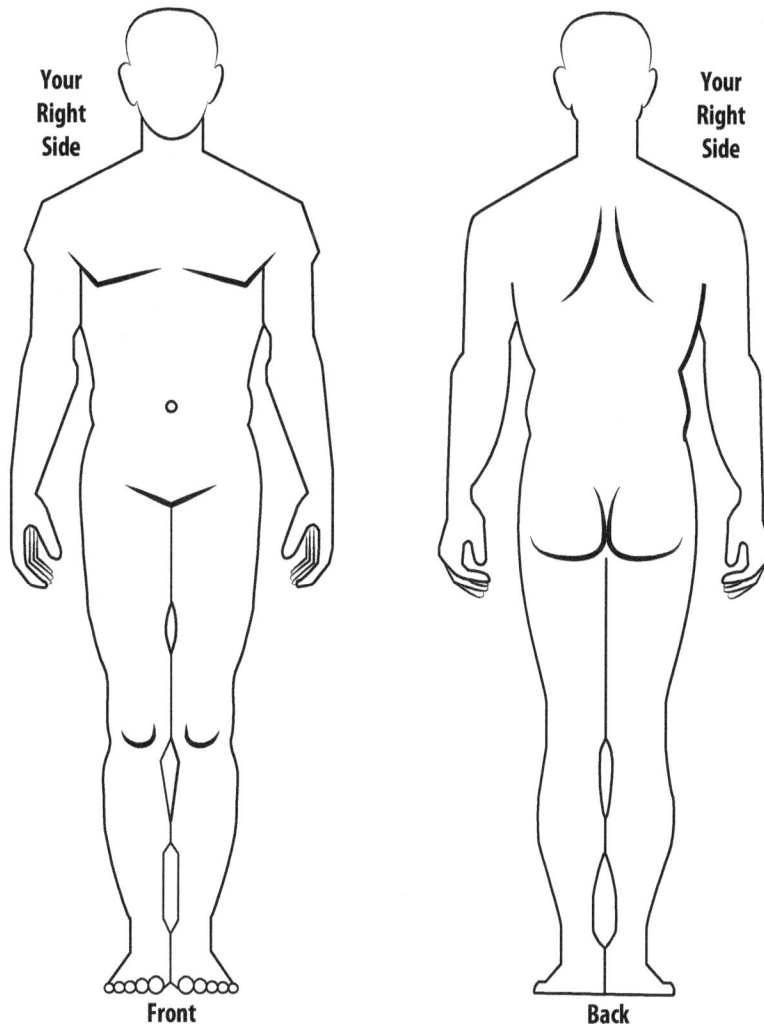

Your Right Side

Your Right Side

11

Front

Back

6 DAILY PAIN SUMMARY

Were there times during the day that you experienced unrelieved breakthrough pain? _____NO _____YES

How many times did this happen today?

1 2 3 4 5 6 7 8 9 10 more than 10

Did any specific activity start your breakthrough pain? _____NO _____YES: What activities?

_____

Put an "X" on the body diagram to show each place you've had **BREAKTHROUGH PAIN** today.

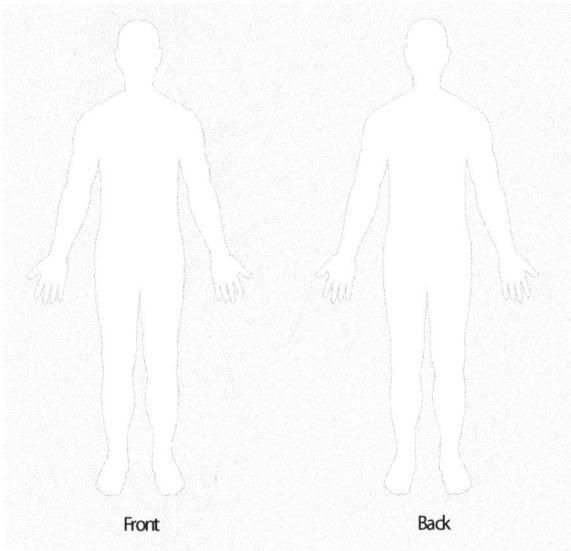

Front   Back

NON-DRUG THERAPIES
(other than prescription or other medicines)

_____

_____

ACTIVITIES/EXERCISE

_____

_____

What was your average level of pain today?

0 1 2 3 4 5 6 7 8 9 10

Other than prescription medicine, did you do anything else today to relieve the pain? _____NO _____YES: (Note any that you used.)
_____ Non-prescription drugs (e.g., acetaminophen, ibuprofen)
_____ Herbal remedies
_____ Hot or cold packs
_____ Exercise
_____ Changing position (such as lying down or elevating your legs)
_____ Physical therapy
_____ Massage
_____ Acupuncture
_____ Rest
_____ Psychological counseling
_____ Talk to trusted friend, family, clergy
_____ Prayer, meditation, guided imagery
_____ Relaxation technique (hypnosis, biofeedback)
_____ Creative technique (art or music therapy)
_____ Other (e.g., specific chiropractic manipulation, osteopathic treatments):

_____

Check any of these common side effects that you've noticed after taking your pain medicine:
_____ Drowsiness, sleepiness
_____ Nausea, vomiting, upset stomach
_____ Constipation
_____ Lack of appetite
_____ Other (describe):

_____

Did you sleep through the night? _____NO_____YES

If not, how many times was your sleep disrupted? _____

How many hours did you sleep during the night? _____

COMMENTS AND MORE INFORMATION: Make notes for and about visits with your healthcare provider, side effects from treatments you may be experiencing, any problems you are having coping with your pain, and more about some of your previous answers or questions.

_____

_____

_____

1 DAILY DIARY

Day_____ Date_____ Weight_____

SATISFACTION CHART Connect the points on your Daily Satisfaction Chart so your medical team can see when and why your mental state changed.

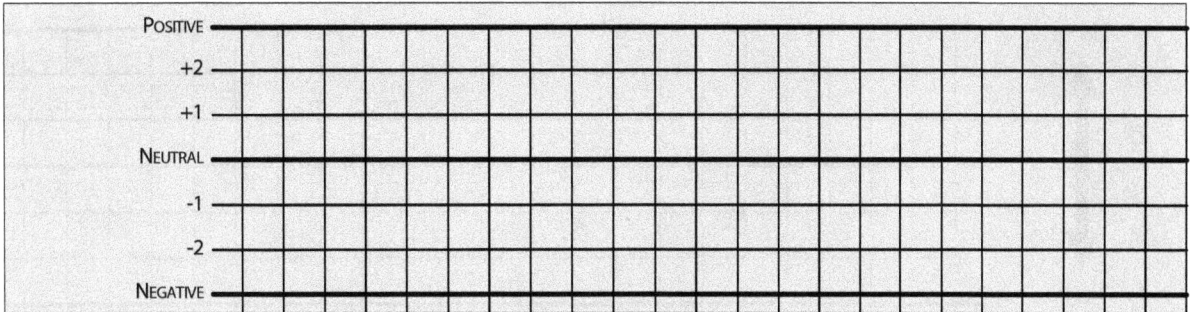

POSITIVE
+2
+1
NEUTRAL
-1
-2
NEGATIVE

2 ACTIVITY LOG

6am 7 8 9 10 11 12pm 1 2 3 4 5 6pm 7 8 9 10 11 12am 1 2 3 4 5

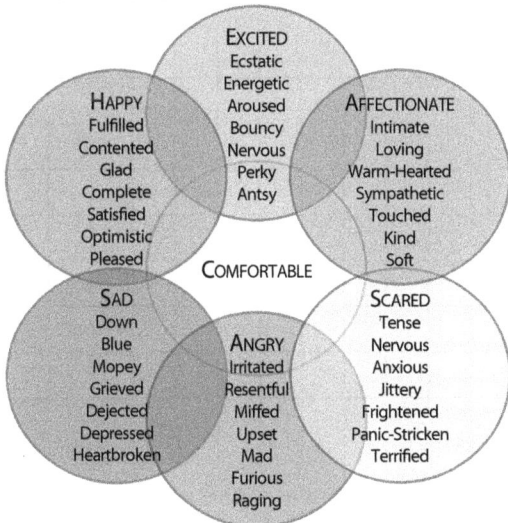

TRIGGERS AND SIGNIFICANT EVENTS

EXCITED
Ecstatic
Energetic
Aroused
Bouncy
Nervous
Perky
Antsy

HAPPY
Fulfilled
Contented
Glad
Complete
Satisfied
Optimistic
Pleased

AFFECTIONATE
Intimate
Loving
Warm-Hearted
Sympathetic
Touched
Kind
Soft

COMFORTABLE

SAD
Down
Blue
Mopey
Grieved
Dejected
Depressed
Heartbroken

ANGRY
Irritated
Resentful
Miffed
Upset
Mad
Furious
Raging

SCARED
Tense
Nervous
Anxious
Jittery
Frightened
Panic-Stricken
Terrified

Describe any changes in your pain today:

_____
_____
_____
_____
_____

Did anything unusual happen today?

_____
_____
_____
_____

11

What did you spend the most time time thinking about today?

Positive Thoughts:

_____

Did your pain increase, decrease, or remain the same when you thought about it?
____ Increased
____ Decreased
____ Stayed the Same

Negative Thoughts:

_____

Did your pain increase, decrease, or remain the same when you thought about it?
____ Increased
____ Decreased
____ Stayed the Same

1 DAILY
MOOD CHART

DAY_____ DATE_____ WEIGHT_____

Connect the points on your Mood Satisfaction Chart so your medical team can see when and why your mental state changed.

MOOD		
HAPPY	+3	
	+2	
	+1	
	0	
	-1	
	-2	
SAD	-3	

2 ACTIVITY LOG

6am 7 8 9 10 11 12pm 1 2 3 4 5 6pm 7 8 9 10 11 12am 1 2 3 4 5

3 MEDICATION LOG
NAME/DOSE

1
2
3
4
5
6
7
8

11

4 PHYSIOLOGY

6am 7 8 9 10 11 12pm 1 2 3 4 5 6pm 7 8 9 10 11 12am 1 2 3 4 5

SLEEP
URINATION
DEFECATION
NAUSEA
EATING
EXERCISE
OTHER (LIST)

1 DAILY RESULTS
OF MEDICATIONS AND TREATMENTS

As you and your medical team develop new treatment plans, it will be especially helpful to record any side effects you experience as you add new treatments. This can help determine which types of treatments will work best for you.

Contact your care provider with any bad reactions or side effects to determine if you should discontinue the medication or treatment.

MEDICATION / TREATMENT	AMOUNT / TIME / COMMENTS

11

1 DAILY
TREATMENT PLAN

As you and your medical team develop new treatment plans, record your plan for the day including new medications, increases or decreases to medications, exercises, physical therapy, or any other treatment efforts.

MEDICATION / TREATMENT	AMOUNT / TIME / COMMENTS

12

1 DAILY
PAIN CHART

DAY_____ DATE_____ WEIGHT_____

Connect the points on your Daily Pain and Satisfaction Charts so your medical team can see when your status changed.

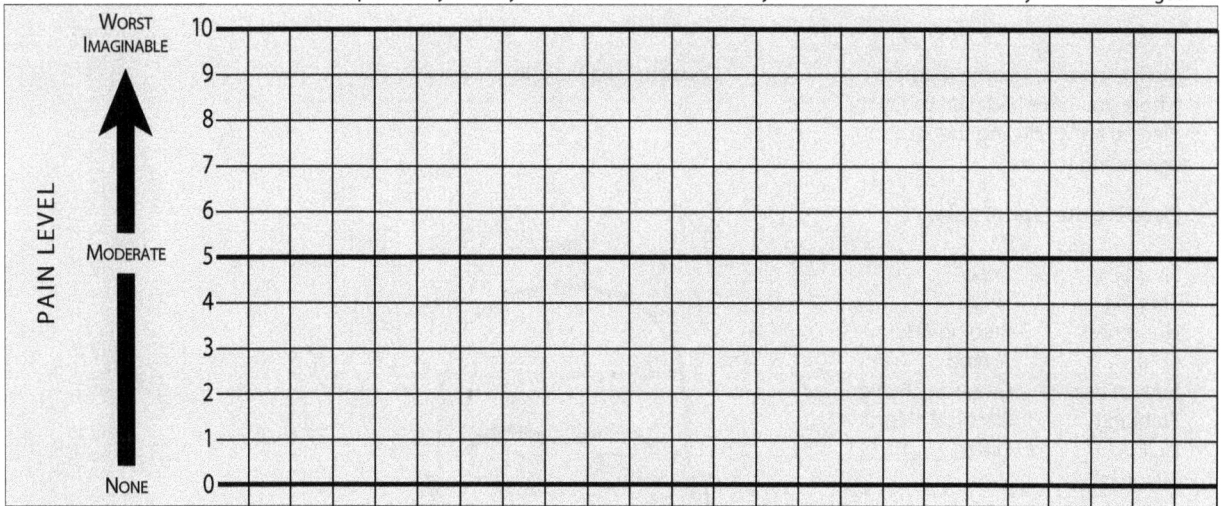

PAIN LEVEL

WORST IMAGINABLE	10
	9
	8
	7
	6
MODERATE	5
	4
	3
	2
	1
NONE	0

2 SATISFACTION

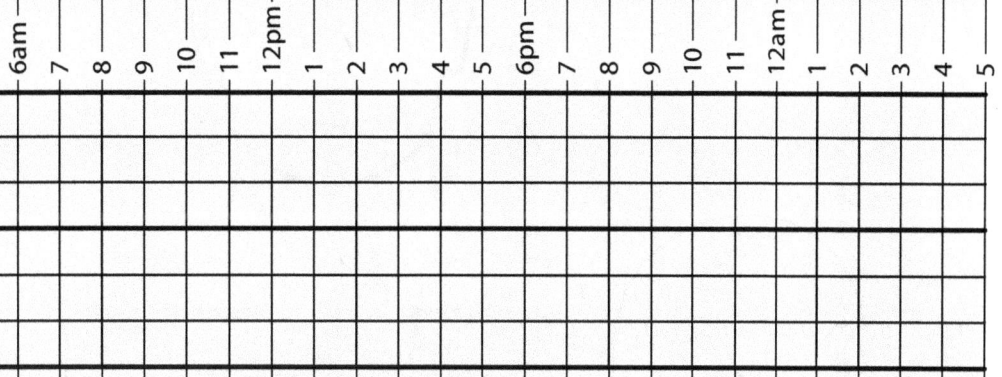

MOOD

Time scale: 6am 7 8 9 10 11 12pm 1 2 3 4 5 6pm 7 8 9 10 11 12am 1 2 3 4 5

(HAPPY)	POSITIVE
	+2
	+1
	NEUTRAL
	-1
	-2
(UNHAPPY)	NEGATIVE

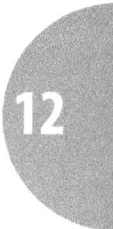

12

3 PHYSIOLOGY

Time scale: 6am 7 8 9 10 11 12pm 1 2 3 4 5 6pm 7 8 9 10 11 12am 1 2 3 4 5

SLEEP

RESTROOM

NAUSEA / DIZZINESS

MEAL / SNACK

EXERCISE

STRESS / ANXIETY

MEDICINE NAME / DOSE

1

2

3

BLOOD PRESSURE

PULSE

4 DAILY HEAD & FACE PAIN DIAGRAM

Mark each place on the diagram where you have had pain today by placing an 'X', circling the location, or shading the area .

Describe the type of pain:

Shooting	Deep
Tingling	Sharp
Numbness	Burning / Hot
Cold	Aching
Surface Pain	Gnawing / Biting
Stabbing	Electrical / Shocks
Dull	Other_____
Stinging	

COMMENTS AND MORE INFORMATION:

Front

Upper Right **Upper Left**

Lower Right **Lower Left**

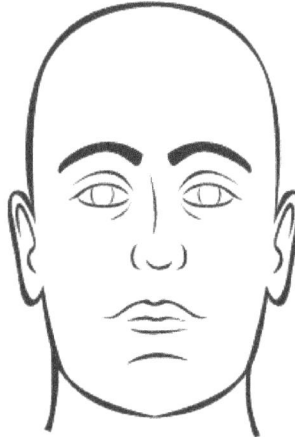

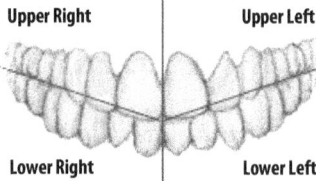

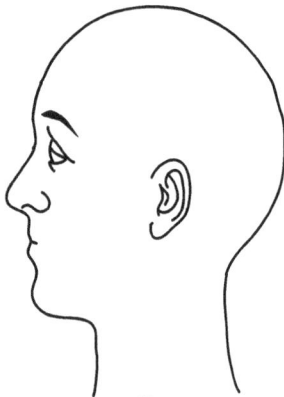

Your Right Side

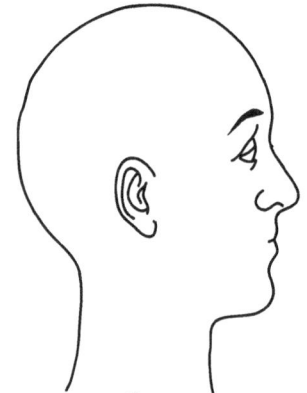

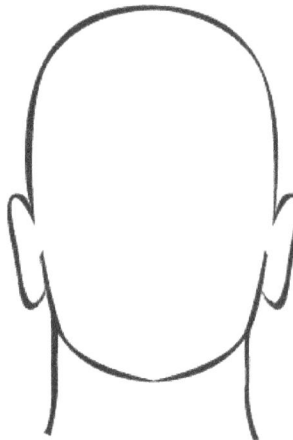

Your Right Side

Back

5 DAILY BODY PAIN DIAGRAM

Mark each place on the diagram where you have had pain today by placing an 'X', circling the location, or shading the area .

Describe the type of pain:

Shooting   Deep
Tingling   Sharp
Numbness   Burning / Hot
Cold   Aching
Surface Pain   Gnawing / Biting
Stabbing   Electrical / Shocks
Dull   Other_____
Stinging

COMMENTS AND MORE INFORMATION:

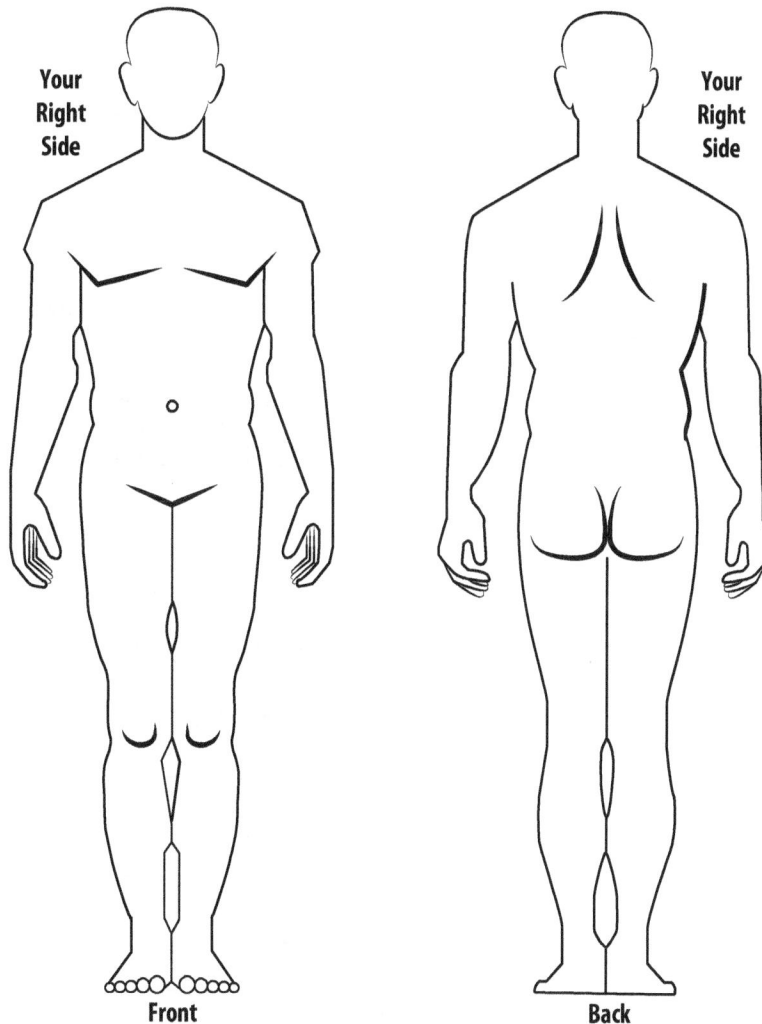

Your Right Side

Your Right Side

Front

Back

12

6 DAILY PAIN SUMMARY

Were there times during the day that you experienced unrelieved breakthrough pain? ____NO ____YES

How many times did this happen today?

1 2 3 4 5 6 7 8 9 10 more than 10

Did any specific activity start your breakthrough pain?
____NO ____YES: What activities?

_____

Put an "X" on the body diagram to show each place you've had **BREAKTHROUGH PAIN** today.

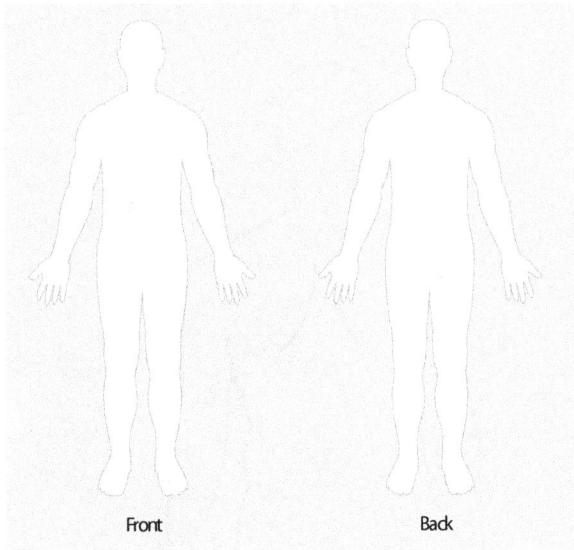

Front   Back

NON-DRUG THERAPIES
(other than prescription or other medicines)

_____

_____

ACTIVITIES/EXERCISE

_____

_____

What was your average level of pain today?

0 1 2 3 4 5 6 7 8 9 10

Other than prescription medicine, did you do anything else today to relieve the pain? ____NO ____YES:
(Note any that you used.)
____ Non-prescription drugs (e.g., acetaminophen, ibuprofen)
____ Herbal remedies
____ Hot or cold packs
____ Exercise
____ Changing position (such as lying down or elevating your legs)
____ Physical therapy
____ Massage
____ Acupuncture
____ Rest
____ Psychological counseling
____ Talk to trusted friend, family, clergy
____ Prayer, meditation, guided imagery
____ Relaxation technique (hypnosis, biofeedback)
____ Creative technique (art or music therapy)
____ Other (e.g., specific chiropractic manipulation, osteopathic treatments):

_____

Check any of these common side effects that you've noticed after taking your pain medicine:
____ Drowsiness, sleepiness
____ Nausea, vomiting, upset stomach
____ Constipation
____ Lack of appetite
____ Other (describe):

_____

Did you sleep through the night? ____NO____YES

If not, how many times was your sleep disrupted? _____

How many hours did you sleep during the night? _____

COMMENTS AND MORE INFORMATION: Make notes for and about visits with your healthcare provider, side effects from treatments you may be experiencing, any problems you are having coping with your pain, and more about some of your previous answers or questions.

_____

_____

_____

1 DAILY DIARY

SATISFACTION CHART Connect the points on your Daily Satisfaction Chart so your medical team can see when and why your mental state changed.

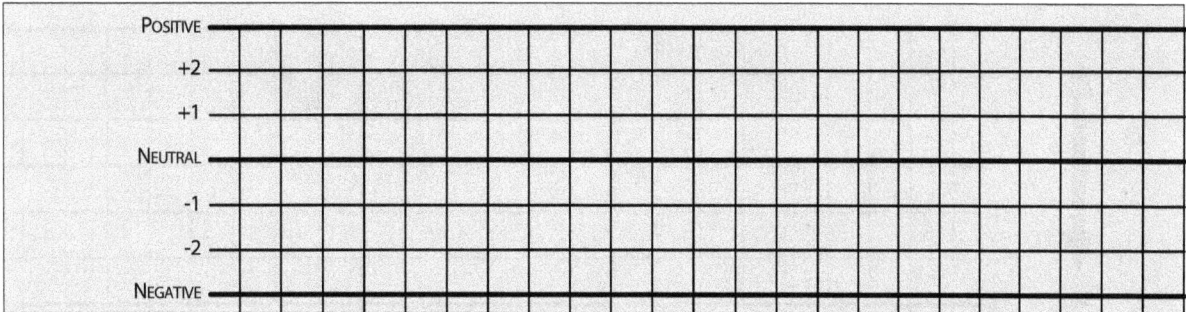

DAY_____ DATE_____ WEIGHT_____

POSITIVE	
+2	
+1	
NEUTRAL	
-1	
-2	
NEGATIVE	

2 ACTIVITY LOG

6am 7 8 9 10 11 12pm 1 2 3 4 5 6pm 7 8 9 10 11 12am 1 2 3 4 5

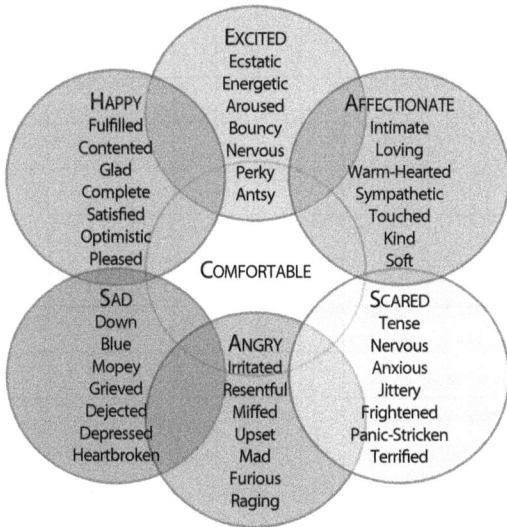

TRIGGERS AND SIGNIFICANT EVENTS

EXCITED
Ecstatic
Energetic
Aroused
Bouncy
Nervous
Perky
Antsy

HAPPY
Fulfilled
Contented
Glad
Complete
Satisfied
Optimistic
Pleased

AFFECTIONATE
Intimate
Loving
Warm-Hearted
Sympathetic
Touched
Kind
Soft

COMFORTABLE

SAD
Down
Blue
Mopey
Grieved
Dejected
Depressed
Heartbroken

ANGRY
Irritated
Resentful
Miffed
Upset
Mad
Furious
Raging

SCARED
Tense
Nervous
Anxious
Jittery
Frightened
Panic-Stricken
Terrified

Describe any changes in your pain today:
_____
_____
_____
_____
_____

Did anything unusual happen today?
_____
_____
_____
_____
_____

What did you spend the most time time thinking about today?

Positive Thoughts:
_____

Did your pain increase, decrease, or remain the same when you thought about it?
____ Increased
____ Decreased
____ Stayed the Same

Negative Thoughts:
_____

Did your pain increase, decrease, or remain the same when you thought about it?
____ Increased
____ Decreased
____ Stayed the Same

12

1 DAILY
MOOD CHART

DAY_____ DATE_____ WEIGHT_____

Connect the points on your Mood Satisfaction Chart so your medical team can see when and why your mental state changed.

HAPPY +3
+2
+1
MOOD 0
-1
-2
SAD -3

2 ACTIVITY LOG

6am 7 8 9 10 11 12pm 1 2 3 4 5 6pm 7 8 9 10 11 12am 1 2 3 4 5

3 MEDICATION LOG
NAME/DOSE

1
2
3
4
5
6
7
8

4 PHYSIOLOGY

6am 7 8 9 10 11 12pm 1 2 3 4 5 6pm 7 8 9 10 11 12am 1 2 3 4 5

SLEEP
URINATION
DEFECATION
NAUSEA
EATING
EXERCISE
OTHER (LIST)

12

1 DAILY RESULTS
OF MEDICATIONS AND TREATMENTS

As you and your medical team develop new treatment plans, it will be especially helpful to record any side effects you experience as you add new treatments. This can help determine which types of treatments will work best for you.

Contact your care provider with any bad reactions or side effects to determine if you should discontinue the medication or treatment.

MEDICATION / TREATMENT	AMOUNT / TIME / COMMENTS

12

1 DAILY
TREATMENT PLAN

As you and your medical team develop new treatment plans, record your plan for the day including new medications, increases or decreases to medications, exercises, physical therapy, or any other treatment efforts.

MEDICATION / TREATMENT	AMOUNT / TIME / COMMENTS

13

1 DAILY
PAIN CHART

DAY_____ DATE_____ WEIGHT_____

Connect the points on your Daily Pain and Satisfaction Charts so your medical team can see when your status changed.

PAIN LEVEL

WORST IMAGINABLE — 10

9

8

7

6

MODERATE — 5

4

3

2

1

NONE — 0

2 SATISFACTION

Time scale: 6am 7 8 9 10 11 12pm 1 2 3 4 5 6pm 7 8 9 10 11 12am 1 2 3 4 5

MOOD

(HAPPY) POSITIVE

+2

+1

NEUTRAL

-1

-2

(UNHAPPY) NEGATIVE

3 PHYSIOLOGY

Time scale: 6am 7 8 9 10 11 12pm 1 2 3 4 5 6pm 7 8 9 10 11 12am 1 2 3 4 5

SLEEP

RESTROOM

NAUSEA / DIZZINESS

MEAL / SNACK

EXERCISE

STRESS / ANXIETY

MEDICINE NAME / DOSE

1

2

3

BLOOD PRESSURE

PULSE

13

4 DAILY HEAD & FACE PAIN DIAGRAM

Mark each place on the diagram where you have had pain today by placing an 'X', circling the location, or shading the area .

COMMENTS AND MORE INFORMATION:

Describe the type of pain:

Shooting	Deep
Tingling	Sharp
Numbness	Burning / Hot
Cold	Aching
Surface Pain	Gnawing / Biting
Stabbing	Electrical / Shocks
Dull	Other_____
Stinging	

Front

Upper Right   **Upper Left**

Lower Right   **Lower Left**

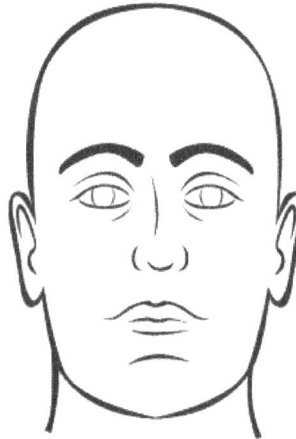

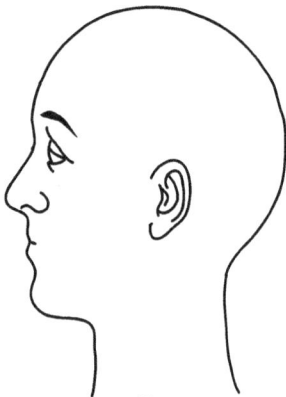

Your Right Side

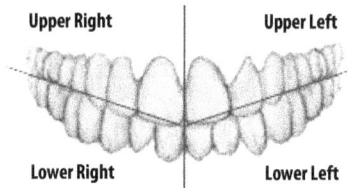

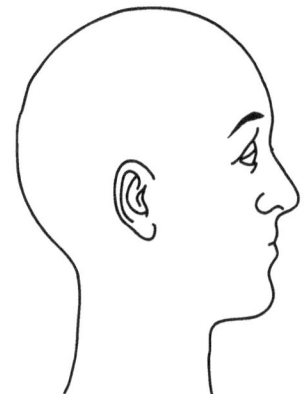

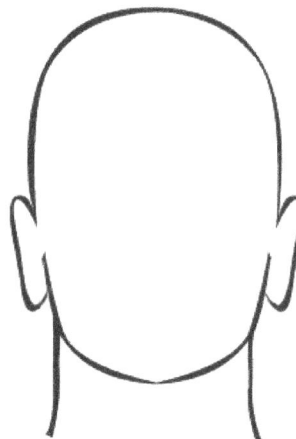

Your Right Side

Back

13

5 DAILY BODY PAIN DIAGRAM

Mark each place on the diagram where you have had pain today by placing an 'X', circling the location, or shading the area .

Describe the type of pain:

Shooting	Deep
Tingling	Sharp
Numbness	Burning / Hot
Cold	Aching
Surface Pain	Gnawing / Biting
Stabbing	Electrical / Shocks
Dull	Other_____
Stinging	

COMMENTS AND MORE INFORMATION:

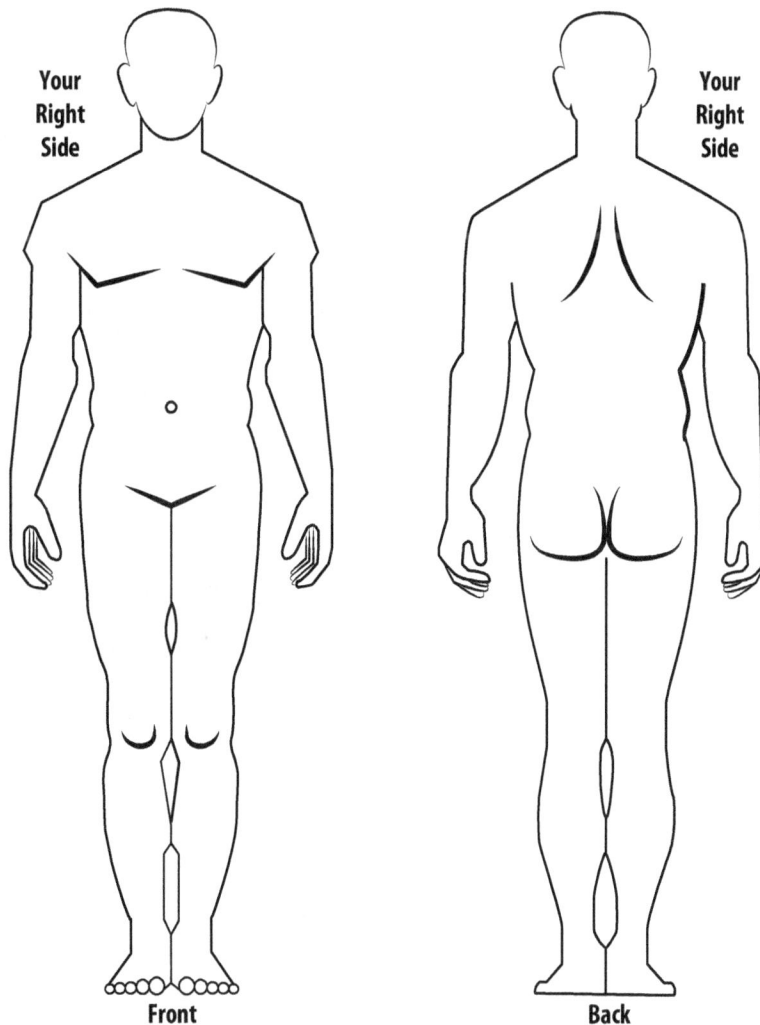

Your Right Side

Your Right Side

Front

Back

13

6 DAILY PAIN SUMMARY

Were there times during the day that you experienced unrelieved breakthrough pain? _____NO _____YES

How many times did this happen today?

1 2 3 4 5 6 7 8 9 10 more than 10

Did any specific activity start your breakthrough pain? _____NO _____YES: What activities?

_____

Put an "X" on the body diagram to show each place you've had **BREAKTHROUGH PAIN** today.

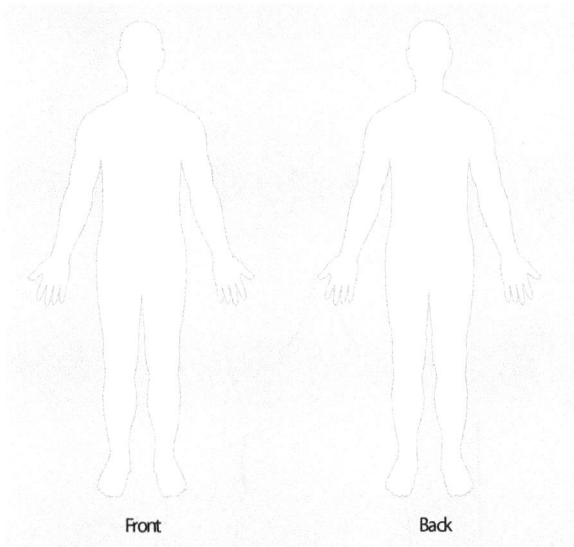

Front   Back

NON-DRUG THERAPIES
(other than prescription or other medicines)

_____

_____

ACTIVITIES/EXERCISE

_____

What was your average level of pain today?

0 1 2 3 4 5 6 7 8 9 10

Other than prescription medicine, did you do anything else today to relieve the pain? _____NO _____YES: (Note any that you used.)
_____ Non-prescription drugs (e.g., acetaminophen, ibuprofen)
_____ Herbal remedies
_____ Hot or cold packs
_____ Exercise
_____ Changing position (such as lying down or elevating your legs)
_____ Physical therapy
_____ Massage
_____ Acupuncture
_____ Rest
_____ Psychological counseling
_____ Talk to trusted friend, family, clergy
_____ Prayer, meditation, guided imagery
_____ Relaxation technique (hypnosis, biofeedback)
_____ Creative technique (art or music therapy)
_____ Other (e.g., specific chiropractic manipulation, osteopathic treatments):

_____

Check any of these common side effects that you've noticed after taking your pain medicine:
_____ Drowsiness, sleepiness
_____ Nausea, vomiting, upset stomach
_____ Constipation
_____ Lack of appetite
_____ Other (describe):

_____

Did you sleep through the night? _____NO_____YES

If not, how many times was your sleep disrupted? _____

How many hours did you sleep during the night? _____

COMMENTS AND MORE INFORMATION: Make notes for and about visits with your healthcare provider, side effects from treatments you may be experiencing, any problems you are having coping with your pain, and more about some of your previous answers or questions.

_____

_____

_____

13

1 DAILY DIARY

SATISFACTION CHART Connect the points on your Daily Satisfaction Chart so your medical team can see when and why your mental state changed.

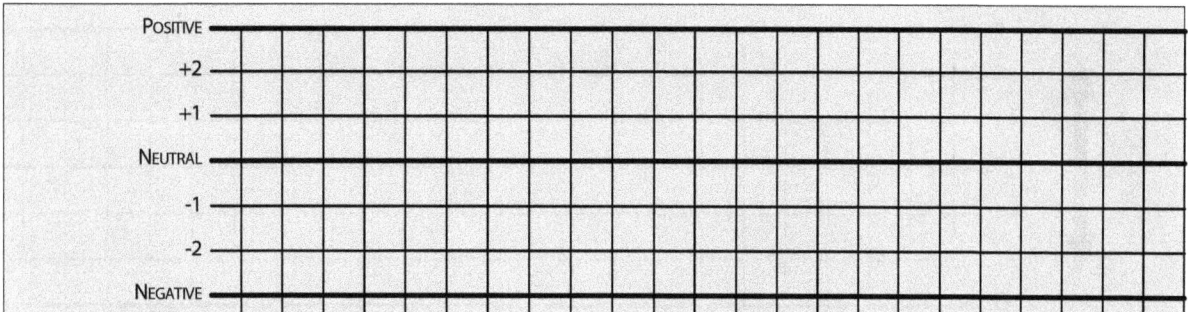

DAY_____ DATE_____ WEIGHT_____

POSITIVE	
+2	
+1	
NEUTRAL	
-1	
-2	
NEGATIVE	

2 ACTIVITY LOG

TRIGGERS AND SIGNIFICANT EVENTS

6am 7 8 9 10 11 12pm 1 2 3 4 5 6pm 7 8 9 10 11 12am 1 2 3 4 5

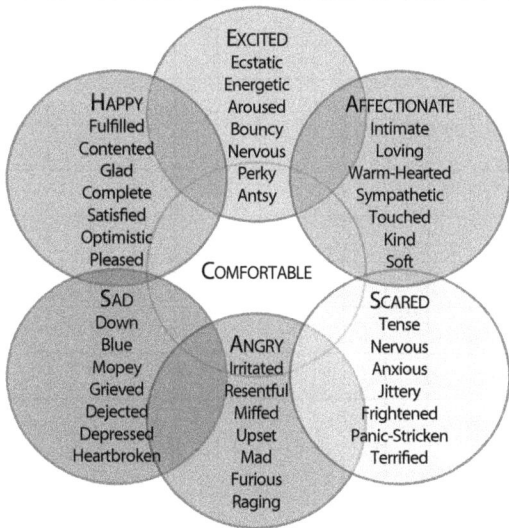

EXCITED
Ecstatic
Energetic
Aroused
Bouncy
Nervous
Perky
Antsy

HAPPY
Fulfilled
Contented
Glad
Complete
Satisfied
Optimistic
Pleased

AFFECTIONATE
Intimate
Loving
Warm-Hearted
Sympathetic
Touched
Kind
Soft

COMFORTABLE

SAD
Down
Blue
Mopey
Grieved
Dejected
Depressed
Heartbroken

ANGRY
Irritated
Resentful
Miffed
Upset
Mad
Furious
Raging

SCARED
Tense
Nervous
Anxious
Jittery
Frightened
Panic-Stricken
Terrified

Describe any changes in your pain today:

_____
_____
_____
_____

Did anything unusual happen today?

_____
_____
_____
_____

13

What did you spend the most time time thinking about today?

Positive Thoughts:

_____

Did your pain increase, decrease, or remain the same when you thought about it?
____ Increased
____ Decreased
____ Stayed the Same

Negative Thoughts:

_____

Did your pain increase, decrease, or remain the same when you thought about it?
____ Increased
____ Decreased
____ Stayed the Same

1 DAILY
MOOD CHART

DAY_____ DATE_____ WEIGHT_____

Connect the points on your Mood Satisfaction Chart so your medical team can see when and why your mental state changed.

MOOD

HAPPY +3
       +2
       +1
        0
       -1
       -2
SAD   -3

2 ACTIVITY LOG

6am 7 8 9 10 11 12pm 1 2 3 4 5 6pm 7 8 9 10 11 12am 1 2 3 4 5

3 MEDICATION LOG
NAME/DOSE

1
2
3
4
5
6
7
8

4 PHYSIOLOGY

6am 7 8 9 10 11 12pm 1 2 3 4 5 6pm 7 8 9 10 11 12am 1 2 3 4 5

SLEEP
URINATION
DEFECATION
NAUSEA
EATING
EXERCISE
OTHER (LIST)

13

1 DAILY RESULTS
OF MEDICATIONS AND TREATMENTS

As you and your medical team develop new treatment plans, it will be especially helpful to record any side effects you experience as you add new treatments. This can help determine which types of treatments will work best for you.

Contact your care provider with any bad reactions or side effects to determine if you should discontinue the medication or treatment.

MEDICATION / TREATMENT	AMOUNT / TIME / COMMENTS

13

1 DAILY
TREATMENT PLAN

As you and your medical team develop new treatment plans, record your plan for the day including new medications, increases or decreases to medications, exercises, physical therapy, or any other treatment efforts.

MEDICATION / TREATMENT	AMOUNT / TIME / COMMENTS

1 DAILY
PAIN CHART

DAY_____ DATE_____ WEIGHT_____

Connect the points on your Daily Pain and Satisfaction Charts so your medical team can see when your status changed.

PAIN LEVEL

WORST IMAGINABLE	10
	9
	8
	7
	6
MODERATE	5
	4
	3
	2
	1
NONE	0

Time axis: 6am 7 8 9 10 11 12pm 1 2 3 4 5 6pm 7 8 9 10 11 12am 1 2 3 4 5

2 SATISFACTION

MOOD

(HAPPY)	POSITIVE
	+2
	+1
	NEUTRAL
	-1
	-2
(UNHAPPY)	NEGATIVE

Time axis: 6am 7 8 9 10 11 12pm 1 2 3 4 5 6pm 7 8 9 10 11 12am 1 2 3 4 5

3 PHYSIOLOGY

Time axis: 6am 7 8 9 10 11 12pm 1 2 3 4 5 6pm 7 8 9 10 11 12am 1 2 3 4 5

- SLEEP
- RESTROOM
- NAUSEA / DIZZINESS
- MEAL / SNACK
- EXERCISE
- STRESS / ANXIETY

MEDICINE NAME / DOSE
1
2
3

BLOOD PRESSURE

PULSE

14

4 DAILY HEAD & FACE PAIN DIAGRAM

Mark each place on the diagram where you have had pain today by placing an 'X', circling the location, or shading the area .

Describe the type of pain:

Shooting	Deep
Tingling	Sharp
Numbness	Burning / Hot
Cold	Aching
Surface Pain	Gnawing / Biting
Stabbing	Electrical / Shocks
Dull	Other_____
Stinging	

COMMENTS AND MORE INFORMATION:

Front

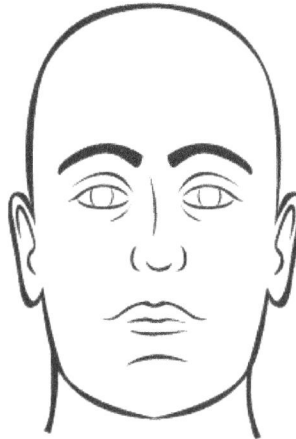

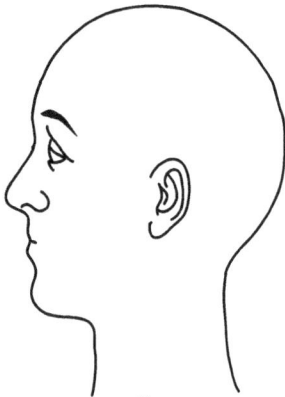

Your Right Side

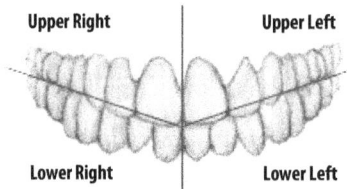

Upper Right   Upper Left

Lower Right   Lower Left

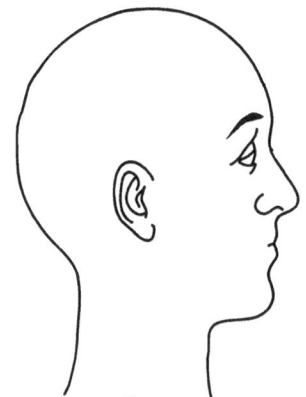

Your Right Side

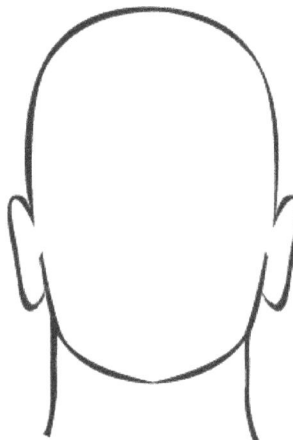

Back

5 DAILY BODY PAIN DIAGRAM

Mark each place on the diagram where you have had pain today by placing an 'X', circling the location, or shading the area .

Describe the type of pain:

Shooting	Deep
Tingling	Sharp
Numbness	Burning / Hot
Cold	Aching
Surface Pain	Gnawing / Biting
Stabbing	Electrical / Shocks
Dull	Other_____
Stinging	

COMMENTS AND MORE INFORMATION:

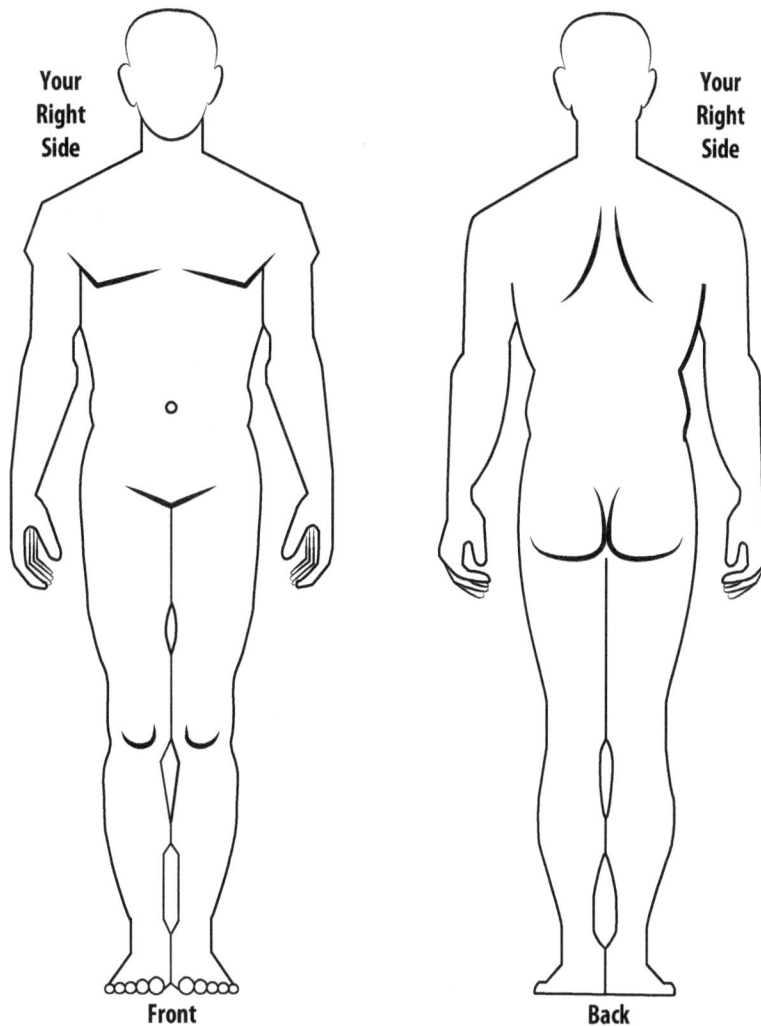

Your Right Side

Your Right Side

Front

Back

14

6 DAILY PAIN SUMMARY

Were there times during the day that you experienced unrelieved breakthrough pain? ____NO ____YES

How many times did this happen today?

1 2 3 4 5 6 7 8 9 10 more than 10

Did any specific activity start your breakthrough pain? ____NO ____YES: What activities?

_____

Put an "X" on the body diagram to show each place you've had **BREAKTHROUGH PAIN** today.

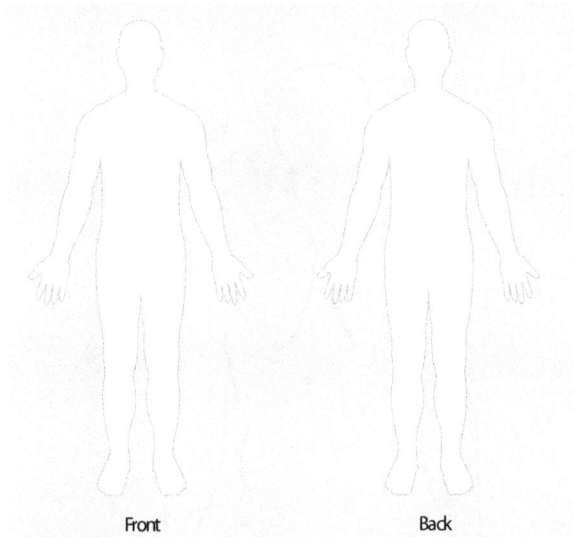

Front   Back

NON-DRUG THERAPIES
(other than prescription or other medicines)

_____

_____

ACTIVITIES/EXERCISE

_____

What was your average level of pain today?

0   1   2   3   4   5   6   7   8   9   10

Other than prescription medicine, did you do anything else today to relieve the pain? ____NO ____YES:
(Note any that you used.)
____ Non-prescription drugs (e.g., acetaminophen, ibuprofen)
____ Herbal remedies
____ Hot or cold packs
____ Exercise
____ Changing position (such as lying down or elevating your legs)
____ Physical therapy
____ Massage
____ Acupuncture
____ Rest
____ Psychological counseling
____ Talk to trusted friend, family, clergy
____ Prayer, meditation, guided imagery
____ Relaxation technique (hypnosis, biofeedback)
____ Creative technique (art or music therapy)
____ Other (e.g., specific chiropractic manipulation, osteopathic treatments):

_____

Check any of these common side effects that you've noticed after taking your pain medicine:
____ Drowsiness, sleepiness
____ Nausea, vomiting, upset stomach
____ Constipation
____ Lack of appetite
____ Other (describe):

_____

Did you sleep through the night? ____NO____YES

If not, how many times was your sleep disrupted? _____

How many hours did you sleep during the night? _____

COMMENTS AND MORE INFORMATION: Make notes for and about visits with your healthcare provider, side effects from treatments you may be experiencing, any problems you are having coping with your pain, and more about some of your previous answers or questions.

_____

_____

_____

14

1 DAILY DIARY

DAY_____ DATE_____ WEIGHT_____

SATISFACTION CHART Connect the points on your Daily Satisfaction Chart so your medical team can see when and why your mental state changed.

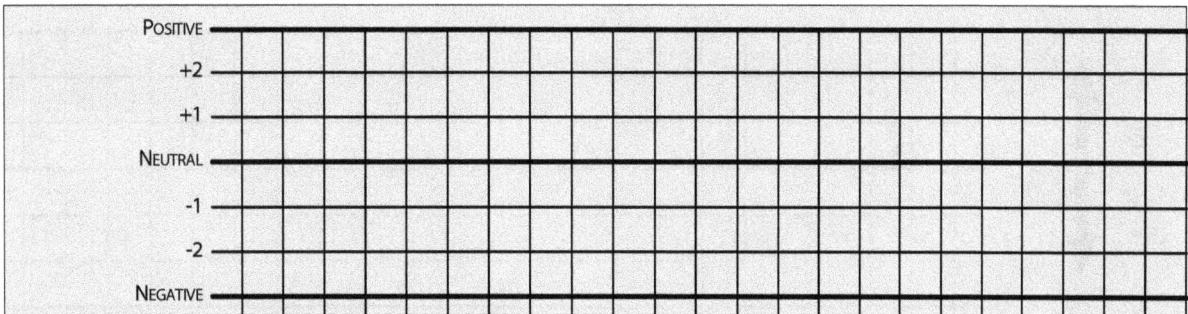

	POSITIVE
+2	
+1	
NEUTRAL	
-1	
-2	
NEGATIVE	

2 ACTIVITY LOG

6am 7 8 9 10 11 12pm 1 2 3 4 5 6pm 7 8 9 10 11 12am 1 2 3 4 5

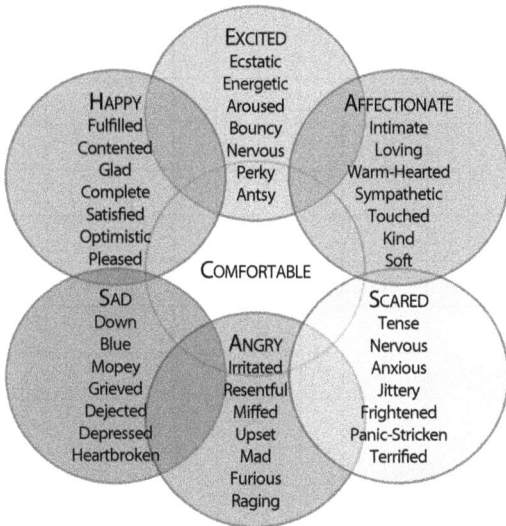

TRIGGERS AND SIGNIFICANT EVENTS

EXCITED
Ecstatic
Energetic
Aroused
Bouncy
Nervous
Perky
Antsy

HAPPY
Fulfilled
Contented
Glad
Complete
Satisfied
Optimistic
Pleased

AFFECTIONATE
Intimate
Loving
Warm-Hearted
Sympathetic
Touched
Kind
Soft

COMFORTABLE

SAD
Down
Blue
Mopey
Grieved
Dejected
Depressed
Heartbroken

ANGRY
Irritated
Resentful
Miffed
Upset
Mad
Furious
Raging

SCARED
Tense
Nervous
Anxious
Jittery
Frightened
Panic-Stricken
Terrified

Describe any changes in your pain today:

_____

_____

_____

_____

Did anything unusual happen today?

_____

_____

_____

_____

What did you spend the most time time thinking about today?

Positive Thoughts:

_____

Did your pain increase, decrease, or remain the same when you thought about it?
____ Increased
____ Decreased
____ Stayed the Same

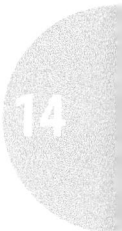

Negative Thoughts:

_____

Did your pain increase, decrease, or remain the same when you thought about it?
____ Increased
____ Decreased
____ Stayed the Same

14

DAY_____ DATE_____ WEIGHT_____

1 DAILY
MOOD CHART

Connect the points on your Mood Satisfaction Chart so your medical team can see when and why your mental state changed.

MOOD		
HAPPY	+3	
	+2	
	+1	
	0	
	-1	
	-2	
SAD	-3	

2 ACTIVITY LOG

6am 7 8 9 10 11 12pm 1 2 3 4 5 6pm 7 8 9 10 11 12am 1 2 3 4 5

3 MEDICATION LOG
NAME/DOSE

1
2
3
4
5
6
7
8

4 PHYSIOLOGY

6am 7 8 9 10 11 12pm 1 2 3 4 5 6pm 7 8 9 10 11 12am 1 2 3 4 5

SLEEP
URINATION
DEFECATION
NAUSEA
EATING
EXERCISE
OTHER (LIST)

1 DAILY RESULTS
OF MEDICATIONS AND TREATMENTS

As you and your medical team develop new treatment plans, it will be especially helpful to record any side effects you experience as you add new treatments. This can help determine which types of treatments will work best for you.

Contact your care provider with any bad reactions or side effects to determine if you should discontinue the medication or treatment.

MEDICATION / TREATMENT	AMOUNT / TIME / COMMENTS

14

15

1 DAILY
TREATMENT PLAN

As you and your medical team develop new treatment plans, record your plan for the day including new medications, increases or decreases to medications, exercises, physical therapy, or any other treatment efforts.

MEDICATION / TREATMENT	AMOUNT / TIME / COMMENTS

1 DAILY
PAIN CHART

DAY_____ DATE_____ WEIGHT_____

Connect the points on your Daily Pain and Satisfaction Charts so your medical team can see when your status changed.

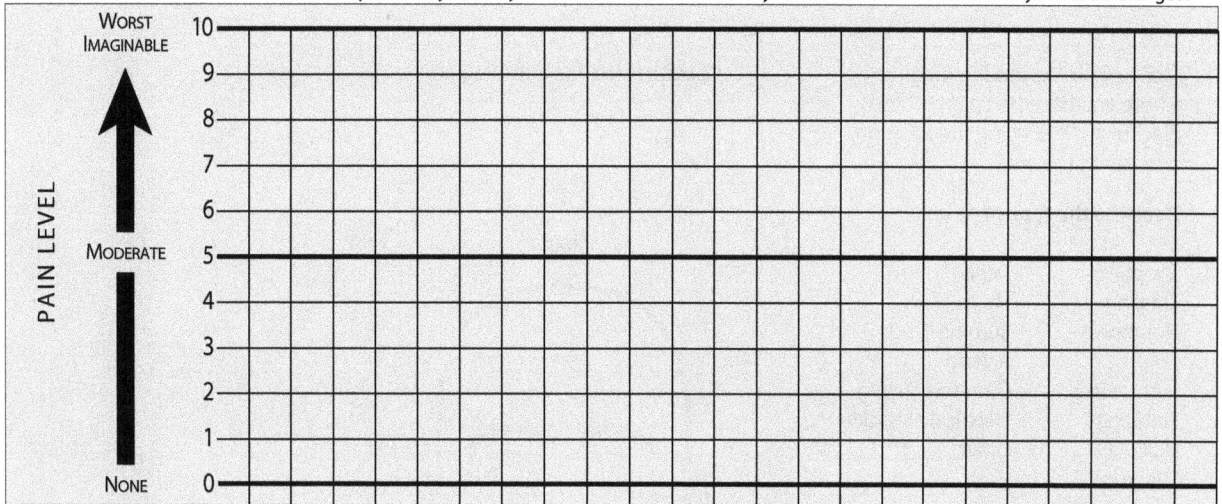

PAIN LEVEL

WORST IMAGINABLE — 10
9
8
7
6
MODERATE — 5
4
3
2
1
NONE — 0

2 SATISFACTION

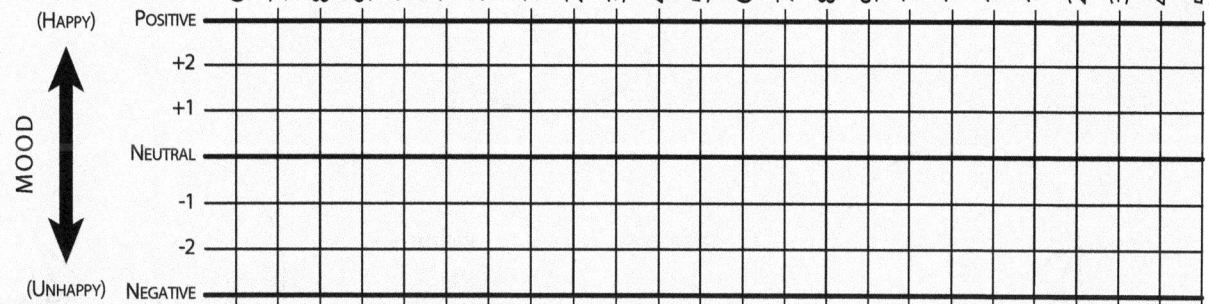

6am 7 8 9 10 11 12pm 1 2 3 4 5 6pm 7 8 9 10 11 12am 1 2 3 4 5

MOOD

(HAPPY) POSITIVE
+2
+1
NEUTRAL
-1
-2
(UNHAPPY) NEGATIVE

3 PHYSIOLOGY

6am 7 8 9 10 11 12pm 1 2 3 4 5 6pm 7 8 9 10 11 12am 1 2 3 4 5

SLEEP
RESTROOM
NAUSEA / DIZZINESS
MEAL / SNACK
EXERCISE
STRESS / ANXIETY

MEDICINE NAME / DOSE
1
2
3

BLOOD PRESSURE
PULSE

15

15

4 DAILY HEAD & FACE PAIN DIAGRAM

Mark each place on the diagram where you have had pain today by placing an 'X', circling the location, or shading the area .

COMMENTS AND MORE INFORMATION:

Describe the type of pain:

Shooting	Deep
Tingling	Sharp
Numbness	Burning / Hot
Cold	Aching
Surface Pain	Gnawing / Biting
Stabbing	Electrical / Shocks
Dull	Other_____
Stinging	

Front

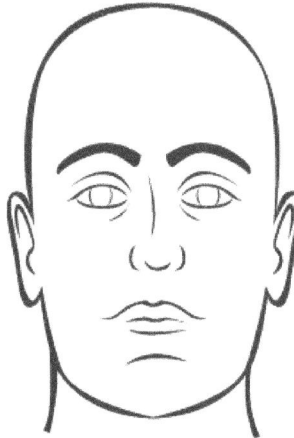

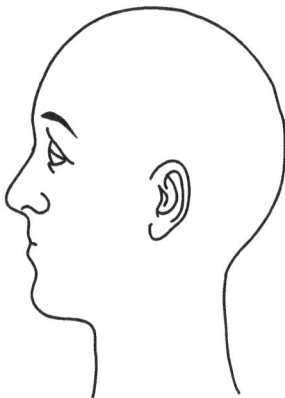

Your Right Side

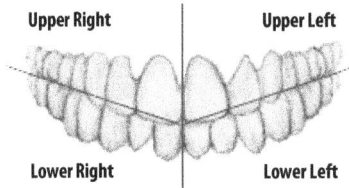

Upper Right   Upper Left

Lower Right   Lower Left

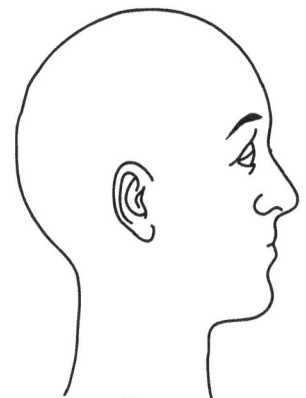

Your Right Side

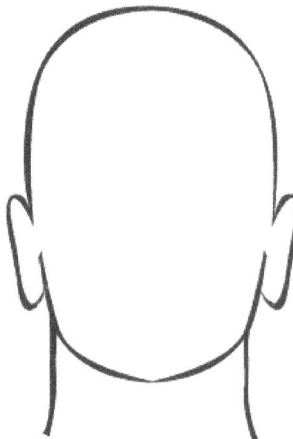

Back

15

5 DAILY BODY PAIN DIAGRAM

Mark each place on the diagram where you have had pain today by placing an 'X', circling the location, or shading the area .

Describe the type of pain:

Shooting	Deep
Tingling	Sharp
Numbness	Burning / Hot
Cold	Aching
Surface Pain	Gnawing / Biting
Stabbing	Electrical / Shocks
Dull	Other_____
Stinging	

COMMENTS AND MORE INFORMATION:

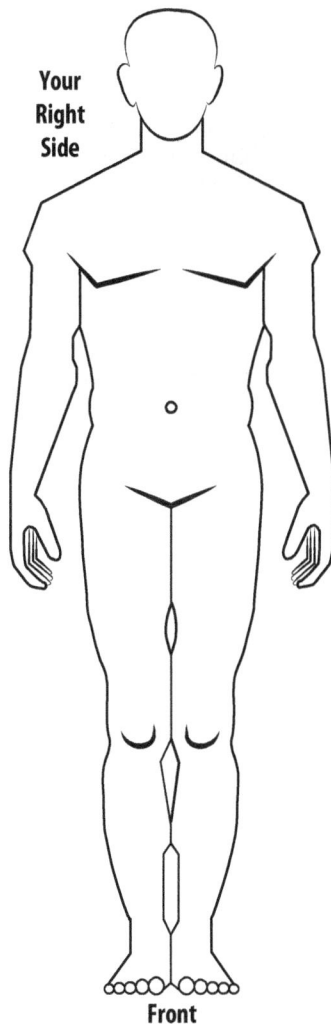

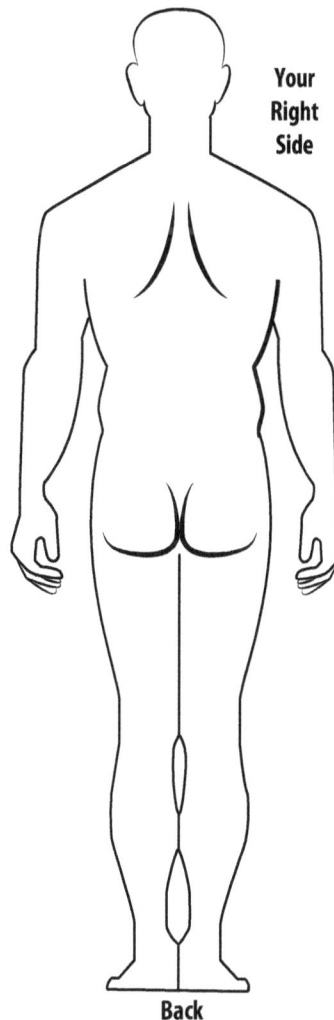

Your
Right
Side

Your
Right
Side

Front

Back

6 DAILY PAIN SUMMARY

Were there times during the day that you experienced unrelieved breakthrough pain? ____NO ____YES

How many times did this happen today?

1 2 3 4 5 6 7 8 9 10 more than 10

Did any specific activity start your breakthrough pain? ____NO ____YES: What activities?

_____

Put an "X" on the body diagram to show each place you've had **BREAKTHROUGH PAIN** today.

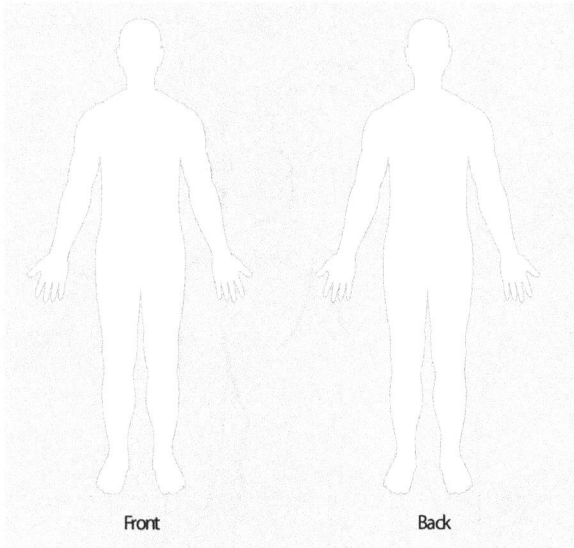

Front   Back

NON-DRUG THERAPIES
(other than prescription or other medicines)

_____

_____

ACTIVITIES/EXERCISE

_____

What was your average level of pain today?

0 1 2 3 4 5 6 7 8 9 10

Other than prescription medicine, did you do anything else today to relieve the pain? ____NO ____YES:
(Note any that you used.)
____ Non-prescription drugs (e.g., acetaminophen, ibuprofen)
____ Herbal remedies
____ Hot or cold packs
____ Exercise
____ Changing position (such as lying down or elevating your legs)
____ Physical therapy
____ Massage
____ Acupuncture
____ Rest
____ Psychological counseling
____ Talk to trusted friend, family, clergy
____ Prayer, meditation, guided imagery
____ Relaxation technique (hypnosis, biofeedback)
____ Creative technique (art or music therapy)
____ Other (e.g., specific chiropractic manipulation, osteopathic treatments):

_____

Check any of these common side effects that you've noticed after taking your pain medicine:
____ Drowsiness, sleepiness
____ Nausea, vomiting, upset stomach
____ Constipation
____ Lack of appetite
____ Other (describe):

_____

Did you sleep through the night? ____NO____YES

If not, how many times was your sleep disrupted? _____

How many hours did you sleep during the night? _____

COMMENTS AND MORE INFORMATION: Make notes for and about visits with your healthcare provider, side effects from treatments you may be experiencing, any problems you are having coping with your pain, and more about some of your previous answers or questions.

_____

_____

_____

1 DAILY DIARY

DAY_____ DATE_____ WEIGHT_____

SATISFACTION CHART Connect the points on your Daily Satisfaction Chart so your medical team can see when and why your mental state changed.

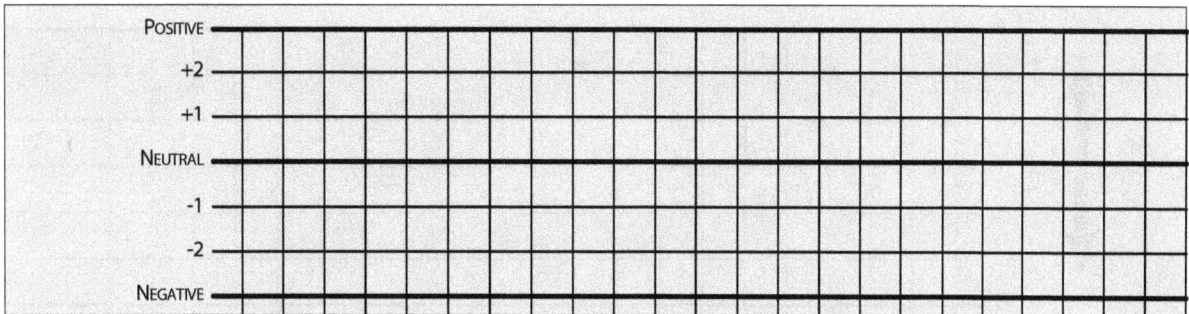

15

POSITIVE	
+2	
+1	
NEUTRAL	
-1	
-2	
NEGATIVE	

2 ACTIVITY LOG

6am 7 8 9 10 11 12pm 1 2 3 4 5 6pm 7 8 9 10 11 12am 1 2 3 4 5

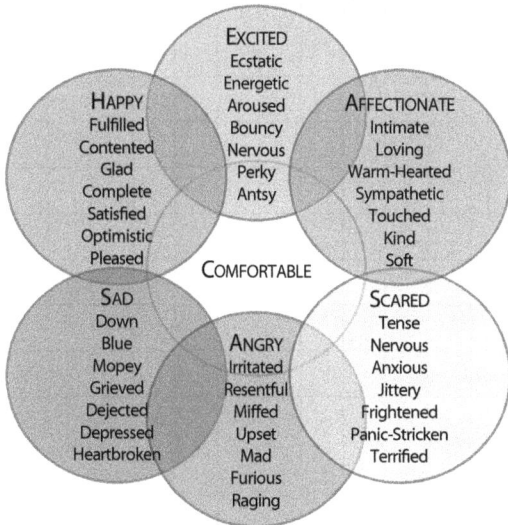

TRIGGERS AND SIGNIFICANT EVENTS

EXCITED
Ecstatic
Energetic
Aroused
Bouncy
Nervous
Perky
Antsy

HAPPY
Fulfilled
Contented
Glad
Complete
Satisfied
Optimistic
Pleased

AFFECTIONATE
Intimate
Loving
Warm-Hearted
Sympathetic
Touched
Kind
Soft

COMFORTABLE

SAD
Down
Blue
Mopey
Grieved
Dejected
Depressed
Heartbroken

ANGRY
Irritated
Resentful
Miffed
Upset
Mad
Furious
Raging

SCARED
Tense
Nervous
Anxious
Jittery
Frightened
Panic-Stricken
Terrified

Describe any changes in your pain today:

_____

_____

_____

_____

_____

Did anything unusual happen today?

_____

_____

_____

_____

What did you spend the most time time thinking about today?

Positive Thoughts:

_____

Did your pain increase, decrease, or remain the same when you thought about it?
____ Increased
____ Decreased
____ Stayed the Same

Negative Thoughts:

_____

Did your pain increase, decrease, or remain the same when you thought about it?
____ Increased
____ Decreased
____ Stayed the Same

15

DAY_____ DATE_____ WEIGHT_____

1 DAILY
MOOD CHART

Connect the points on your Mood Satisfaction Chart so your medical team can see when and why your mental state changed.

MOOD		
HAPPY	+3	
	+2	
	+1	
	0	
	-1	
	-2	
SAD	-3	

2 ACTIVITY LOG

6am 7 8 9 10 11 12pm 1 2 3 4 5 6pm 7 8 9 10 11 12am 1 2 3 4 5

3 MEDICATION LOG
NAME/DOSE

1
2
3
4
5
6
7
8

4 PHYSIOLOGY

6am 7 8 9 10 11 12pm 1 2 3 4 5 6pm 7 8 9 10 11 12am 1 2 3 4 5

SLEEP

URINATION

DEFECATION

NAUSEA

EATING

EXERCISE

OTHER (LIST)

1 DAILY RESULTS
OF MEDICATIONS AND TREATMENTS

As you and your medical team develop new treatment plans, it will be especially helpful to record any side effects you experience as you add new treatments. This can help determine which types of treatments will work best for you.

Contact your care provider with any bad reactions or side effects to determine if you should discontinue the medication or treatment.

MEDICATION / TREATMENT	AMOUNT / TIME / COMMENTS

1 DAILY
TREATMENT PLAN

As you and your medical team develop new treatment plans, record your plan for the day including new medications, increases or decreases to medications, exercises, physical therapy, or any other treatment efforts.

16

MEDICATION / TREATMENT	AMOUNT / TIME / COMMENTS

1 DAILY PAIN CHART

DAY_____ DATE_____ WEIGHT_____

Connect the points on your Daily Pain and Satisfaction Charts so your medical team can see when your status changed.

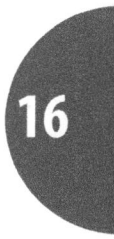

16

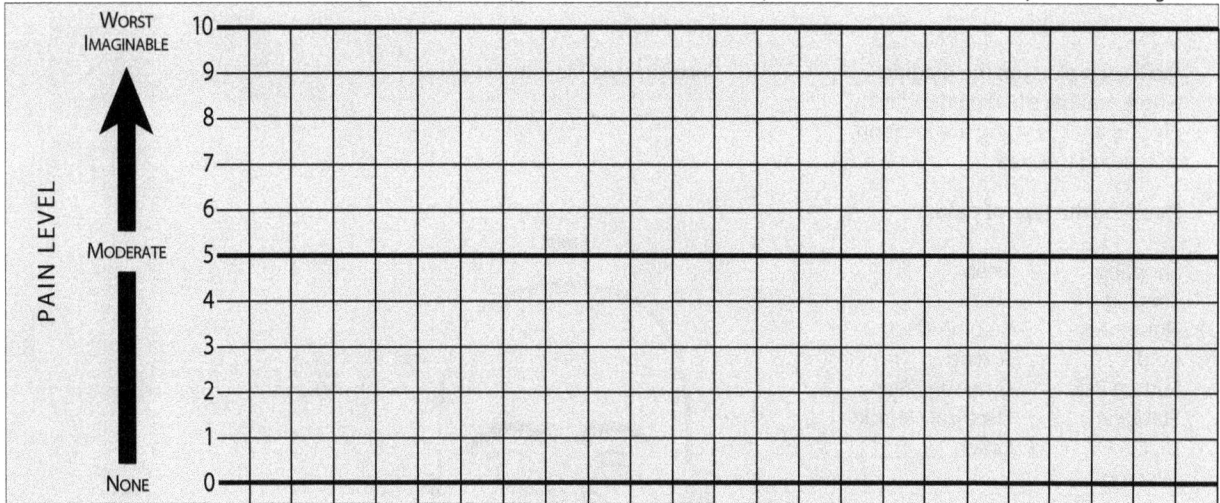

PAIN LEVEL

WORST IMAGINABLE — 10
9
8
7
6
MODERATE — 5
4
3
2
1
NONE — 0

2 SATISFACTION

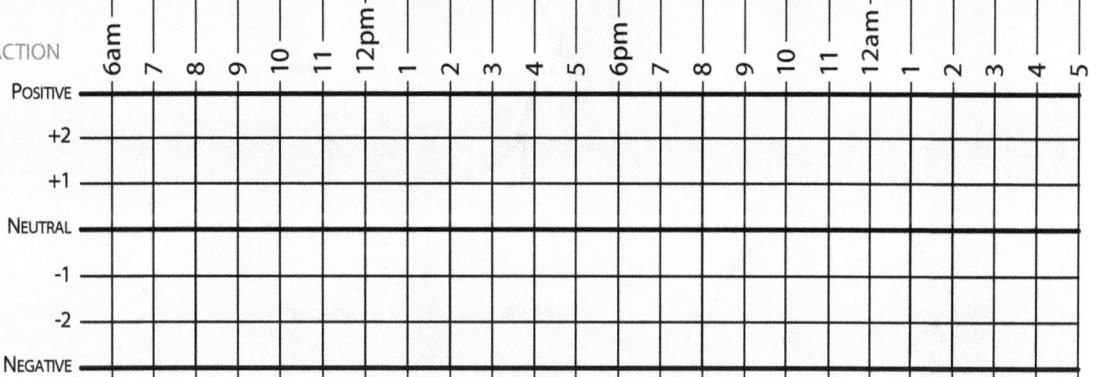

MOOD

(HAPPY) POSITIVE
+2
+1
NEUTRAL
-1
-2
(UNHAPPY) NEGATIVE

6am 7 8 9 10 11 12pm 1 2 3 4 5 6pm 7 8 9 10 11 12am 1 2 3 4 5

3 PHYSIOLOGY

6am 7 8 9 10 11 12pm 1 2 3 4 5 6pm 7 8 9 10 11 12am 1 2 3 4 5

SLEEP
RESTROOM
NAUSEA / DIZZINESS
MEAL / SNACK
EXERCISE
STRESS / ANXIETY

MEDICINE NAME / DOSE
1_____
2_____
3_____

BLOOD PRESSURE
PULSE

4 DAILY HEAD & FACE PAIN DIAGRAM

16

Mark each place on the diagram where you have had pain today by placing an 'X', circling the location, or shading the area .

COMMENTS AND MORE INFORMATION:

Describe the type of pain:

Shooting	Deep
Tingling	Sharp
Numbness	Burning / Hot
Cold	Aching
Surface Pain	Gnawing / Biting
Stabbing	Electrical / Shocks
Dull	Other_____
Stinging	

Front

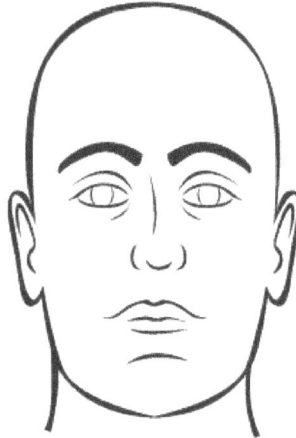

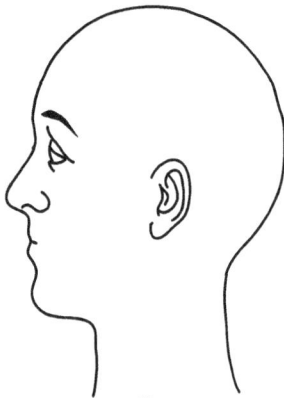

Your Right Side

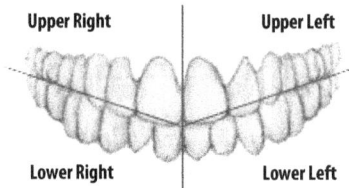

Upper Right   Upper Left

Lower Right   Lower Left

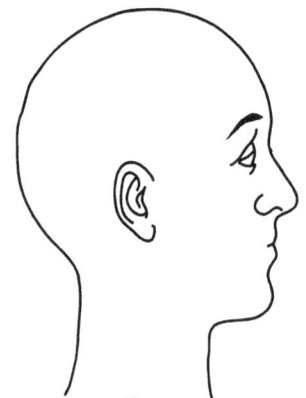

Your Right Side

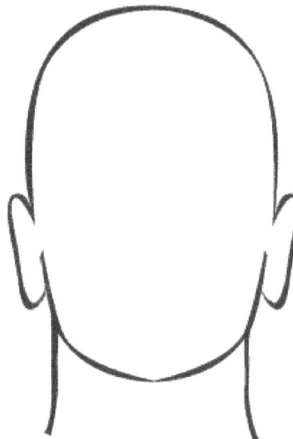

Back

5 DAILY BODY PAIN DIAGRAM

Mark each place on the diagram where you have had pain today by placing an 'X', circling the location, or shading the area .

Describe the type of pain:

Shooting	Deep
Tingling	Sharp
Numbness	Burning / Hot
Cold	Aching
Surface Pain	Gnawing / Biting
Stabbing	Electrical / Shocks
Dull	Other_____
Stinging	

COMMENTS AND MORE INFORMATION:

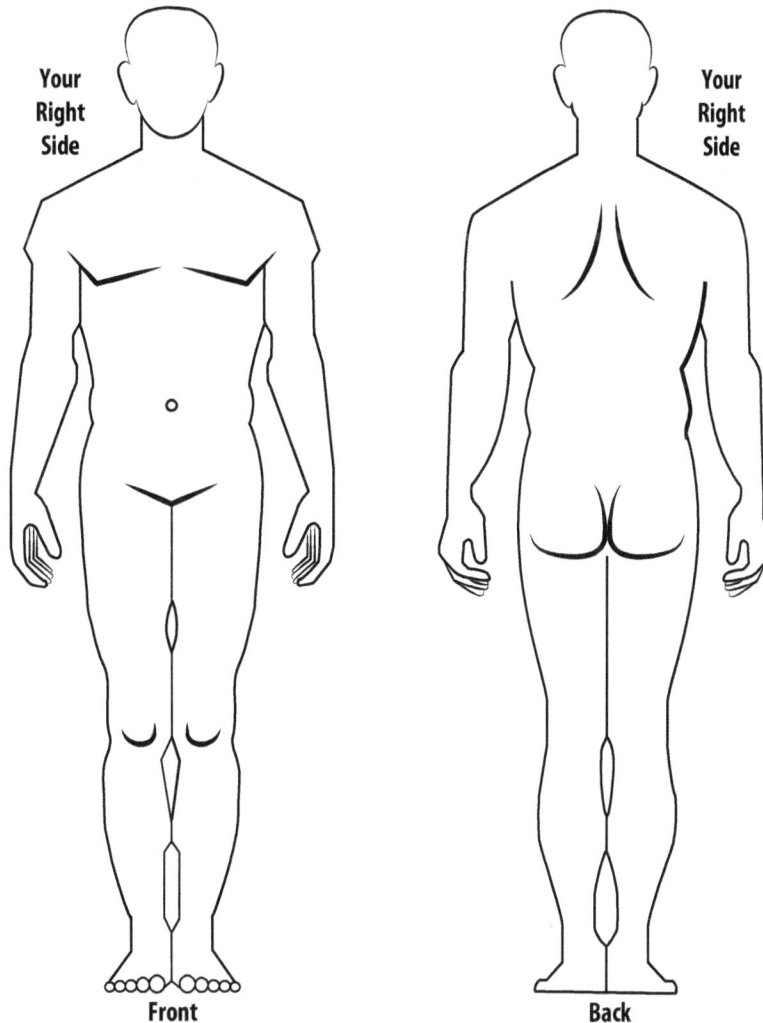

16

Your Right Side

Your Right Side

Front

Back

6 DAILY PAIN SUMMARY

Were there times during the day that you experienced unrelieved breakthrough pain? ____NO ____YES

How many times did this happen today?

1 2 3 4 5 6 7 8 9 10   more than 10

Did any specific activity start your breakthrough pain?
____NO ____YES: What activities?

_____

Put an "X" on the body diagram to show each place you've had **BREAKTHROUGH PAIN** today.

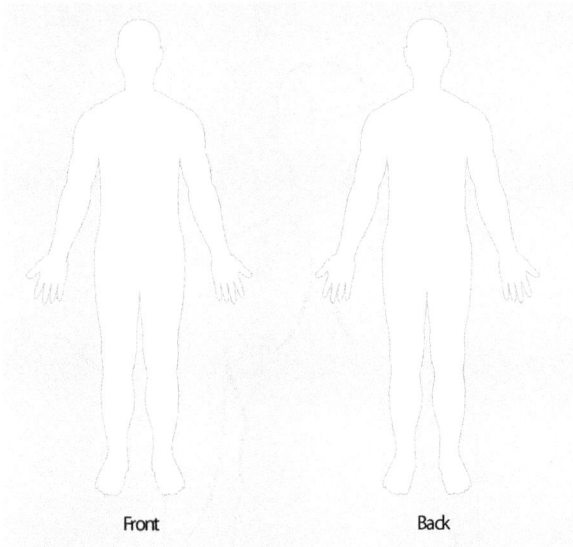

Front   Back

NON-DRUG THERAPIES
(other than prescription or other medicines)

_____

_____

ACTIVITIES/EXERCISE

_____

_____

What was your average level of pain today?

0 1 2 3 4 5 6 7 8 9 10

Other than prescription medicine, did you do anything else today to relieve the pain? ____NO ____YES:
(Note any that you used.)
____ Non-prescription drugs (e.g., acetaminophen, ibuprofen)
____ Herbal remedies
____ Hot or cold packs
____ Exercise
____ Changing position (such as lying down or elevating your legs)
____ Physical therapy
____ Massage
____ Acupuncture
____ Rest
____ Psychological counseling
____ Talk to trusted friend, family, clergy
____ Prayer, meditation, guided imagery
____ Relaxation technique (hypnosis, biofeedback)
____ Creative technique (art or music therapy)
____ Other (e.g., specific chiropractic manipulation, osteopathic treatments):

_____

Check any of these common side effects that you've noticed after taking your pain medicine:
____ Drowsiness, sleepiness
____ Nausea, vomiting, upset stomach
____ Constipation
____ Lack of appetite
____ Other (describe):

_____

Did you sleep through the night? ____NO____YES

If not, how many times was your sleep disrupted? _____

How many hours did you sleep during the night? _____

COMMENTS AND MORE INFORMATION: Make notes for and about visits with your healthcare provider, side effects from treatments you may be experiencing, any problems you are having coping with your pain, and more about some of your previous answers or questions.

_____

_____

_____

1 DAILY DIARY

DAY_____ DATE_____ WEIGHT_____

SATISFACTION CHART Connect the points on your Daily Satisfaction Chart so your medical team can see when and why your mental state changed.

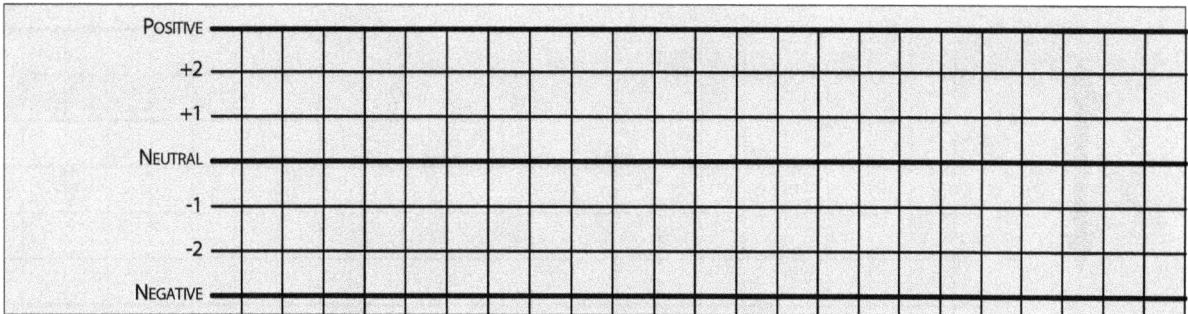

POSITIVE		
+2		
+1		
NEUTRAL		
-1		
-2		
NEGATIVE		

2 ACTIVITY LOG

TRIGGERS AND SIGNIFICANT EVENTS

6am 7 8 9 10 11 12pm 1 2 3 4 5 6pm 7 8 9 10 11 12am 1 2 3 4 5

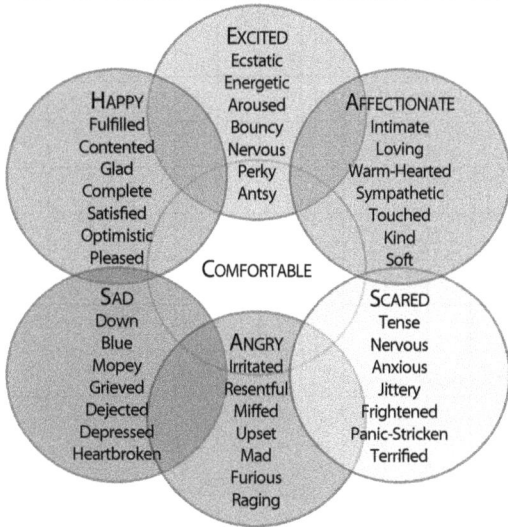

EXCITED
Ecstatic
Energetic
Aroused
Bouncy
Nervous
Perky
Antsy

HAPPY
Fulfilled
Contented
Glad
Complete
Satisfied
Optimistic
Pleased

AFFECTIONATE
Intimate
Loving
Warm-Hearted
Sympathetic
Touched
Kind
Soft

COMFORTABLE

SAD
Down
Blue
Mopey
Grieved
Dejected
Depressed
Heartbroken

ANGRY
Irritated
Resentful
Miffed
Upset
Mad
Furious
Raging

SCARED
Tense
Nervous
Anxious
Jittery
Frightened
Panic-Stricken
Terrified

Describe any changes in your pain today:

_____

_____

_____

_____

_____

Did anything unusual happen today?

_____

_____

_____

_____

_____

What did you spend the most time time thinking about today?

Positive Thoughts:

Negative Thoughts:

_____   _____

Did your pain increase, decrease, or remain the same when you thought about it?
____ Increased
____ Decreased
____ Stayed the Same

Did your pain increase, decrease, or remain the same when you thought about it?
____ Increased
____ Decreased
____ Stayed the Same

16

DAY_____ DATE_____ WEIGHT_____

1 DAILY
MOOD CHART

Connect the points on your Mood Satisfaction Chart so your medical team can see when and why your mental state changed.

MOOD		
HAPPY	+3	
	+2	
	+1	
	0	
	-1	
	-2	
SAD	-3	

2 ACTIVITY LOG

6am 7 8 9 10 11 12pm 1 2 3 4 5 6pm 7 8 9 10 11 12am 1 2 3 4 5

3 MEDICATION LOG
NAME/DOSE

1
2
3
4
5
6
7
8

4 PHYSIOLOGY

6am 7 8 9 10 11 12pm 1 2 3 4 5 6pm 7 8 9 10 11 12am 1 2 3 4 5

SLEEP

URINATION

DEFECATION

NAUSEA

EATING

EXERCISE

OTHER (LIST)

16

1 DAILY RESULTS
OF MEDICATIONS AND TREATMENTS

As you and your medical team develop new treatment plans, it will be especially helpful to record any side effects you experience as you add new treatments. This can help determine which types of treatments will work best for you.

Contact your care provider with any bad reactions or side effects to determine if you should discontinue the medication or treatment.

16

MEDICATION / TREATMENT	AMOUNT / TIME / COMMENTS

1 DAILY
TREATMENT PLAN

As you and your medical team develop new treatment plans, record your plan for the day including new medications, increases or decreases to medications, exercises, physical therapy, or any other treatment efforts.

MEDICATION / TREATMENT	AMOUNT / TIME / COMMENTS

17

1 DAILY
PAIN CHART

DAY_____ DATE_____ WEIGHT_____

Connect the points on your Daily Pain and Satisfaction Charts so your medical team can see when your status changed.

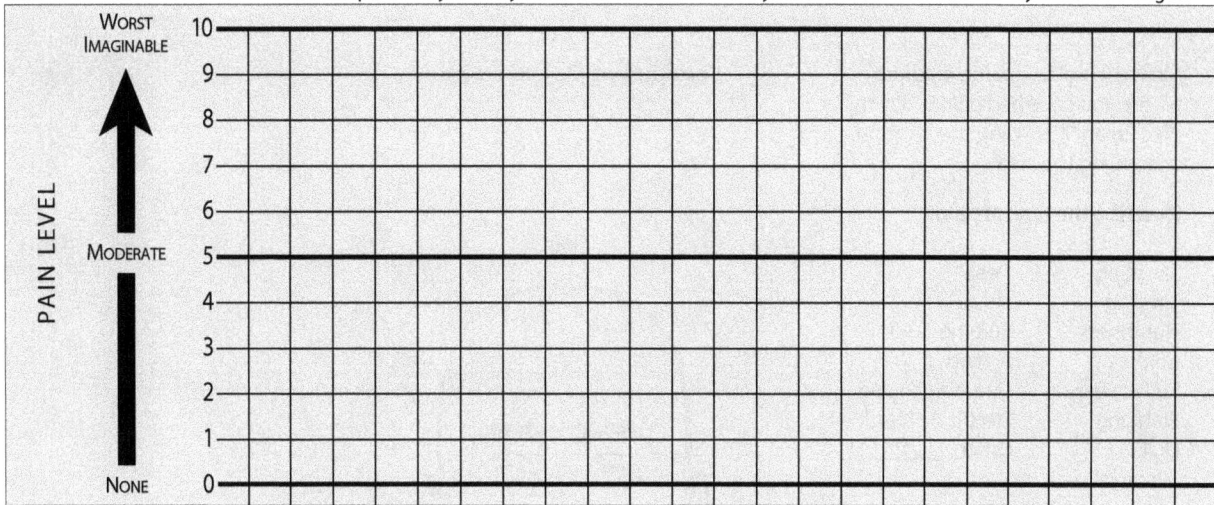

PAIN LEVEL

WORST IMAGINABLE — 10
9
8
7
6
MODERATE — 5
4
3
2
1
NONE — 0

2 SATISFACTION

MOOD

(HAPPY) POSITIVE
+2
+1
NEUTRAL
-1
-2
(UNHAPPY) NEGATIVE

6am 7 8 9 10 11 12pm 1 2 3 4 5 6pm 7 8 9 10 11 12am 1 2 3 4 5

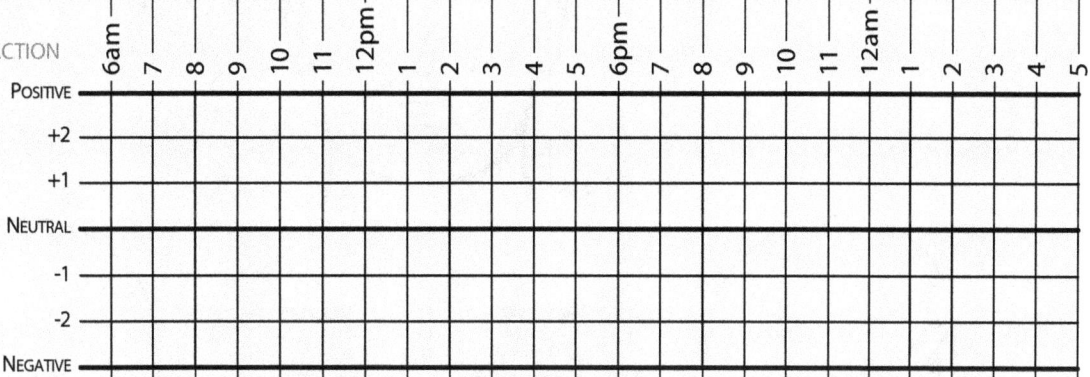

3 PHYSIOLOGY

6am 7 8 9 10 11 12pm 1 2 3 4 5 6pm 7 8 9 10 11 12am 1 2 3 4 5

SLEEP
RESTROOM
NAUSEA / DIZZINESS
MEAL / SNACK
EXERCISE
STRESS / ANXIETY
MEDICINE NAME / DOSE
1
2
3

BLOOD PRESSURE
PULSE

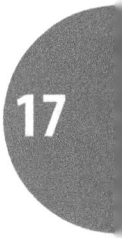

17

4 DAILY HEAD & FACE PAIN DIAGRAM

Mark each place on the diagram where you have had pain today by placing an 'X', circling the location, or shading the area.

Describe the type of pain:

Shooting	Deep
Tingling	Sharp
Numbness	Burning / Hot
Cold	Aching
Surface Pain	Gnawing / Biting
Stabbing	Electrical / Shocks
Dull	Other_____
Stinging	

17

COMMENTS AND MORE INFORMATION:

Front

Upper Right   **Upper Left**

Lower Right   **Lower Left**

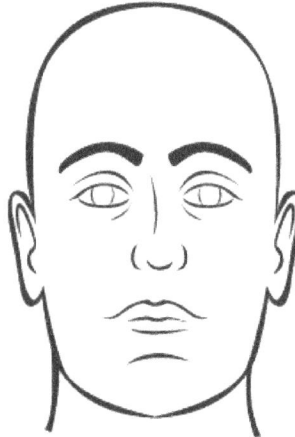

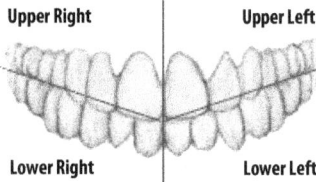

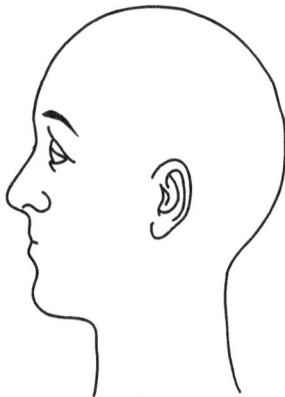

Your Right Side

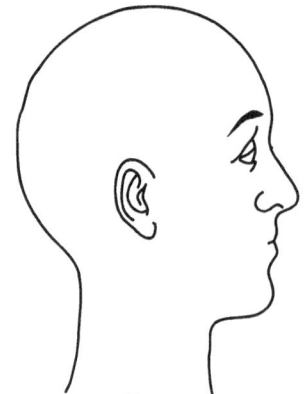

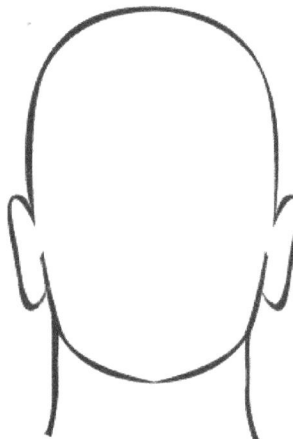

Your Right Side

Back

5 DAILY BODY PAIN DIAGRAM

Mark each place on the diagram where you have had pain today by placing an 'X', circling the location, or shading the area .

Describe the type of pain:

Shooting	Deep
Tingling	Sharp
Numbness	Burning / Hot
Cold	Aching
Surface Pain	Gnawing / Biting
Stabbing	Electrical / Shocks
Dull	Other_____
Stinging	

COMMENTS AND MORE INFORMATION:

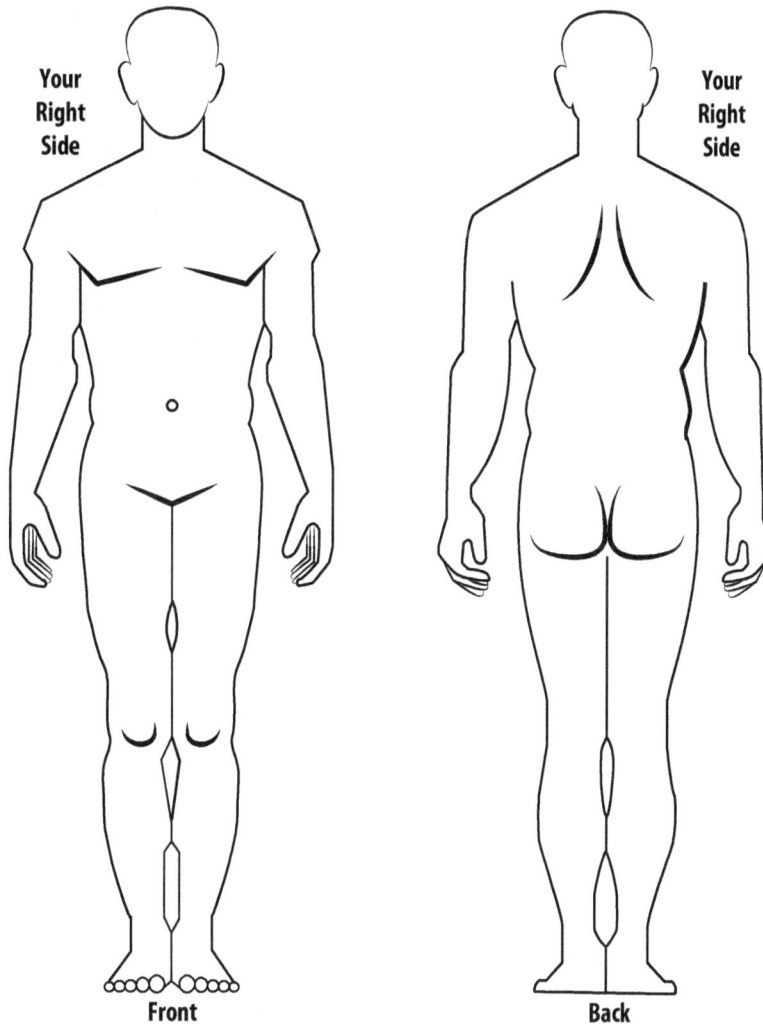

17

Your Right Side

Your Right Side

Front

Back

6 DAILY PAIN SUMMARY

Were there times during the day that you experienced unrelieved breakthrough pain? ____NO ____YES

How many times did this happen today?

1 2 3 4 5 6 7 8 9 10 more than 10

Did any specific activity start your breakthrough pain? ____NO ____YES: What activities?

_____

Put an "X" on the body diagram to show each place you've had **BREAKTHROUGH PAIN** today.

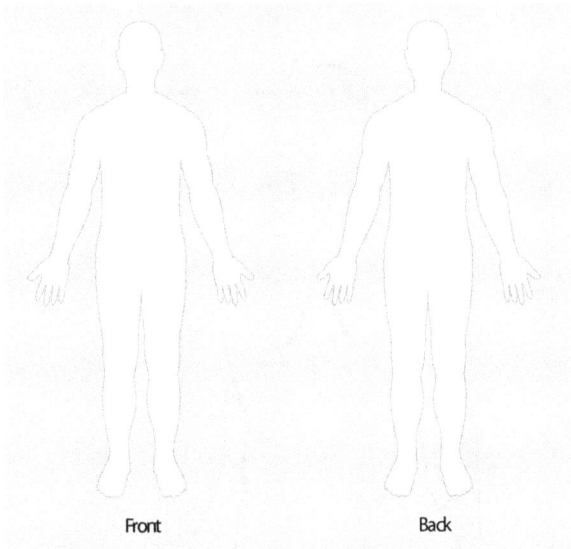

Front   Back

NON-DRUG THERAPIES
(other than prescription or other medicines)

_____

_____

ACTIVITIES/EXERCISE

_____

What was your average level of pain today?

0 1 2 3 4 5 6 7 8 9 10

Other than prescription medicine, did you do anything else today to relieve the pain? ____NO ____YES: (Note any that you used.)
____ Non-prescription drugs (e.g., acetaminophen, ibuprofen)
____ Herbal remedies
____ Hot or cold packs
____ Exercise
____ Changing position (such as lying down or elevating your legs)
____ Physical therapy
____ Massage
____ Acupuncture
____ Rest
____ Psychological counseling
____ Talk to trusted friend, family, clergy
____ Prayer, meditation, guided imagery
____ Relaxation technique (hypnosis, biofeedback)
____ Creative technique (art or music therapy)
____ Other (e.g., specific chiropractic manipulation, osteopathic treatments):

_____

Check any of these common side effects that you've noticed after taking your pain medicine:
____ Drowsiness, sleepiness
____ Nausea, vomiting, upset stomach
____ Constipation
____ Lack of appetite
____ Other (describe):

_____

Did you sleep through the night? ____NO____YES

If not, how many times was your sleep disrupted? _____

How many hours did you sleep during the night? _____

COMMENTS AND MORE INFORMATION: Make notes for and about visits with your healthcare provider, side effects from treatments you may be experiencing, any problems you are having coping with your pain, and more about some of your previous answers or questions.

1 DAILY DIARY

SATISFACTION CHART DAY_____ DATE_____ WEIGHT_____

Connect the points on your Daily Satisfaction Chart so your medical team can see when and why your mental state changed.

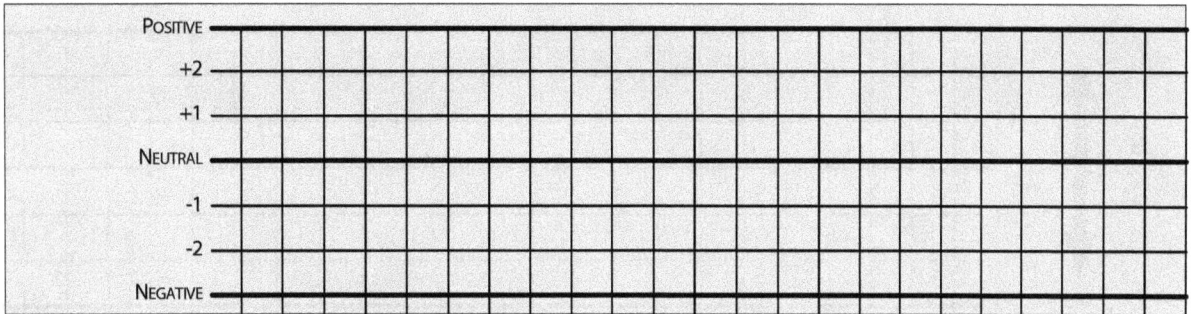

POSITIVE	
+2	
+1	
NEUTRAL	
-1	
-2	
NEGATIVE	

2 ACTIVITY LOG

TRIGGERS AND SIGNIFICANT EVENTS

6am 7 8 9 10 11 12pm 1 2 3 4 5 6pm 7 8 9 10 11 12am 1 2 3 4 5

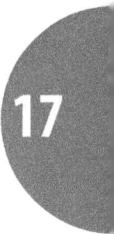

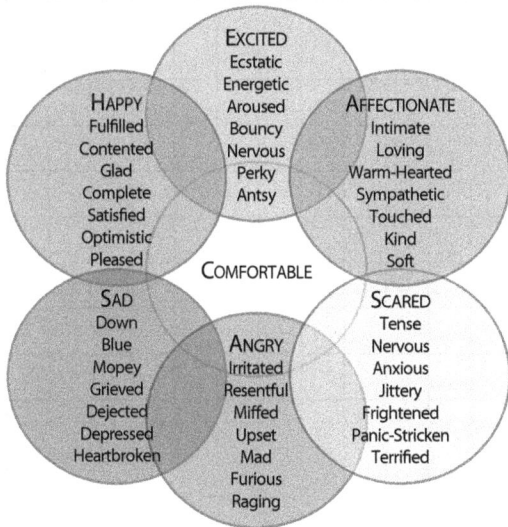

17

EXCITED Ecstatic Energetic Aroused Bouncy Nervous Perky Antsy

HAPPY Fulfilled Contented Glad Complete Satisfied Optimistic Pleased

AFFECTIONATE Intimate Loving Warm-Hearted Sympathetic Touched Kind Soft

COMFORTABLE

SAD Down Blue Mopey Grieved Dejected Depressed Heartbroken

ANGRY Irritated Resentful Miffed Upset Mad Furious Raging

SCARED Tense Nervous Anxious Jittery Frightened Panic-Stricken Terrified

Describe any changes in your pain today:

_____
_____
_____
_____

Did anything unusual happen today?

_____
_____
_____
_____

What did you spend the most time time thinking about today?

Positive Thoughts:

_____

Did your pain increase, decrease, or remain the same when you thought about it?
____ Increased
____ Decreased
____ Stayed the Same

Negative Thoughts:

_____

Did your pain increase, decrease, or remain the same when you thought about it?
____ Increased
____ Decreased
____ Stayed the Same

1 DAILY
MOOD CHART

DAY_____ DATE_____ WEIGHT_____

Connect the points on your Mood Satisfaction Chart so your medical team can see when and why your mental state changed.

HAPPY +3
+2
+1
MOOD 0
-1
-2
SAD -3

2 ACTIVITY LOG

6am 7 8 9 10 11 12pm 1 2 3 4 5 6pm 7 8 9 10 11 12am 1 2 3 4 5

17

3 MEDICATION LOG
NAME/DOSE

1
2
3
4
5
6
7
8

4 PHYSIOLOGY

6am 7 8 9 10 11 12pm 1 2 3 4 5 6pm 7 8 9 10 11 12am 1 2 3 4 5

SLEEP

URINATION

DEFECATION

NAUSEA

EATING

EXERCISE

OTHER (LIST)

1 DAILY RESULTS
OF MEDICATIONS AND TREATMENTS

As you and your medical team develop new treatment plans, it will be especially helpful to record any side effects you experience as you add new treatments. This can help determine which types of treatments will work best for you.

Contact your care provider with any bad reactions or side effects to determine if you should discontinue the medication or treatment.

MEDICATION / TREATMENT	AMOUNT / TIME / COMMENTS

17

1 DAILY
TREATMENT PLAN

As you and your medical team develop new treatment plans, record your plan for the day including new medications, increases or decreases to medications, exercises, physical therapy, or any other treatment efforts.

MEDICATION / TREATMENT	AMOUNT / TIME / COMMENTS

18

1 DAILY
PAIN CHART

DAY_____ DATE_____ WEIGHT_____

Connect the points on your Daily Pain and Satisfaction Charts so your medical team can see when your status changed.

PAIN LEVEL

WORST IMAGINABLE — 10
9
8
7
6
MODERATE — 5
4
3
2
1
NONE — 0

2 SATISFACTION

Time axis: 6am 7 8 9 10 11 12pm 1 2 3 4 5 6pm 7 8 9 10 11 12am 1 2 3 4 5

MOOD

(HAPPY) POSITIVE
+2
+1
NEUTRAL
-1
-2
(UNHAPPY) NEGATIVE

3 PHYSIOLOGY

Time axis: 6am 7 8 9 10 11 12pm 1 2 3 4 5 6pm 7 8 9 10 11 12am 1 2 3 4 5

SLEEP
RESTROOM
NAUSEA / DIZZINESS
MEAL / SNACK
EXERCISE
STRESS / ANXIETY

MEDICINE NAME / DOSE
1
2
3

BLOOD PRESSURE
PULSE

4 DAILY HEAD & FACE PAIN DIAGRAM

Mark each place on the diagram where you have had pain today by placing an 'X', circling the location, or shading the area .

Describe the type of pain:

Shooting	Deep
Tingling	Sharp
Numbness	Burning / Hot
Cold	Aching
Surface Pain	Gnawing / Biting
Stabbing	Electrical / Shocks
Dull	Other_____
Stinging	

COMMENTS AND MORE INFORMATION:

Front

Upper Right **Upper Left**

Lower Right **Lower Left**

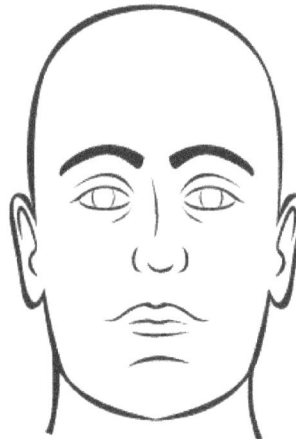

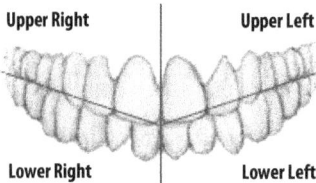

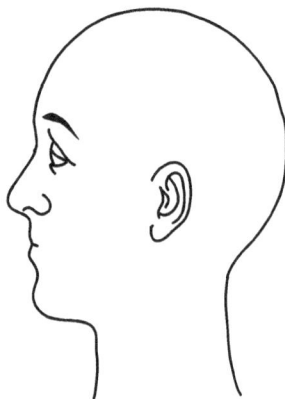

Your Right Side

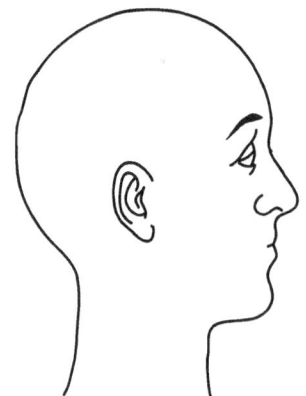

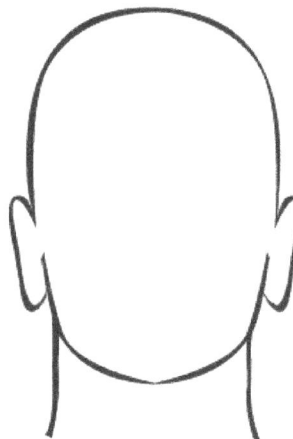

Your Right Side

Back

5 DAILY BODY PAIN DIAGRAM

Mark each place on the diagram where you have had pain today by placing an 'X', circling the location, or shading the area .

Describe the type of pain:

Shooting	Deep
Tingling	Sharp
Numbness	Burning / Hot
Cold	Aching
Surface Pain	Gnawing / Biting
Stabbing	Electrical / Shocks
Dull	Other_____
Stinging	

COMMENTS AND MORE INFORMATION:

Your Right Side

Your Right Side

18

Front

Back

6 DAILY PAIN SUMMARY

Were there times during the day that you experienced unrelieved breakthrough pain? ____NO ____YES

How many times did this happen today?

1   2   3   4   5   6   7   8   9   10   more than 10

Did any specific activity start your breakthrough pain?
____NO   ____YES: What activities?

_____

Put an "X" on the body diagram to show each place you've had **BREAKTHROUGH PAIN** today.

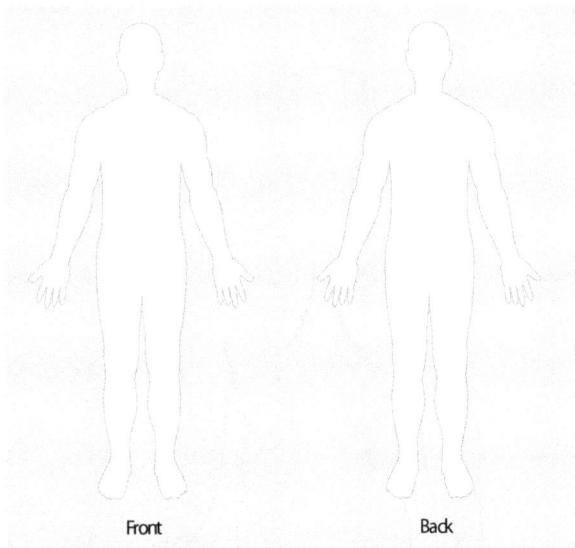

Front   Back

NON-DRUG THERAPIES
(other than prescription or other medicines)

_____

_____

ACTIVITIES/EXERCISE

_____

_____

What was your average level of pain today?

0   1   2   3   4   5   6   7   8   9   10

Other than prescription medicine, did you do anything else today to relieve the pain? ____NO ____YES:
(Note any that you used.)
____ Non-prescription drugs (e.g., acetaminophen, ibuprofen)
____ Herbal remedies
____ Hot or cold packs
____ Exercise
____ Changing position (such as lying down or elevating your legs)
____ Physical therapy
____ Massage
____ Acupuncture
____ Rest
____ Psychological counseling
____ Talk to trusted friend, family, clergy
____ Prayer, meditation, guided imagery
____ Relaxation technique (hypnosis, biofeedback)
____ Creative technique (art or music therapy)
____ Other (e.g., specific chiropractic manipulation, osteopathic treatments):

_____

Check any of these common side effects that you've noticed after taking your pain medicine:
____ Drowsiness, sleepiness
____ Nausea, vomiting, upset stomach
____ Constipation
____ Lack of appetite
____ Other (describe):

_____

Did you sleep through the night? ____NO____YES

If not, how many times was your sleep disrupted? _____

How many hours did you sleep during the night? _____

COMMENTS AND MORE INFORMATION: Make notes for and about visits with your healthcare provider, side effects from treatments you may be experiencing, any problems you are having coping with your pain, and more about some of your previous answers or questions.

_____

_____

_____

18

1 DAILY DIARY

SATISFACTION CHART

DAY_____ DATE_____ WEIGHT_____

Connect the points on your Daily Satisfaction Chart so your medical team can see when and why your mental state changed.

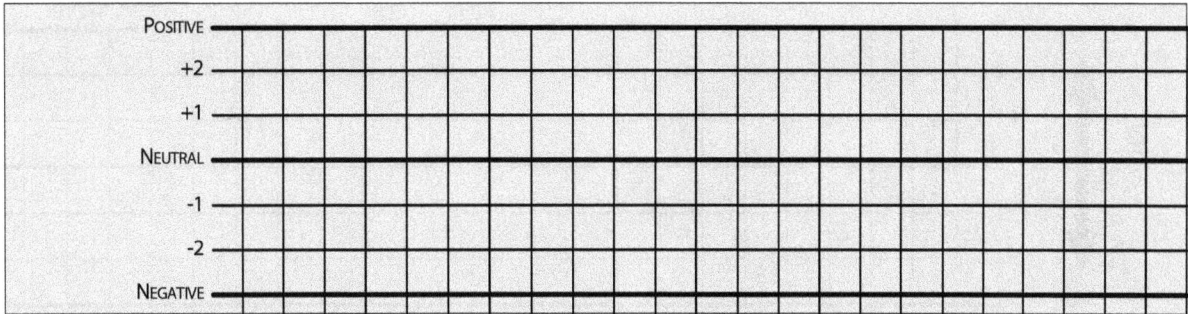

POSITIVE

+2

+1

NEUTRAL

-1

-2

NEGATIVE

2 ACTIVITY LOG

6am 7 8 9 10 11 12pm 1 2 3 4 5 6pm 7 8 9 10 11 12am 1 2 3 4 5

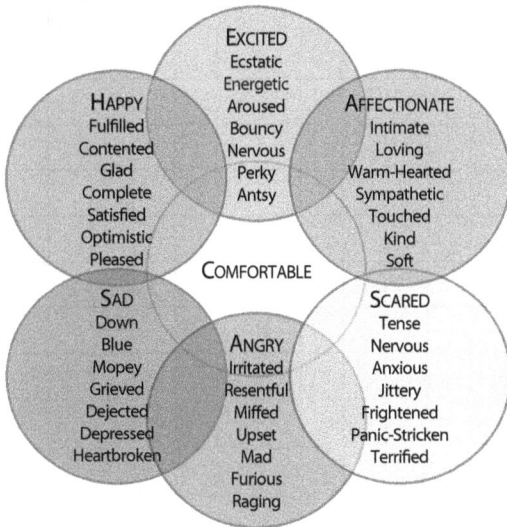

TRIGGERS AND SIGNIFICANT EVENTS

EXCITED
Ecstatic
Energetic
Aroused
Bouncy
Nervous
Perky
Antsy

HAPPY
Fulfilled
Contented
Glad
Complete
Satisfied
Optimistic
Pleased

AFFECTIONATE
Intimate
Loving
Warm-Hearted
Sympathetic
Touched
Kind
Soft

COMFORTABLE

SAD
Down
Blue
Mopey
Grieved
Dejected
Depressed
Heartbroken

ANGRY
Irritated
Resentful
Miffed
Upset
Mad
Furious
Raging

SCARED
Tense
Nervous
Anxious
Jittery
Frightened
Panic-Stricken
Terrified

Describe any changes in your pain today:

_____

_____

_____

_____

_____

Did anything unusual happen today?

_____

_____

_____

_____

18

What did you spend the most time time thinking about today?

Positive Thoughts:

_____

Did your pain increase, decrease, or remain the same when you thought about it?
____ Increased
____ Decreased
____ Stayed the Same

Negative Thoughts:

_____

Did your pain increase, decrease, or remain the same when you thought about it?
____ Increased
____ Decreased
____ Stayed the Same

DAY_____ DATE_____ WEIGHT_____

1 DAILY
MOOD CHART

Connect the points on your Mood Satisfaction Chart so your medical team can see when and why your mental state changed.

HAPPY +3
       +2
       +1
MOOD   0
       -1
       -2
SAD   -3

2 ACTIVITY LOG

6am 7 8 9 10 11 12pm 1 2 3 4 5 6pm 7 8 9 10 11 12am 1 2 3 4 5

3 MEDICATION LOG
NAME/DOSE

1
2
3
4
5
6
7
8

4 PHYSIOLOGY

6am 7 8 9 10 11 12pm 1 2 3 4 5 6pm 7 8 9 10 11 12am 1 2 3 4 5

SLEEP
URINATION
DEFECATION
NAUSEA
EATING
EXERCISE
OTHER (LIST)

18

1 DAILY RESULTS
OF MEDICATIONS AND TREATMENTS

As you and your medical team develop new treatment plans, it will be especially helpful to record any side effects you experience as you add new treatments. This can help determine which types of treatments will work best for you.

Contact your care provider with any bad reactions or side effects to determine if you should discontinue the medication or treatment.

MEDICATION / TREATMENT	AMOUNT / TIME / COMMENTS

18

1 DAILY
TREATMENT PLAN

As you and your medical team develop new treatment plans, record your plan for the day including new medications, increases or decreases to medications, exercises, physical therapy, or any other treatment efforts.

MEDICATION / TREATMENT	AMOUNT / TIME / COMMENTS

19

1 DAILY
PAIN CHART

DAY_____ DATE_____ WEIGHT_____

Connect the points on your Daily Pain and Satisfaction Charts so your medical team can see when your status changed.

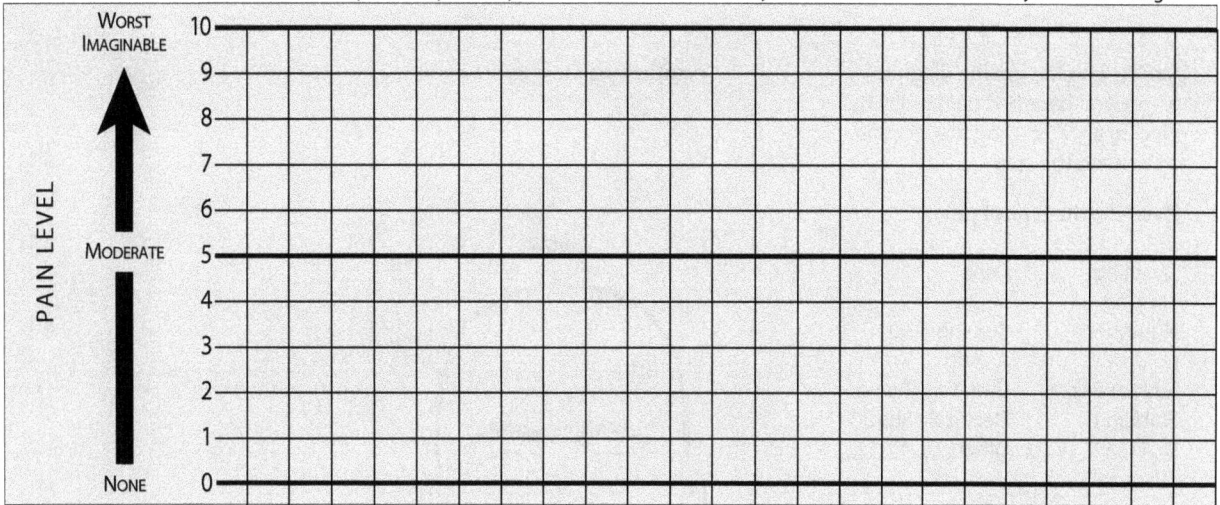

2 SATISFACTION

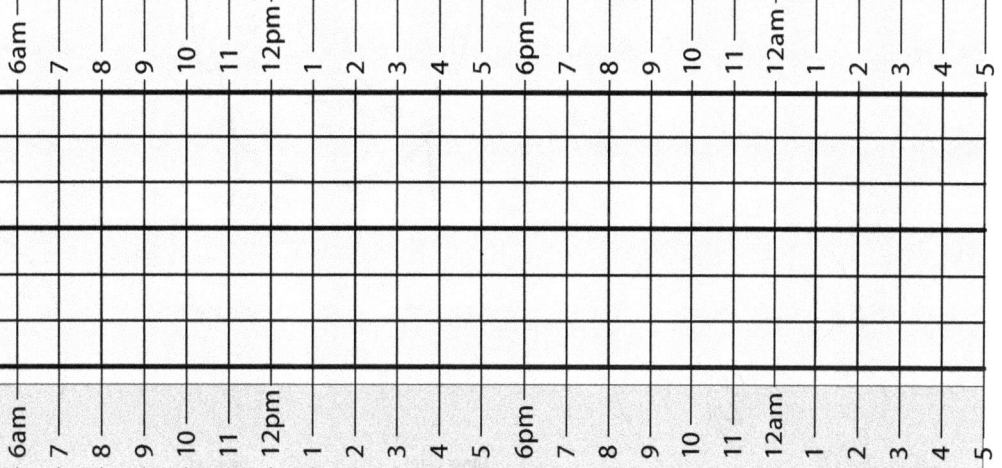

3 PHYSIOLOGY

SLEEP

RESTROOM

NAUSEA / DIZZINESS

MEAL / SNACK

EXERCISE

STRESS / ANXIETY

MEDICINE NAME / DOSE

1

2

3

BLOOD PRESSURE

PULSE

19

4 DAILY HEAD & FACE PAIN DIAGRAM

Mark each place on the diagram where you have had pain today by placing an 'X', circling the location, or shading the area .

Describe the type of pain:

Shooting	Deep
Tingling	Sharp
Numbness	Burning / Hot
Cold	Aching
Surface Pain	Gnawing / Biting
Stabbing	Electrical / Shocks
Dull	Other_____
Stinging	

COMMENTS AND MORE INFORMATION:

Front

Upper Right   **Upper Left**

Lower Right   **Lower Left**

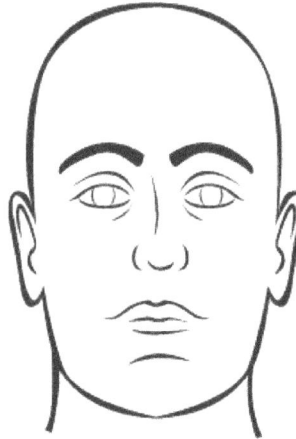

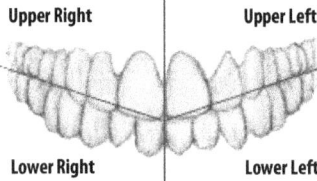

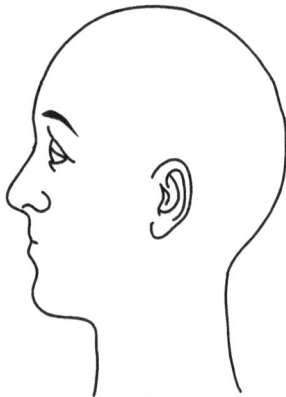

Your Right Side

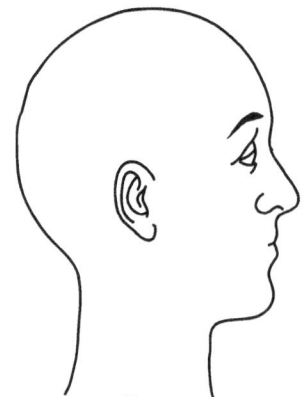

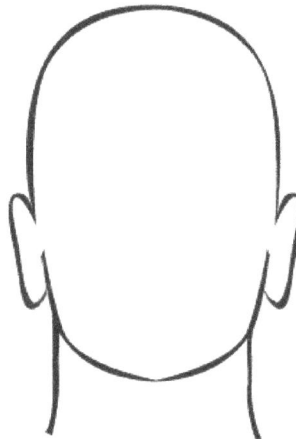

Your Right Side

Back

19

5 DAILY BODY PAIN DIAGRAM

Mark each place on the diagram where you have had pain today by placing an 'X', circling the location, or shading the area .

Describe the type of pain:

Shooting	Deep
Tingling	Sharp
Numbness	Burning / Hot
Cold	Aching
Surface Pain	Gnawing / Biting
Stabbing	Electrical / Shocks
Dull	Other_____
Stinging	

COMMENTS AND MORE INFORMATION:

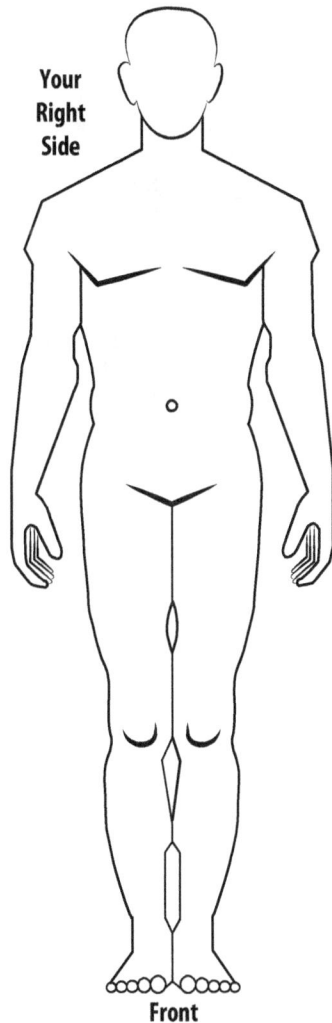

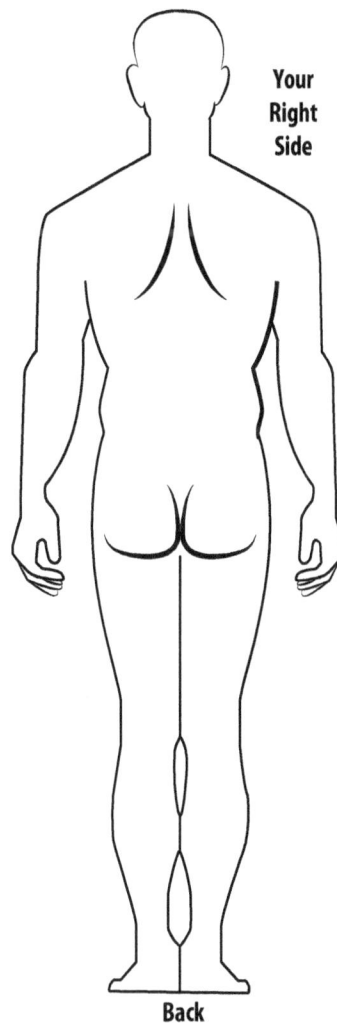

Your Right Side

Your Right Side

Front

Back

19

6 DAILY PAIN SUMMARY

Were there times during the day that you experienced unrelieved breakthrough pain? _____NO _____YES

How many times did this happen today?

1 2 3 4 5 6 7 8 9 10   more than 10

Did any specific activity start your breakthrough pain? _____NO _____YES: What activities?

_____

Put an "X" on the body diagram to show each place you've had **BREAKTHROUGH PAIN** today.

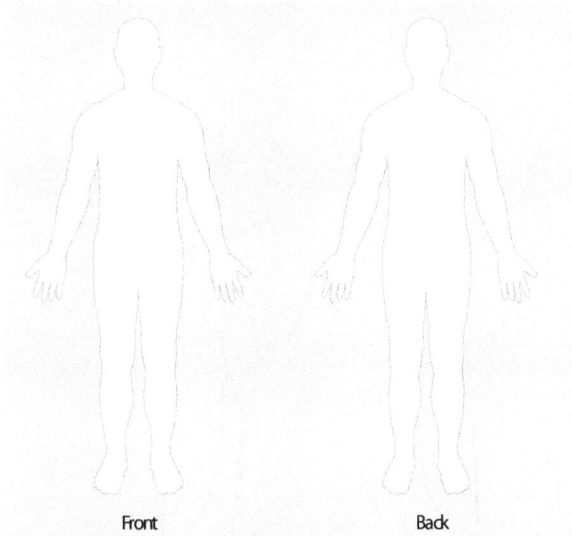

Front   Back

NON-DRUG THERAPIES
(other than prescription or other medicines)

_____

_____

ACTIVITIES/EXERCISE

_____

_____

What was your average level of pain today?

0 1 2 3 4 5 6 7 8 9 10

Other than prescription medicine, did you do anything else today to relieve the pain? _____NO _____YES:
(Note any that you used.)
_____ Non-prescription drugs (e.g., acetaminophen, ibuprofen)
_____ Herbal remedies
_____ Hot or cold packs
_____ Exercise
_____ Changing position (such as lying down or elevating your legs)
_____ Physical therapy
_____ Massage
_____ Acupuncture
_____ Rest
_____ Psychological counseling
_____ Talk to trusted friend, family, clergy
_____ Prayer, meditation, guided imagery
_____ Relaxation technique (hypnosis, biofeedback)
_____ Creative technique (art or music therapy)
_____ Other (e.g., specific chiropractic manipulation, osteopathic treatments):

_____

Check any of these common side effects that you've noticed after taking your pain medicine:
_____ Drowsiness, sleepiness
_____ Nausea, vomiting, upset stomach
_____ Constipation
_____ Lack of appetite
_____ Other (describe):

_____

Did you sleep through the night? _____NO_____YES

If not, how many times was your sleep disrupted? _____

How many hours did you sleep during the night? _____

COMMENTS AND MORE INFORMATION: Make notes for and about visits with your healthcare provider, side effects from treatments you may be experiencing, any problems you are having coping with your pain, and more about some of your previous answers or questions.

_____

_____

_____

_____

19

1 DAILY DIARY

DAY_____ DATE_____ WEIGHT_____

SATISFACTION CHART Connect the points on your Daily Satisfaction Chart so your medical team can see when and why your mental state changed.

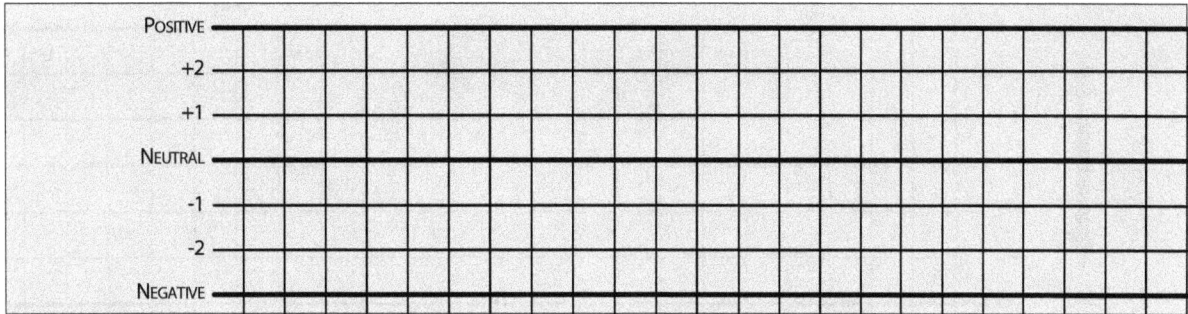

POSITIVE

+2

+1

NEUTRAL

-1

-2

NEGATIVE

2 ACTIVITY LOG

TRIGGERS AND SIGNIFICANT EVENTS

6am 7 8 9 10 11 12pm 1 2 3 4 5 6pm 7 8 9 10 11 12am 1 2 3 4 5

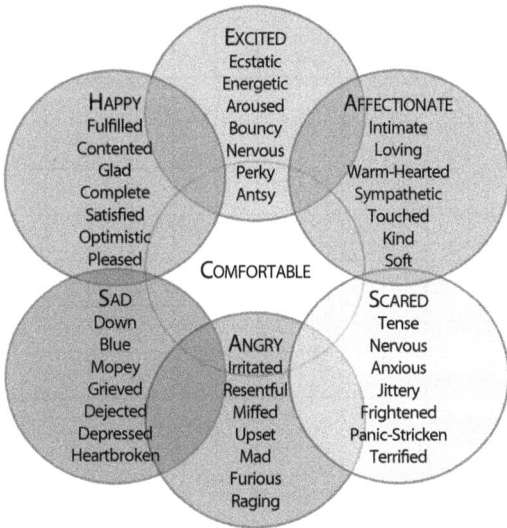

EXCITED
Ecstatic
Energetic
Aroused
Bouncy
Nervous
Perky
Antsy

HAPPY
Fulfilled
Contented
Glad
Complete
Satisfied
Optimistic
Pleased

AFFECTIONATE
Intimate
Loving
Warm-Hearted
Sympathetic
Touched
Kind
Soft

COMFORTABLE

SAD
Down
Blue
Mopey
Grieved
Dejected
Depressed
Heartbroken

ANGRY
Irritated
Resentful
Miffed
Upset
Mad
Furious
Raging

SCARED
Tense
Nervous
Anxious
Jittery
Frightened
Panic-Stricken
Terrified

Describe any changes in your pain today:

_____
_____
_____
_____
_____

Did anything unusual happen today?

_____
_____
_____
_____

19

What did you spend the most time time thinking about today?

Positive Thoughts:

_____

Did your pain increase, decrease, or remain the same when you thought about it?
____ Increased
____ Decreased
____ Stayed the Same

Negative Thoughts:

_____

Did your pain increase, decrease, or remain the same when you thought about it?
____ Increased
____ Decreased
____ Stayed the Same

1 DAILY
MOOD CHART

DAY_____ DATE_____ WEIGHT_____

Connect the points on your Mood Satisfaction Chart so your medical team can see when and why your mental state changed.

MOOD	HAPPY	+3																						
		+2																						
		+1																						
		0																						
		-1																						
		-2																						
	SAD	-3																						

2 ACTIVITY LOG

6am 7 8 9 10 11 12pm 1 2 3 4 5 6pm 7 8 9 10 11 12am 1 2 3 4 5

3 MEDICATION LOG
NAME/DOSE

1——————
2——————
3——————
4——————
5——————
6——————
7——————
8——————

4 PHYSIOLOGY

6am 7 8 9 10 11 12pm 1 2 3 4 5 6pm 7 8 9 10 11 12am 1 2 3 4 5

SLEEP —
URINATION —
DEFECATION —
NAUSEA —
EATING —
EXERCISE —
OTHER (LIST) —

19

1 DAILY RESULTS
OF MEDICATIONS AND TREATMENTS

As you and your medical team develop new treatment plans, it will be especially helpful to record any side effects you experience as you add new treatments. This can help determine which types of treatments will work best for you.

Contact your care provider with any bad reactions or side effects to determine if you should discontinue the medication or treatment.

MEDICATION / TREATMENT	AMOUNT / TIME / COMMENTS

19

1 DAILY
TREATMENT PLAN

As you and your medical team develop new treatment plans, record your plan for the day including new medications, increases or decreases to medications, exercises, physical therapy, or any other treatment efforts.

MEDICATION / TREATMENT	AMOUNT / TIME / COMMENTS

20

1 DAILY
PAIN CHART

DAY_____ DATE_____ WEIGHT_____

Connect the points on your Daily Pain and Satisfaction Charts so your medical team can see when your status changed.

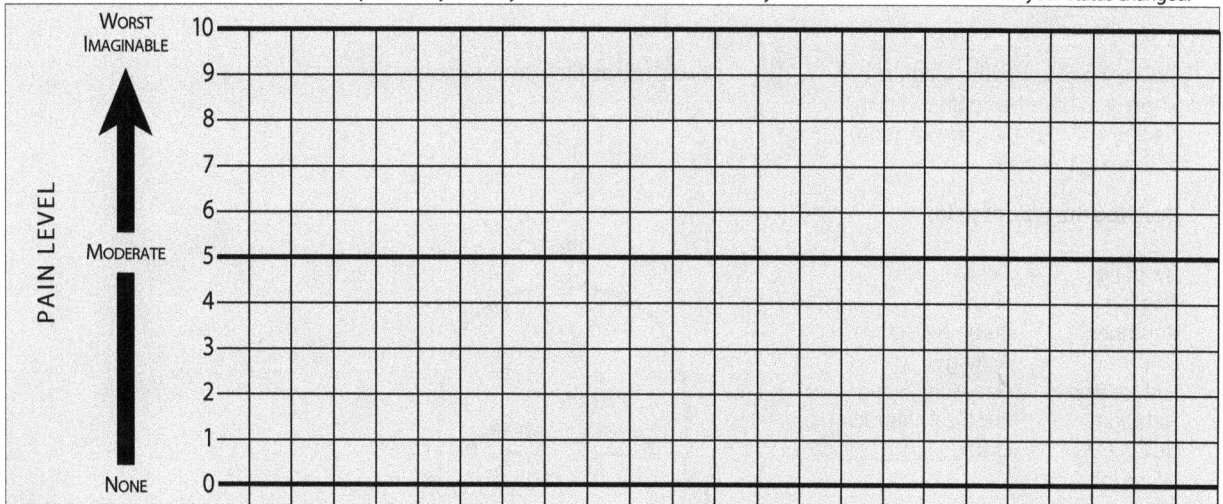

PAIN LEVEL

WORST IMAGINABLE — 10
9
8
7
6
MODERATE — 5
4
3
2
1
NONE — 0

2 SATISFACTION

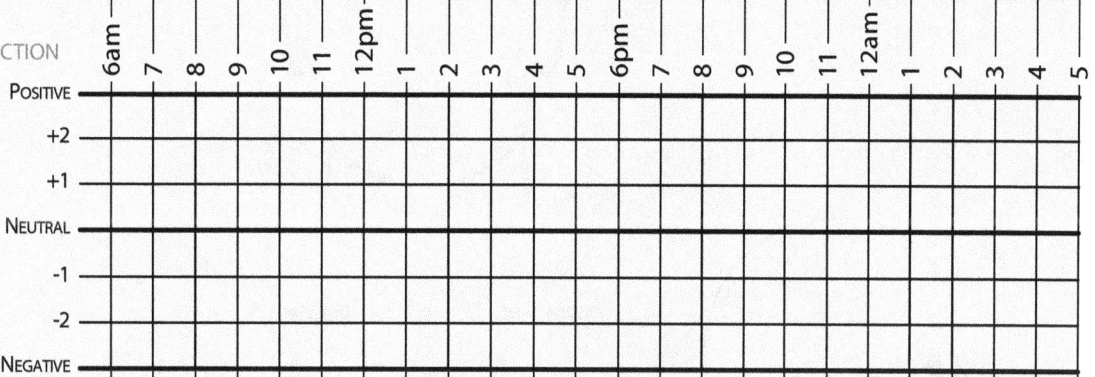

6am 7 8 9 10 11 12pm 1 2 3 4 5 6pm 7 8 9 10 11 12am 1 2 3 4 5

MOOD

(HAPPY) POSITIVE
+2
+1
NEUTRAL
-1
-2
(UNHAPPY) NEGATIVE

3 PHYSIOLOGY

6am 7 8 9 10 11 12pm 1 2 3 4 5 6pm 7 8 9 10 11 12am 1 2 3 4 5

SLEEP
RESTROOM
NAUSEA / DIZZINESS
MEAL / SNACK
EXERCISE
STRESS / ANXIETY
MEDICINE NAME / DOSE
1
2
3
BLOOD PRESSURE
PULSE

20

4 DAILY HEAD & FACE PAIN DIAGRAM

Mark each place on the diagram where you have had pain today by placing an 'X', circling the location, or shading the area.

Describe the type of pain:

Shooting	Deep
Tingling	Sharp
Numbness	Burning / Hot
Cold	Aching
Surface Pain	Gnawing / Biting
Stabbing	Electrical / Shocks
Dull	Other_____
Stinging	

COMMENTS AND MORE INFORMATION:

Front

Upper Right   Upper Left

Lower Right   Lower Left

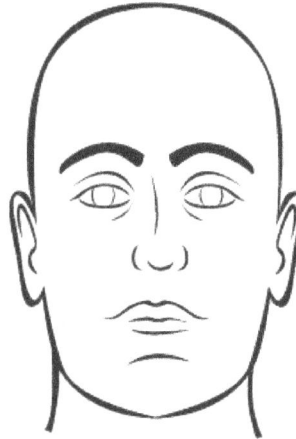

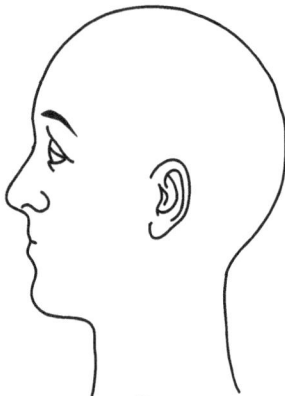

Your Right Side

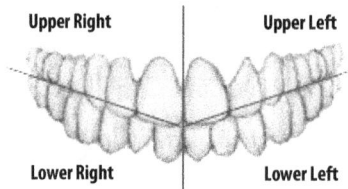

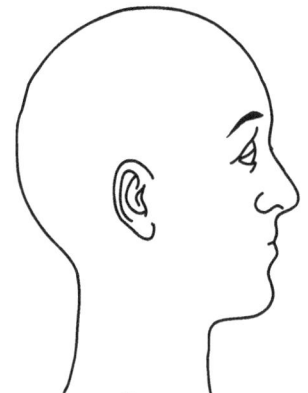

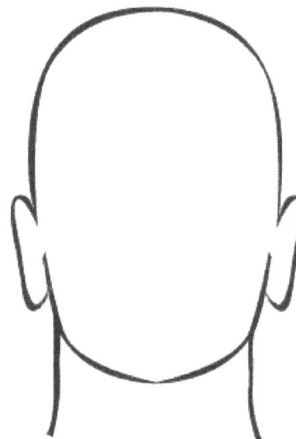

Your Right Side

Back

20

5 DAILY BODY PAIN DIAGRAM

Mark each place on the diagram where you have had pain today by placing an 'X', circling the location, or shading the area .

Describe the type of pain:

Shooting	Deep
Tingling	Sharp
Numbness	Burning / Hot
Cold	Aching
Surface Pain	Gnawing / Biting
Stabbing	Electrical / Shocks
Dull	Other_____
Stinging	

COMMENTS AND MORE INFORMATION:

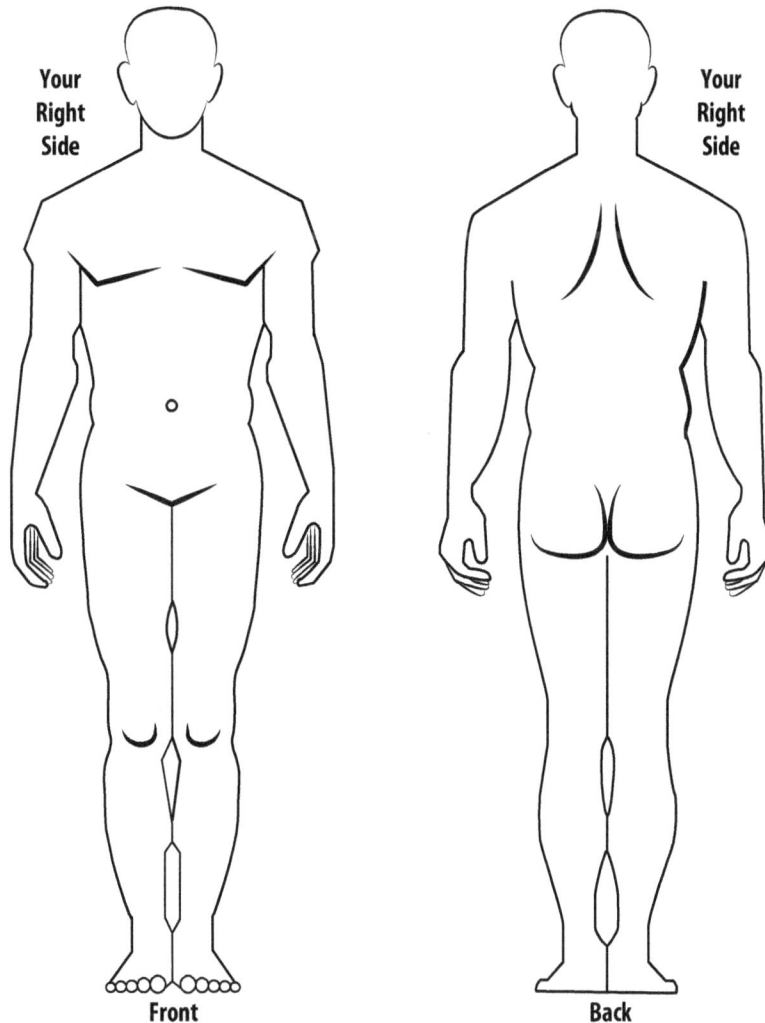

Your
Right
Side

Your
Right
Side

Front

Back

20

6 DAILY PAIN SUMMARY

Were there times during the day that you experienced unrelieved breakthrough pain? _____NO _____YES

How many times did this happen today?

1 2 3 4 5 6 7 8 9 10 more than 10

Did any specific activity start your breakthrough pain? _____NO _____YES: What activities?

_____

Put an "X" on the body diagram to show each place you've had *BREAKTHROUGH PAIN* today.

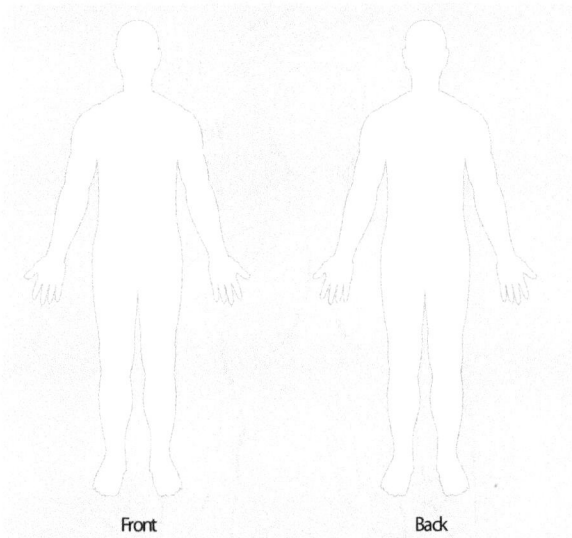

Front   Back

NON-DRUG THERAPIES
(other than prescription or other medicines)

_____

_____

ACTIVITIES/EXERCISE

_____

_____

What was your average level of pain today?

0 1 2 3 4 5 6 7 8 9 10

Other than prescription medicine, did you do anything else today to relieve the pain? _____NO _____YES: (Note any that you used.)
_____ Non-prescription drugs (e.g., acetaminophen, ibuprofen)
_____ Herbal remedies
_____ Hot or cold packs
_____ Exercise
_____ Changing position (such as lying down or elevating your legs)
_____ Physical therapy
_____ Massage
_____ Acupuncture
_____ Rest
_____ Psychological counseling
_____ Talk to trusted friend, family, clergy
_____ Prayer, meditation, guided imagery
_____ Relaxation technique (hypnosis, biofeedback)
_____ Creative technique (art or music therapy)
_____ Other (e.g., specific chiropractic manipulation, osteopathic treatments):

_____

Check any of these common side effects that you've noticed after taking your pain medicine:
_____ Drowsiness, sleepiness
_____ Nausea, vomiting, upset stomach
_____ Constipation
_____ Lack of appetite
_____ Other (describe):

_____

Did you sleep through the night? _____NO_____YES

If not, how many times was your sleep disrupted? _____

How many hours did you sleep during the night? _____

COMMENTS AND MORE INFORMATION: Make notes for and about visits with your healthcare provider, side effects from treatments you may be experiencing, any problems you are having coping with your pain, and more about some of your previous answers or questions.

_____

_____

_____

20

1 DAILY DIARY

DAY_____ DATE_____ WEIGHT_____

SATISFACTION CHART Connect the points on your Daily Satisfaction Chart so your medical team can see when and why your mental state changed.

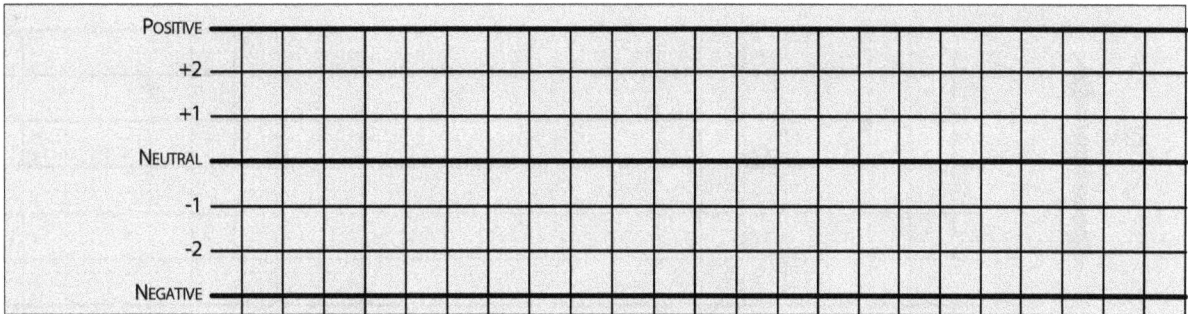

POSITIVE
+2
+1
NEUTRAL
-1
-2
NEGATIVE

2 ACTIVITY LOG

6am 7 8 9 10 11 12pm 1 2 3 4 5 6pm 7 8 9 10 11 12am 1 2 3 4 5

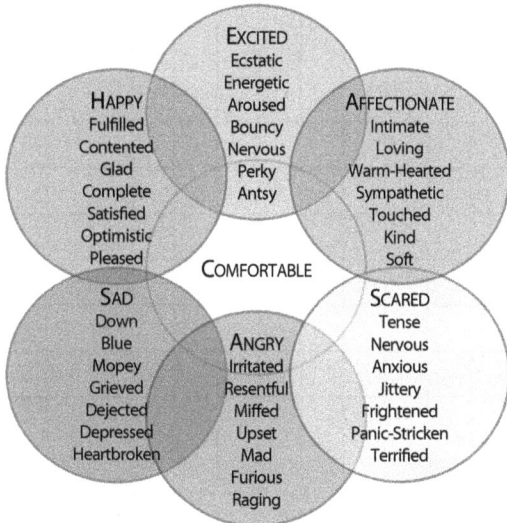

TRIGGERS AND SIGNIFICANT EVENTS

EXCITED
Ecstatic
Energetic
Aroused
Bouncy
Nervous
Perky
Antsy

HAPPY
Fulfilled
Contented
Glad
Complete
Satisfied
Optimistic
Pleased

AFFECTIONATE
Intimate
Loving
Warm-Hearted
Sympathetic
Touched
Kind
Soft

COMFORTABLE

SAD
Down
Blue
Mopey
Grieved
Dejected
Depressed
Heartbroken

ANGRY
Irritated
Resentful
Miffed
Upset
Mad
Furious
Raging

SCARED
Tense
Nervous
Anxious
Jittery
Frightened
Panic-Stricken
Terrified

Describe any changes in your pain today:

_____
_____
_____
_____

Did anything unusual happen today?

_____
_____
_____
_____

What did you spend the most time time thinking about today?

Positive Thoughts:

_____

Did your pain increase, decrease, or remain the same when you thought about it?
____ Increased
____ Decreased
____ Stayed the Same

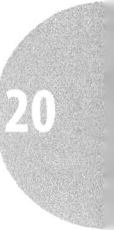

Negative Thoughts:

_____

Did your pain increase, decrease, or remain the same when you thought about it?
____ Increased
____ Decreased
____ Stayed the Same

20

1 DAILY
MOOD CHART

DAY_____ DATE_____ WEIGHT_____

Connect the points on your Mood Satisfaction Chart so your medical team can see when and why your mental state changed.

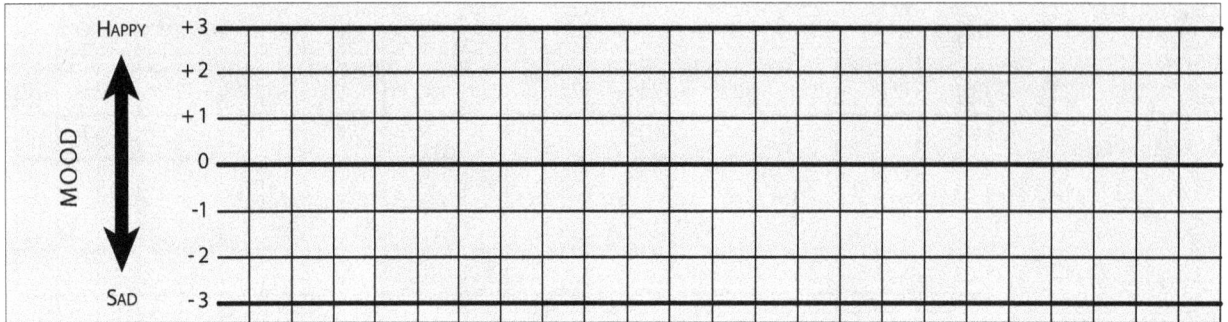

HAPPY +3
+2
+1
MOOD 0
-1
-2
SAD -3

2 ACTIVITY LOG

6am 7 8 9 10 11 12pm 1 2 3 4 5 6pm 7 8 9 10 11 12am 1 2 3 4 5

3 MEDICATION LOG
NAME/DOSE

1
2
3
4
5
6
7
8

4 PHYSIOLOGY

6am 7 8 9 10 11 12pm 1 2 3 4 5 6pm 7 8 9 10 11 12am 1 2 3 4 5

SLEEP
URINATION
DEFECATION
NAUSEA
EATING
EXERCISE
OTHER (LIST)

20

1 DAILY RESULTS
OF MEDICATIONS AND TREATMENTS

As you and your medical team develop new treatment plans, it will be especially helpful to record any side effects you experience as you add new treatments. This can help determine which types of treatments will work best for you.

Contact your care provider with any bad reactions or side effects to determine if you should discontinue the medication or treatment.

MEDICATION / TREATMENT	AMOUNT / TIME / COMMENTS

20

1 DAILY
TREATMENT PLAN

As you and your medical team develop new treatment plans, record your plan for the day including new medications, increases or decreases to medications, exercises, physical therapy, or any other treatment efforts.

MEDICATION / TREATMENT	AMOUNT / TIME / COMMENTS

21

1 DAILY
PAIN CHART

DAY_____ DATE_____ WEIGHT_____

Connect the points on your Daily Pain and Satisfaction Charts so your medical team can see when your status changed.

PAIN LEVEL

WORST IMAGINABLE — 10

9

8

7

6

MODERATE — 5

4

3

2

1

NONE — 0

| | 6am | 7 | 8 | 9 | 10 | 11 | 12pm | 1 | 2 | 3 | 4 | 5 | 6pm | 7 | 8 | 9 | 10 | 11 | 12am | 1 | 2 | 3 | 4 | 5 |

2 SATISFACTION

MOOD

(HAPPY) POSITIVE

+2

+1

NEUTRAL

-1

-2

(UNHAPPY) NEGATIVE

| | 6am | 7 | 8 | 9 | 10 | 11 | 12pm | 1 | 2 | 3 | 4 | 5 | 6pm | 7 | 8 | 9 | 10 | 11 | 12am | 1 | 2 | 3 | 4 | 5 |

3 PHYSIOLOGY

	6am	7	8	9	10	11	12pm	1	2	3	4	5	6pm	7	8	9	10	11	12am	1	2	3	4	5

SLEEP

RESTROOM

NAUSEA / DIZZINESS

MEAL / SNACK

EXERCISE

STRESS / ANXIETY

MEDICINE NAME / DOSE

1

2

3

BLOOD PRESSURE

PULSE

4 DAILY HEAD & FACE PAIN DIAGRAM

Mark each place on the diagram where you have had pain today by placing an 'X', circling the location, or shading the area .

Describe the type of pain:

Shooting	Deep
Tingling	Sharp
Numbness	Burning / Hot
Cold	Aching
Surface Pain	Gnawing / Biting
Stabbing	Electrical / Shocks
Dull	Other_____
Stinging	

COMMENTS AND MORE INFORMATION:

Front

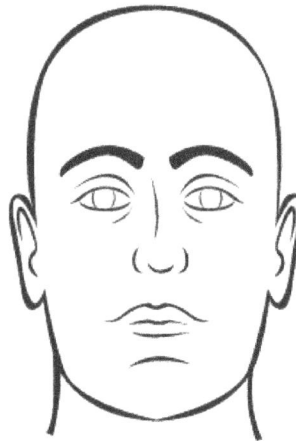

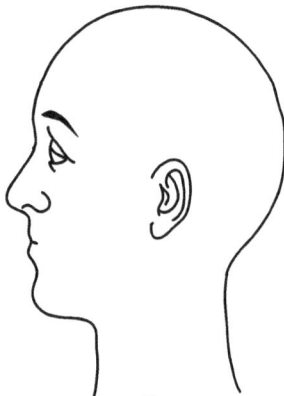

Your
Right
Side

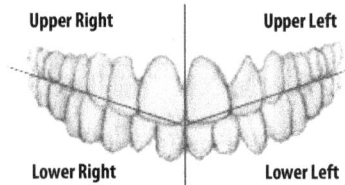

Upper Right Upper Left

Lower Right Lower Left

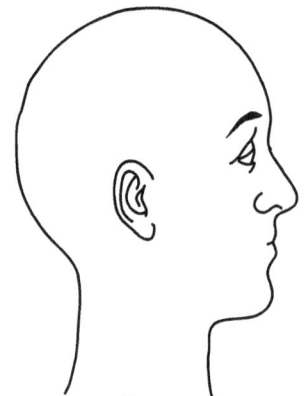

Your
Right
Side

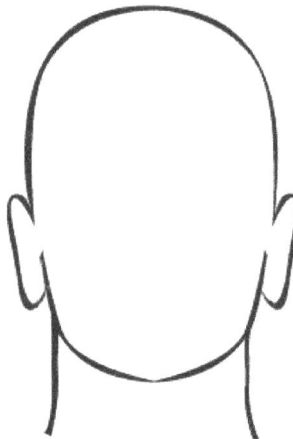

Back

5 DAILY BODY PAIN DIAGRAM

Mark each place on the diagram where you have had pain today by placing an 'X', circling the location, or shading the area .

Describe the type of pain:

Shooting	Deep
Tingling	Sharp
Numbness	Burning / Hot
Cold	Aching
Surface Pain	Gnawing / Biting
Stabbing	Electrical / Shocks
Dull	Other_____
Stinging	

COMMENTS AND MORE INFORMATION:

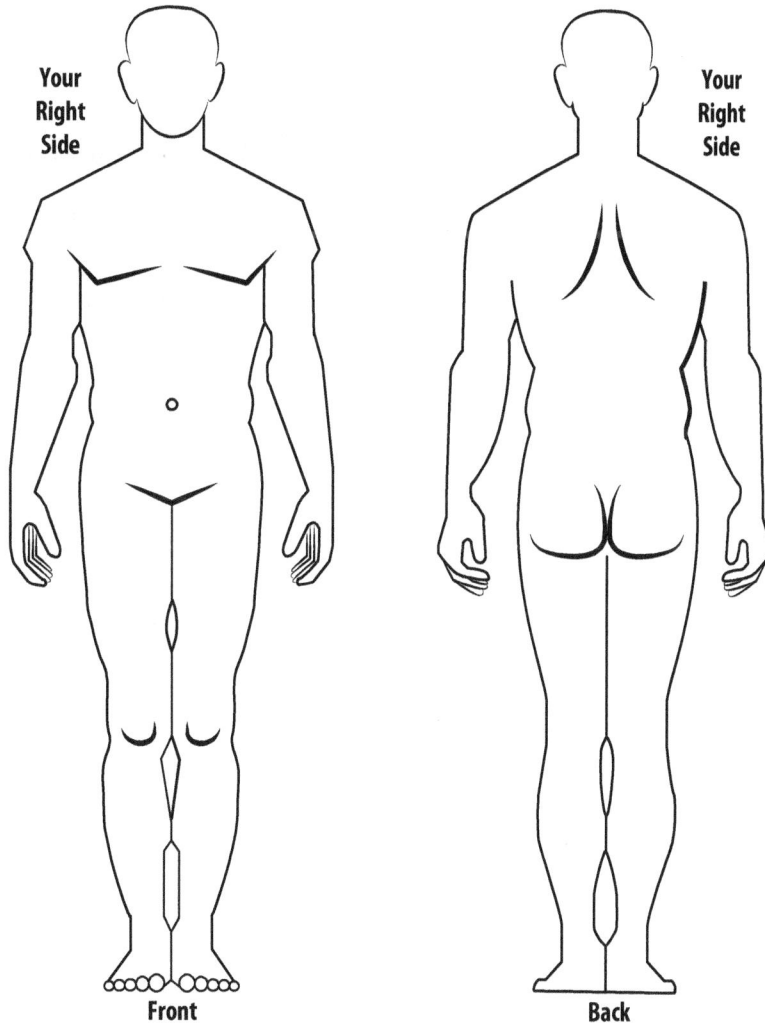

Your Right Side

Your Right Side

Front

Back

21

6 DAILY PAIN SUMMARY

Were there times during the day that you experienced unrelieved breakthrough pain? ____NO ____YES

How many times did this happen today?

1 2 3 4 5 6 7 8 9 10 more than 10

Did any specific activity start your breakthrough pain?
____NO ____YES: What activities?

_____

Put an "X" on the body diagram to show each place you've had *BREAKTHROUGH PAIN* today.

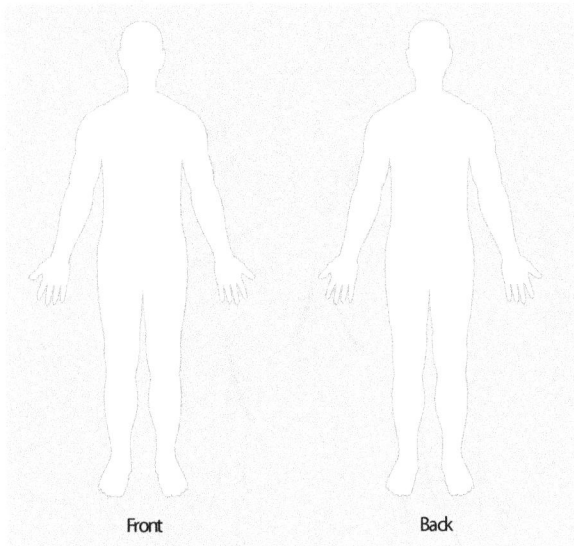

Front   Back

NON-DRUG THERAPIES
(other than prescription or other medicines)

_____
_____

ACTIVITIES/EXERCISE

_____
_____

What was your average level of pain today?

0 1 2 3 4 5 6 7 8 9 10

Other than prescription medicine, did you do anything else today to relieve the pain? ____NO ____YES:
(Note any that you used.)
____ Non-prescription drugs (e.g., acetaminophen, ibuprofen)
____ Herbal remedies
____ Hot or cold packs
____ Exercise
____ Changing position (such as lying down or elevating your legs)
____ Physical therapy
____ Massage
____ Acupuncture
____ Rest
____ Psychological counseling
____ Talk to trusted friend, family, clergy
____ Prayer, meditation, guided imagery
____ Relaxation technique (hypnosis, biofeedback)
____ Creative technique (art or music therapy)
____ Other (e.g., specific chiropractic manipulation, osteopathic treatments):

_____

Check any of these common side effects that you've noticed after taking your pain medicine:
____ Drowsiness, sleepiness
____ Nausea, vomiting, upset stomach
____ Constipation
____ Lack of appetite
____ Other (describe):

_____

Did you sleep through the night? ____NO____YES

If not, how many times was your sleep disrupted? _____

How many hours did you sleep during the night? _____

COMMENTS AND MORE INFORMATION: Make notes for and about visits with your healthcare provider, side effects from treatments you may be experiencing, any problems you are having coping with your pain, and more about some of your previous answers or questions.

_____
_____
_____

1 DAILY DIARY

Day_____ Date_____ Weight_____

SATISFACTION CHART Connect the points on your Daily Satisfaction Chart so your medical team can see when and why your mental state changed.

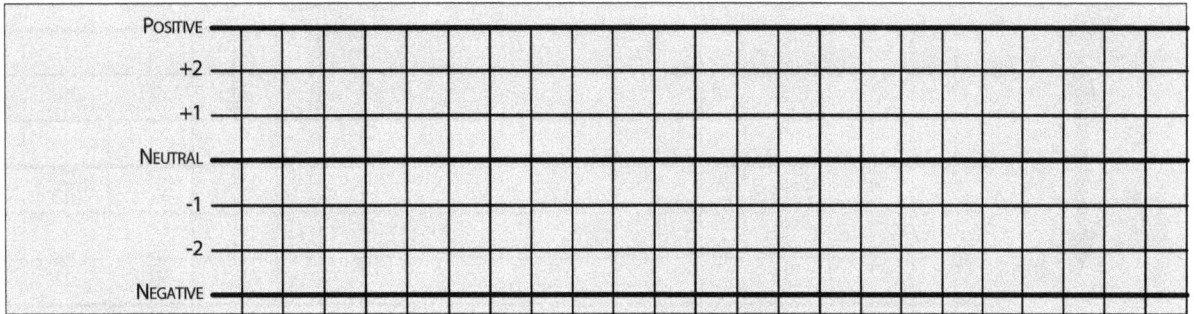

| POSITIVE |
| +2 |
| +1 |
| NEUTRAL |
| -1 |
| -2 |
| NEGATIVE |

2 ACTIVITY LOG

6am 7 8 9 10 11 12pm 1 2 3 4 5 6pm 7 8 9 10 11 12am 1 2 3 4 5

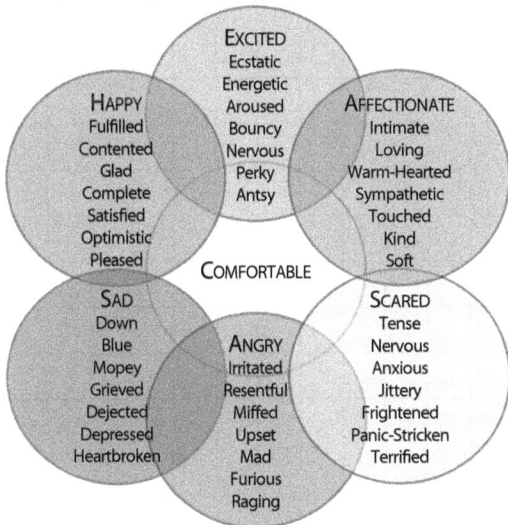

TRIGGERS AND SIGNIFICANT EVENTS

EXCITED
Ecstatic
Energetic
Aroused
Bouncy
Nervous
Perky
Antsy

HAPPY
Fulfilled
Contented
Glad
Complete
Satisfied
Optimistic
Pleased

AFFECTIONATE
Intimate
Loving
Warm-Hearted
Sympathetic
Touched
Kind
Soft

COMFORTABLE

SAD
Down
Blue
Mopey
Grieved
Dejected
Depressed
Heartbroken

ANGRY
Irritated
Resentful
Miffed
Upset
Mad
Furious
Raging

SCARED
Tense
Nervous
Anxious
Jittery
Frightened
Panic-Stricken
Terrified

Describe any changes in your pain today:

_____

_____

_____

_____

Did anything unusual happen today?

_____

_____

_____

_____

What did you spend the most time time thinking about today?

Positive Thoughts:

_____

Did your pain increase, decrease, or remain the same when you thought about it?
____ Increased
____ Decreased
____ Stayed the Same

Negative Thoughts:

_____

Did your pain increase, decrease, or remain the same when you thought about it?
____ Increased
____ Decreased
____ Stayed the Same

1 DAILY
MOOD CHART

DAY_____ DATE_____ WEIGHT_____

Connect the points on your Mood Satisfaction Chart so your medical team can see when and why your mental state changed.

MOOD			
HAPPY	+3		
	+2		
	+1		
	0		
	-1		
	-2		
SAD	-3		

2 ACTIVITY LOG

6am 7 8 9 10 11 12pm 1 2 3 4 5 6pm 7 8 9 10 11 12am 1 2 3 4 5

3 MEDICATION LOG
NAME/DOSE

1
2
3
4
5
6
7
8

4 PHYSIOLOGY

6am 7 8 9 10 11 12pm 1 2 3 4 5 6pm 7 8 9 10 11 12am 1 2 3 4 5

SLEEP

URINATION

DEFECATION

NAUSEA

EATING

EXERCISE

OTHER (LIST)

1 DAILY RESULTS
OF MEDICATIONS AND TREATMENTS

As you and your medical team develop new treatment plans, it will be especially helpful to record any side effects you experience as you add new treatments. This can help determine which types of treatments will work best for you.

Contact your care provider with any bad reactions or side effects to determine if you should discontinue the medication or treatment.

MEDICATION / TREATMENT	AMOUNT / TIME / COMMENTS

1 DAILY
TREATMENT PLAN

22

As you and your medical team develop new treatment plans, record your plan for the day including new medications, increases or decreases to medications, exercises, physical therapy, or any other treatment efforts.

MEDICATION / TREATMENT	AMOUNT / TIME / COMMENTS

1 DAILY PAIN CHART

DAY_____ DATE_____ WEIGHT_____

Connect the points on your Daily Pain and Satisfaction Charts so your medical team can see when your status changed.

22

PAIN LEVEL

WORST IMAGINABLE	10
	9
	8
	7
	6
MODERATE	5
	4
	3
	2
	1
NONE	0

2 SATISFACTION

Time axis: 6am 7 8 9 10 11 12pm 1 2 3 4 5 6pm 7 8 9 10 11 12am 1 2 3 4 5

MOOD

(HAPPY)	POSITIVE
	+2
	+1
	NEUTRAL
	-1
	-2
(UNHAPPY)	NEGATIVE

3 PHYSIOLOGY

Time axis: 6am 7 8 9 10 11 12pm 1 2 3 4 5 6pm 7 8 9 10 11 12am 1 2 3 4 5

- SLEEP
- RESTROOM
- NAUSEA / DIZZINESS
- MEAL / SNACK
- EXERCISE
- STRESS / ANXIETY
- MEDICINE NAME / DOSE
- 1
- 2
- 3
- BLOOD PRESSURE
- PULSE

22

4 DAILY HEAD & FACE PAIN DIAGRAM

Mark each place on the diagram where you have had pain today by placing an 'X', circling the location, or shading the area .

Describe the type of pain:

Shooting	Deep
Tingling	Sharp
Numbness	Burning / Hot
Cold	Aching
Surface Pain	Gnawing / Biting
Stabbing	Electrical / Shocks
Dull	Other_____
Stinging	

COMMENTS AND MORE INFORMATION:

Front

Upper Right   **Upper Left**

Lower Right   **Lower Left**

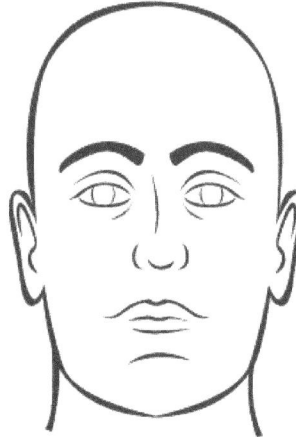

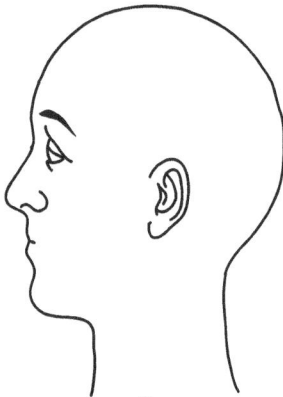

**Your
Right
Side**

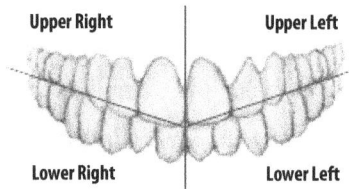

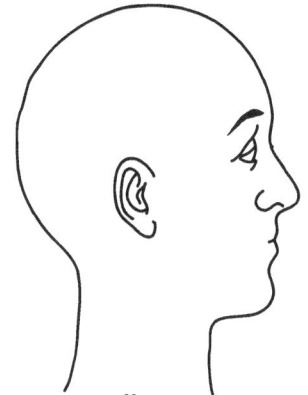

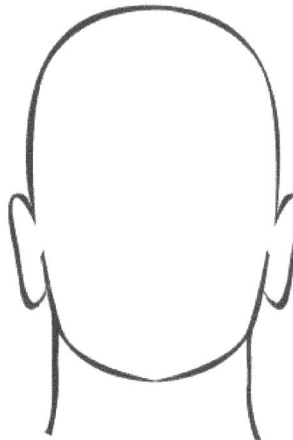

**Your
Right
Side**

Back

5 DAILY BODY PAIN DIAGRAM

Mark each place on the diagram where you have had pain today by placing an 'X', circling the location, or shading the area .

Describe the type of pain:

Shooting   Deep
Tingling   Sharp
Numbness   Burning / Hot
Cold   Aching
Surface Pain   Gnawing / Biting
Stabbing   Electrical / Shocks
Dull   Other_____
Stinging

COMMENTS AND MORE INFORMATION:

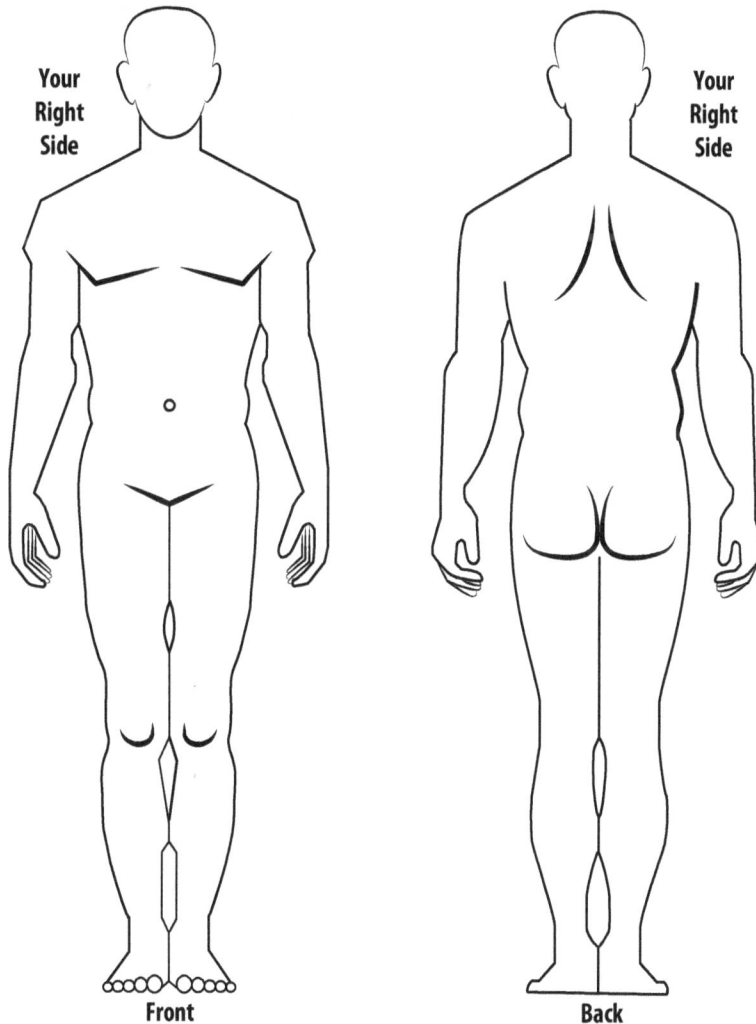

Your Right Side

Your Right Side

Front

Back

6 DAILY PAIN SUMMARY

Were there times during the day that you experienced unrelieved breakthrough pain? ____NO ____YES

How many times did this happen today?

1 2 3 4 5 6 7 8 9 10 more than 10

Did any specific activity start your breakthrough pain? ____NO ____YES: What activities?

_____

Put an "X" on the body diagram to show each place you've had **BREAKTHROUGH PAIN** today.

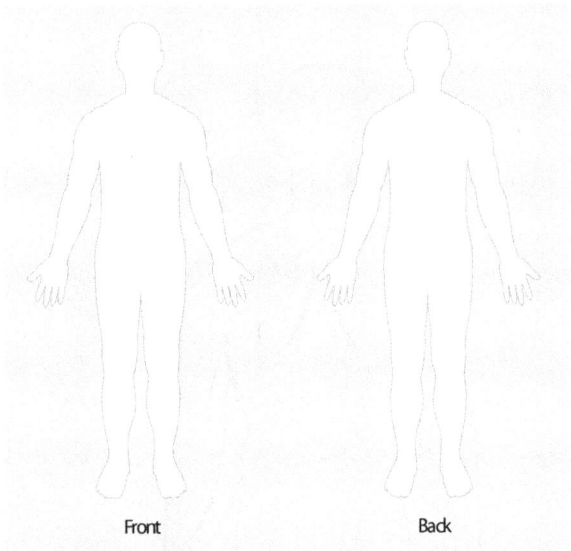

Front   Back

NON-DRUG THERAPIES
(other than prescription or other medicines)

_____

_____

ACTIVITIES/EXERCISE

_____

What was your average level of pain today?

0 1 2 3 4 5 6 7 8 9 10

Other than prescription medicine, did you do anything else today to relieve the pain? ____NO ____YES: (Note any that you used.)
____ Non-prescription drugs (e.g., acetaminophen, ibuprofen)
____ Herbal remedies
____ Hot or cold packs
____ Exercise
____ Changing position (such as lying down or elevating your legs)
____ Physical therapy
____ Massage
____ Acupuncture
____ Rest
____ Psychological counseling
____ Talk to trusted friend, family, clergy
____ Prayer, meditation, guided imagery
____ Relaxation technique (hypnosis, biofeedback)
____ Creative technique (art or music therapy)
____ Other (e.g., specific chiropractic manipulation, osteopathic treatments):

_____

Check any of these common side effects that you've noticed after taking your pain medicine:
____ Drowsiness, sleepiness
____ Nausea, vomiting, upset stomach
____ Constipation
____ Lack of appetite
____ Other (describe):

_____

Did you sleep through the night? ____NO____YES

If not, how many times was your sleep disrupted? _____

How many hours did you sleep during the night? _____

COMMENTS AND MORE INFORMATION: Make notes for and about visits with your healthcare provider, side effects from treatments you may be experiencing, any problems you are having coping with your pain, and more about some of your previous answers or questions.

_____

_____

_____

1 DAILY DIARY
SATISFACTION CHART Connect the points on your Daily Satisfaction Chart so your medical team can see when and why your mental state changed.

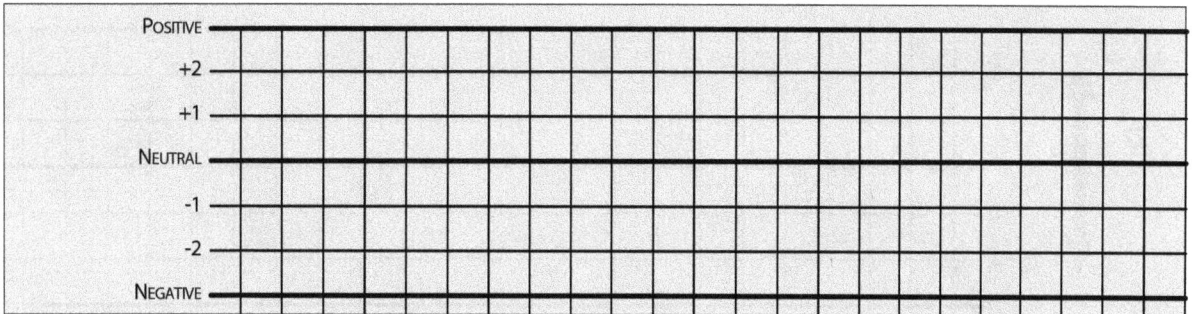

DAY_____ DATE_____ WEIGHT_____

| | |
POSITIVE
+2
+1
NEUTRAL
-1
-2
NEGATIVE

2 ACTIVITY LOG

6am 7 8 9 10 11 12pm 1 2 3 4 5 6pm 7 8 9 10 11 12am 1 2 3 4 5

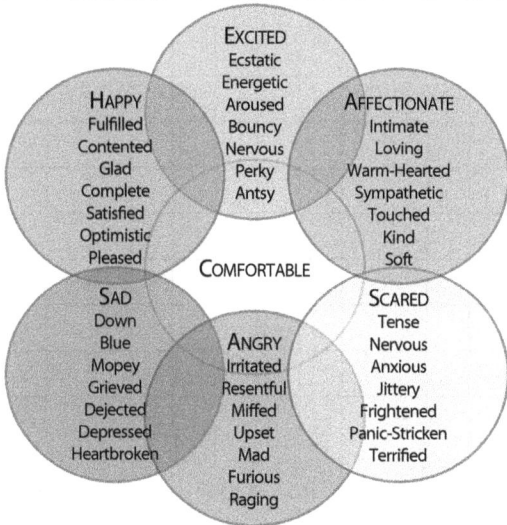

TRIGGERS AND SIGNIFICANT EVENTS

EXCITED Ecstatic Energetic Aroused Bouncy Nervous Perky Antsy

HAPPY Fulfilled Contented Glad Complete Satisfied Optimistic Pleased

AFFECTIONATE Intimate Loving Warm-Hearted Sympathetic Touched Kind Soft

COMFORTABLE

SAD Down Blue Mopey Grieved Dejected Depressed Heartbroken

ANGRY Irritated Resentful Miffed Upset Mad Furious Raging

SCARED Tense Nervous Anxious Jittery Frightened Panic-Stricken Terrified

Describe any changes in your pain today:
_____

Did anything unusual happen today?
_____

What did you spend the most time time thinking about today?

Positive Thoughts:
_____
Did your pain increase, decrease, or remain the same when you thought about it?
____ Increased
____ Decreased
____ Stayed the Same

Negative Thoughts:
_____
Did your pain increase, decrease, or remain the same when you thought about it?
____ Increased
____ Decreased
____ Stayed the Same

22

1 DAILY
MOOD CHART

DAY_____ DATE_____ WEIGHT_____

Connect the points on your Mood Satisfaction Chart so your medical team can see when and why your mental state changed.

MOOD		
HAPPY	+3	
	+2	
	+1	
	0	
	-1	
	-2	
SAD	-3	

2 ACTIVITY LOG

6am 7 8 9 10 11 12pm 1 2 3 4 5 6pm 7 8 9 10 11 12am 1 2 3 4 5

3 MEDICATION LOG
NAME/DOSE

1
2
3
4
5
6
7
8

4 PHYSIOLOGY

6am 7 8 9 10 11 12pm 1 2 3 4 5 6pm 7 8 9 10 11 12am 1 2 3 4 5

SLEEP

URINATION

DEFECATION

NAUSEA

EATING

EXERCISE

OTHER (LIST)

1 DAILY RESULTS
OF MEDICATIONS AND TREATMENTS

As you and your medical team develop new treatment plans, it will be especially helpful to record any side effects you experience as you add new treatments. This can help determine which types of treatments will work best for you.

Contact your care provider with any bad reactions or side effects to determine if you should discontinue the medication or treatment.

MEDICATION / TREATMENT	AMOUNT / TIME / COMMENTS

1 DAILY
TREATMENT PLAN

As you and your medical team develop new treatment plans, record your plan for the day including new medications, increases or decreases to medications, exercises, physical therapy, or any other treatment efforts.

23

MEDICATION / TREATMENT	AMOUNT / TIME / COMMENTS

1 DAILY
PAIN CHART

DAY_____ DATE_____ WEIGHT_____

Connect the points on your Daily Pain and Satisfaction Charts so your medical team can see when your status changed.

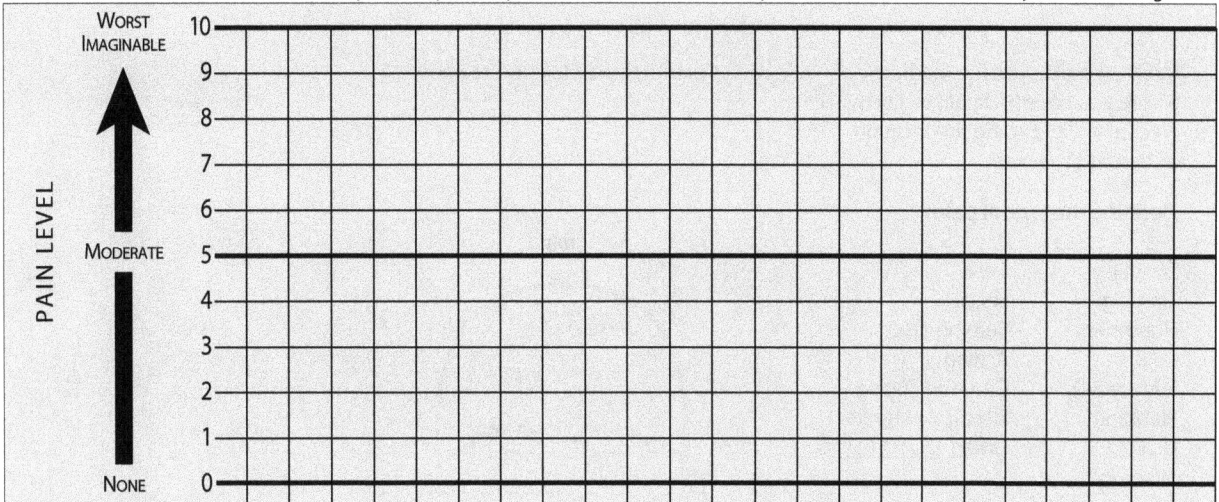

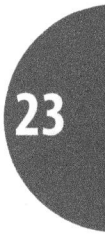

2 SATISFACTION

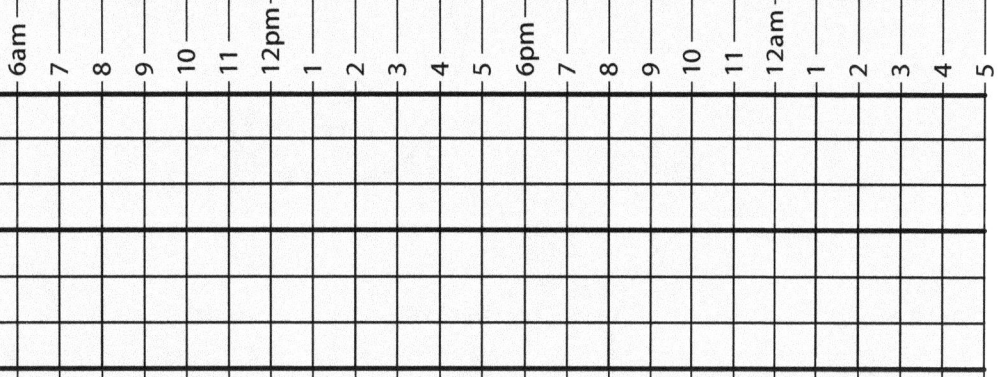

3 PHYSIOLOGY

	6am	7	8	9	10	11	12pm	1	2	3	4	5	6pm	7	8	9	10	11	12am	1	2	3	4	5
SLEEP																								
RESTROOM																								
NAUSEA / DIZZINESS																								
MEAL / SNACK																								
EXERCISE																								
STRESS / ANXIETY																								
MEDICINE NAME / DOSE																								
1																								
2																								
3																								
BLOOD PRESSURE																								
PULSE																								

4 DAILY HEAD & FACE PAIN DIAGRAM

23

Mark each place on the diagram where you have had pain today by placing an 'X', circling the location, or shading the area .

Describe the type of pain:

Shooting	Deep
Tingling	Sharp
Numbness	Burning / Hot
Cold	Aching
Surface Pain	Gnawing / Biting
Stabbing	Electrical / Shocks
Dull	Other_____
Stinging	

COMMENTS AND MORE INFORMATION:

Front

Upper Right   Upper Left

Lower Right   Lower Left

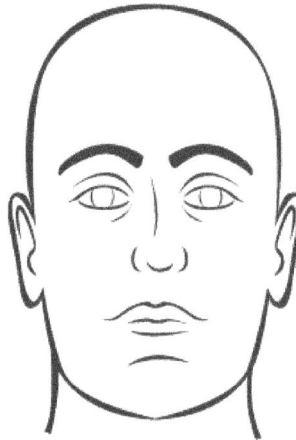

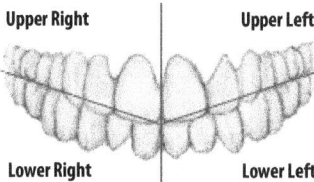

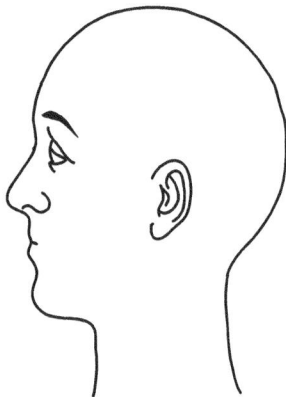

Your Right Side

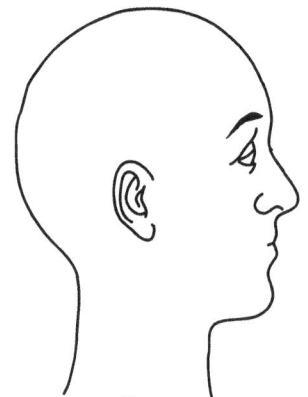

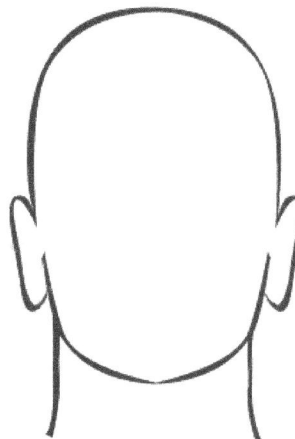

Your Right Side

Back

5 DAILY BODY PAIN DIAGRAM

Mark each place on the diagram where you have had pain today by placing an 'X', circling the location, or shading the area .

Describe the type of pain:

Shooting	Deep
Tingling	Sharp
Numbness	Burning / Hot
Cold	Aching
Surface Pain	Gnawing / Biting
Stabbing	Electrical / Shocks
Dull	Other_____
Stinging	

COMMENTS AND MORE INFORMATION:

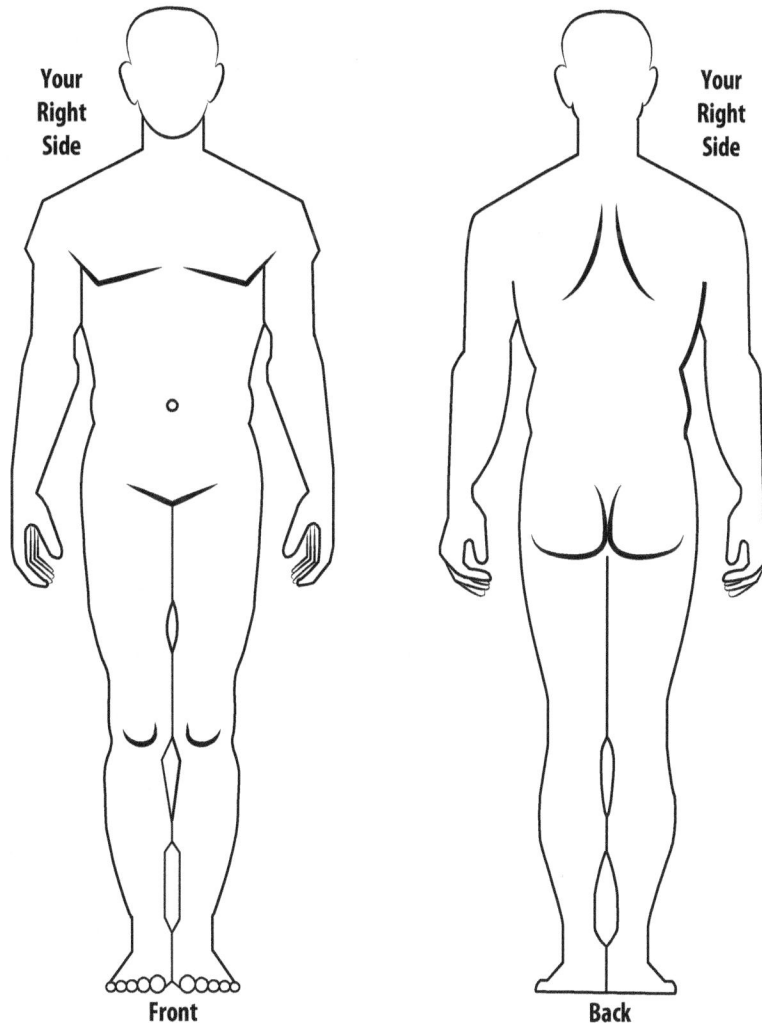

23

Your Right Side

Your Right Side

Front

Back

6 DAILY PAIN SUMMARY

Were there times during the day that you experienced unrelieved breakthrough pain? ____NO ____YES

How many times did this happen today?

1 2 3 4 5 6 7 8 9 10 more than 10

Did any specific activity start your breakthrough pain? ____NO ____YES: What activities?

_____

Put an "X" on the body diagram to show each place you've had *BREAKTHROUGH PAIN* today.

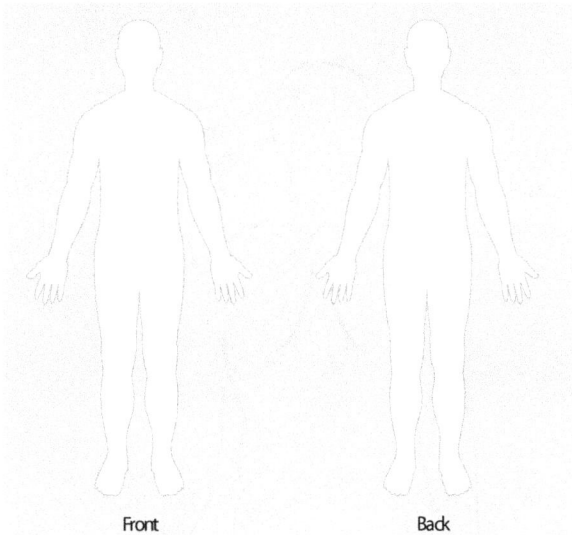

Front   Back

NON-DRUG THERAPIES
(other than prescription or other medicines)

_____

_____

ACTIVITIES/EXERCISE

_____

_____

What was your average level of pain today?

0 1 2 3 4 5 6 7 8 9 10

Other than prescription medicine, did you do anything else today to relieve the pain? ____NO ____YES: (Note any that you used.)
____ Non-prescription drugs (e.g., acetaminophen, ibuprofen)
____ Herbal remedies
____ Hot or cold packs
____ Exercise
____ Changing position (such as lying down or elevating your legs)
____ Physical therapy
____ Massage
____ Acupuncture
____ Rest
____ Psychological counseling
____ Talk to trusted friend, family, clergy
____ Prayer, meditation, guided imagery
____ Relaxation technique (hypnosis, biofeedback)
____ Creative technique (art or music therapy)
____ Other (e.g., specific chiropractic manipulation, osteopathic treatments):

_____

Check any of these common side effects that you've noticed after taking your pain medicine:
____ Drowsiness, sleepiness
____ Nausea, vomiting, upset stomach
____ Constipation
____ Lack of appetite
____ Other (describe):

_____

Did you sleep through the night? ____NO____YES

If not, how many times was your sleep disrupted? _____

How many hours did you sleep during the night? _____

COMMENTS AND MORE INFORMATION: Make notes for and about visits with your healthcare provider, side effects from treatments you may be experiencing, any problems you are having coping with your pain, and more about some of your previous answers or questions.

_____

_____

_____

1 DAILY DIARY

SATISFACTION CHART Connect the points on your Daily Satisfaction Chart so your medical team can see when and why your mental state changed.

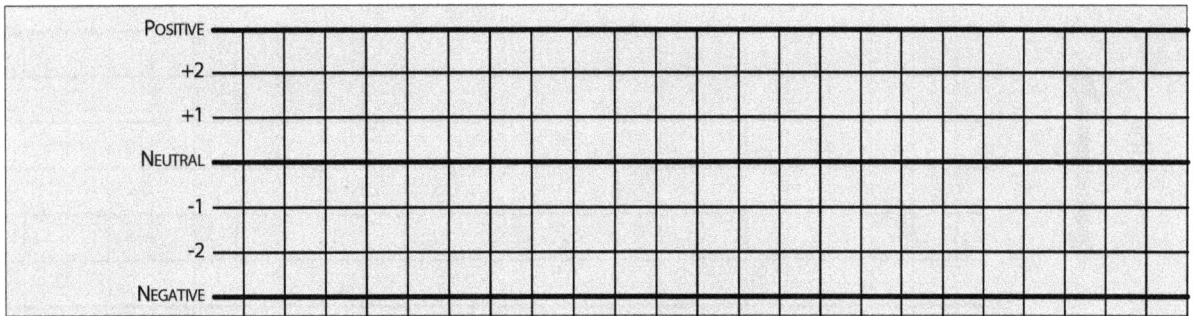

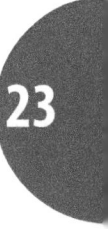

DAY_____ DATE_____ WEIGHT_____

	POSITIVE
	+2
	+1
	NEUTRAL
	-1
	-2
	NEGATIVE

23

2 ACTIVITY LOG

6am 7 8 9 10 11 12pm 1 2 3 4 5 6pm 7 8 9 10 11 12am 1 2 3 4 5

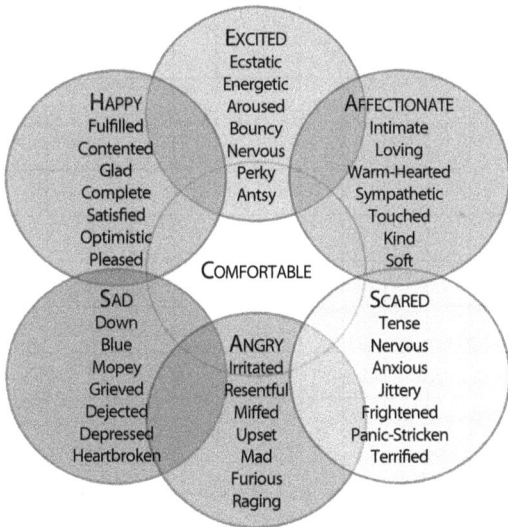

TRIGGERS AND SIGNIFICANT EVENTS

EXCITED
Ecstatic
Energetic
Aroused
Bouncy
Nervous
Perky
Antsy

HAPPY
Fulfilled
Contented
Glad
Complete
Satisfied
Optimistic
Pleased

AFFECTIONATE
Intimate
Loving
Warm-Hearted
Sympathetic
Touched
Kind
Soft

COMFORTABLE

SAD
Down
Blue
Mopey
Grieved
Dejected
Depressed
Heartbroken

ANGRY
Irritated
Resentful
Miffed
Upset
Mad
Furious
Raging

SCARED
Tense
Nervous
Anxious
Jittery
Frightened
Panic-Stricken
Terrified

Describe any changes in your pain today:

_____
_____
_____
_____
_____

Did anything unusual happen today?

_____
_____
_____
_____

What did you spend the most time time thinking about today?

Positive Thoughts:

_____

Did your pain increase, decrease, or remain the same when you thought about it?
____ Increased
____ Decreased
____ Stayed the Same

Negative Thoughts:

_____

Did your pain increase, decrease, or remain the same when you thought about it?
____ Increased
____ Decreased
____ Stayed the Same

1 DAILY
MOOD CHART

DAY_____ DATE_____ WEIGHT_____

Connect the points on your Mood Satisfaction Chart so your medical team can see when and why your mental state changed.

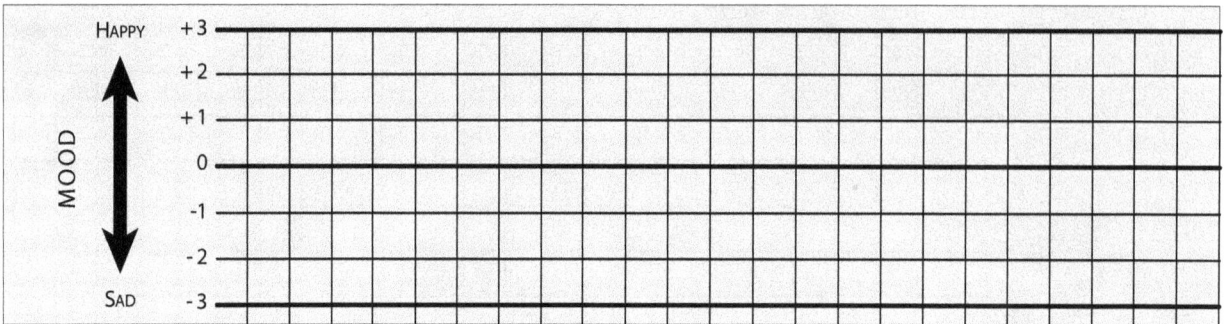

23

HAPPY +3

MOOD +2

+1

0

-1

-2

SAD -3

2 ACTIVITY LOG

6am 7 8 9 10 11 12pm 1 2 3 4 5 6pm 7 8 9 10 11 12am 1 2 3 4 5

3 MEDICATION LOG
NAME/DOSE

1
2
3
4
5
6
7
8

4 PHYSIOLOGY

6am 7 8 9 10 11 12pm 1 2 3 4 5 6pm 7 8 9 10 11 12am 1 2 3 4 5

SLEEP

URINATION

DEFECATION

NAUSEA

EATING

EXERCISE

OTHER (LIST)

1 DAILY RESULTS
OF MEDICATIONS AND TREATMENTS

As you and your medical team develop new treatment plans, it will be especially helpful to record any side effects you experience as you add new treatments. This can help determine which types of treatments will work best for you.

Contact your care provider with any bad reactions or side effects to determine if you should discontinue the medication or treatment.

23

MEDICATION / TREATMENT	AMOUNT / TIME / COMMENTS

1 DAILY
TREATMENT PLAN

As you and your medical team develop new treatment plans, record your plan for the day including new medications, increases or decreases to medications, exercises, physical therapy, or any other treatment efforts.

MEDICATION / TREATMENT	AMOUNT / TIME / COMMENTS

24

1 DAILY
PAIN CHART

DAY_____ DATE_____ WEIGHT_____

Connect the points on your Daily Pain and Satisfaction Charts so your medical team can see when your status changed.

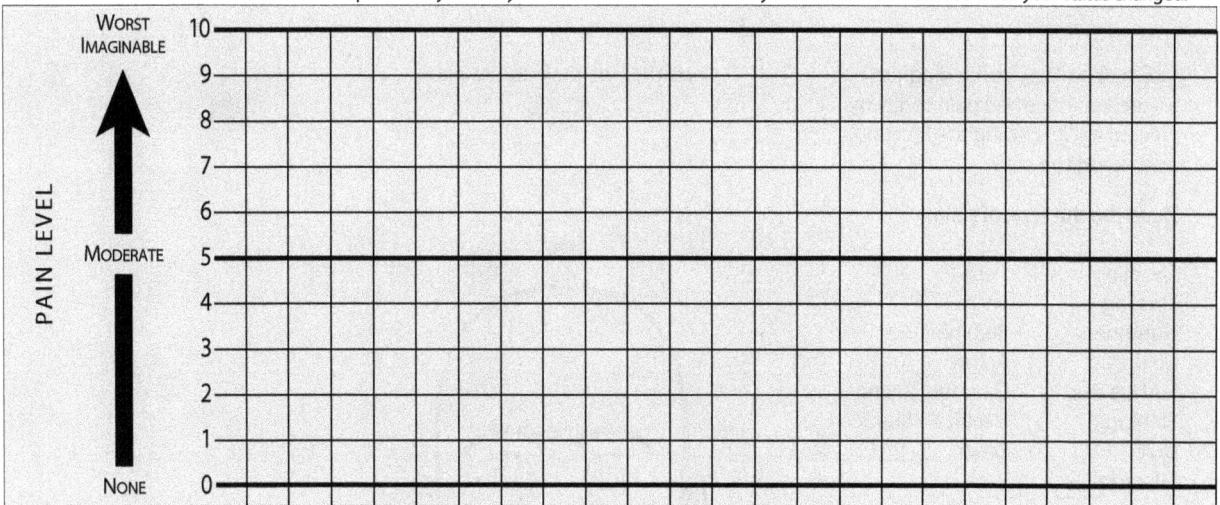

PAIN LEVEL

- WORST IMAGINABLE — 10
- 9
- 8
- 7
- 6
- MODERATE — 5
- 4
- 3
- 2
- 1
- NONE — 0

Times: 6am, 7, 8, 9, 10, 11, 12pm, 1, 2, 3, 4, 5, 6pm, 7, 8, 9, 10, 11, 12am, 1, 2, 3, 4, 5

2 SATISFACTION

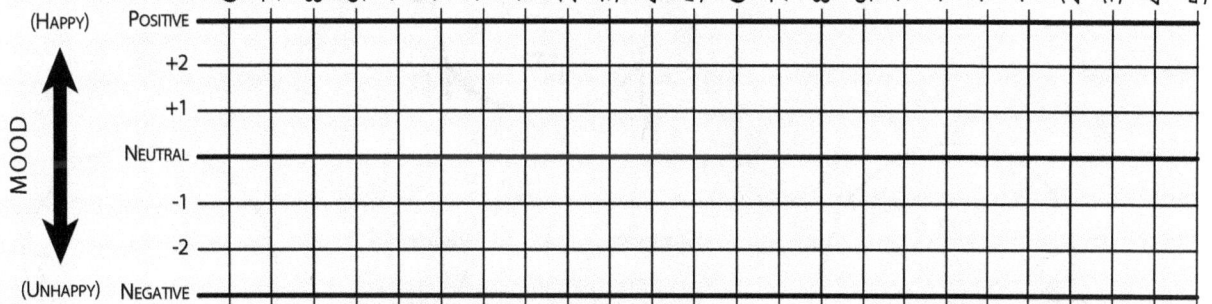

MOOD

- (HAPPY) POSITIVE
- +2
- +1
- NEUTRAL
- -1
- -2
- (UNHAPPY) NEGATIVE

3 PHYSIOLOGY

- SLEEP
- RESTROOM
- NAUSEA / DIZZINESS
- MEAL / SNACK
- EXERCISE
- STRESS / ANXIETY
- MEDICINE NAME / DOSE
  1
  2
  3
- BLOOD PRESSURE
- PULSE

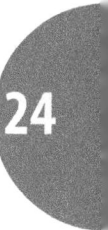

4 DAILY HEAD & FACE PAIN DIAGRAM

Mark each place on the diagram where you have had pain today by placing an 'X', circling the location, or shading the area .

Describe the type of pain:

Shooting	Deep
Tingling	Sharp
Numbness	Burning / Hot
Cold	Aching
Surface Pain	Gnawing / Biting
Stabbing	Electrical / Shocks
Dull	Other_____
Stinging	

24

COMMENTS AND MORE INFORMATION:

Front

Upper Right **Upper Left**

Lower Right **Lower Left**

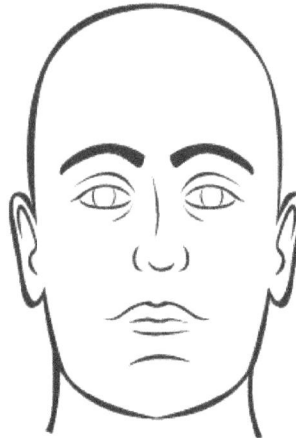

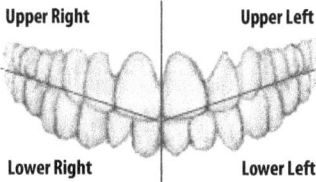

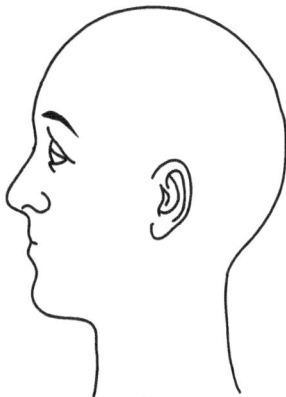

Your Right Side

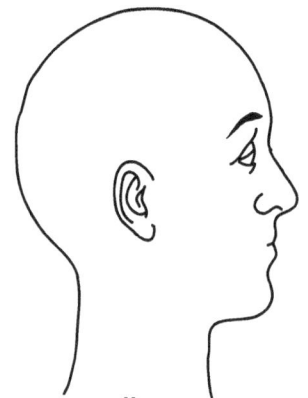

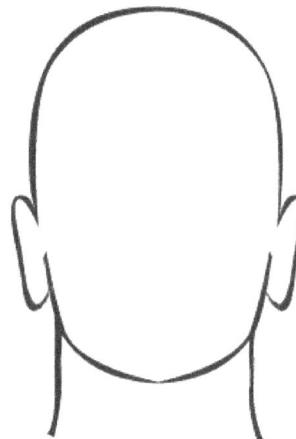

Your Right Side

Back

5 DAILY BODY PAIN DIAGRAM

Mark each place on the diagram where you have had pain today by placing an 'X', circling the location, or shading the area .

Describe the type of pain:

Shooting	Deep
Tingling	Sharp
Numbness	Burning / Hot
Cold	Aching
Surface Pain	Gnawing / Biting
Stabbing	Electrical / Shocks
Dull	Other_____
Stinging	

COMMENTS AND MORE INFORMATION:

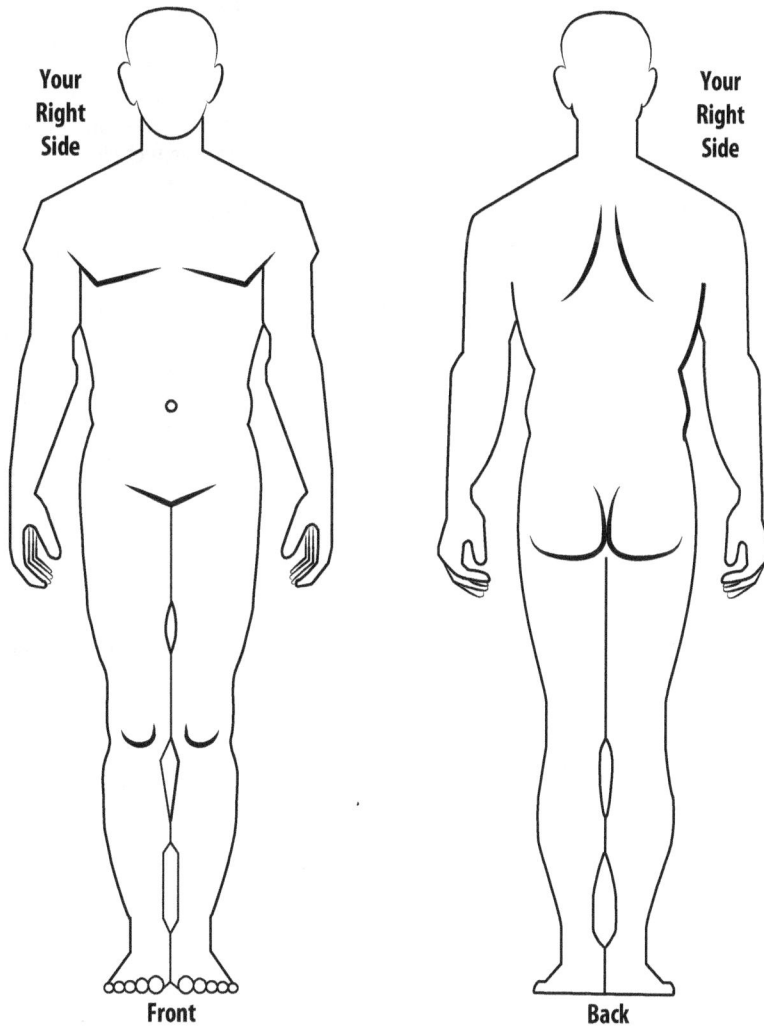

24

Your Right Side

Your Right Side

Front

Back

6 DAILY PAIN SUMMARY

Were there times during the day that you experienced unrelieved breakthrough pain? ____NO ____YES

How many times did this happen today?

  1 2 3 4 5 6 7 8 9 10 more than 10

Did any specific activity start your breakthrough pain?
____NO   ____YES: What activities?

_____

Put an "X" on the body diagram to show each place you've had **BREAKTHROUGH PAIN** today.

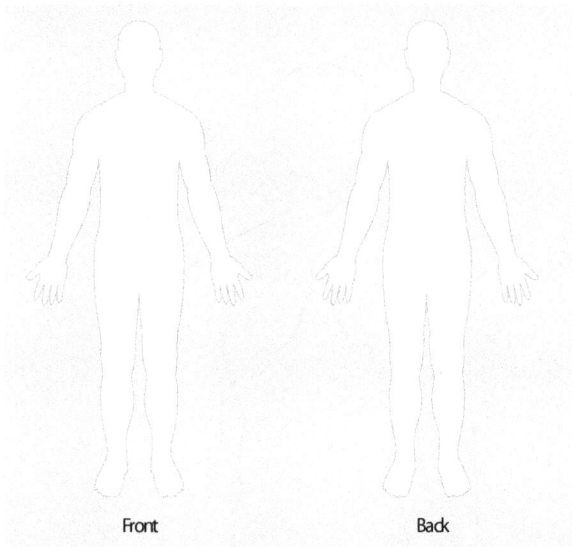

Front   Back

NON-DRUG THERAPIES
(other than prescription or other medicines)

_____

_____

ACTIVITIES/EXERCISE

_____

What was your average level of pain today?

  0 1 2 3 4 5 6 7 8 9 10

Other than prescription medicine, did you do anything else today to relieve the pain? ____NO   ____YES:
(Note any that you used.)
____ Non-prescription drugs (e.g., acetaminophen, ibuprofen)
____ Herbal remedies
____ Hot or cold packs
____ Exercise
____ Changing position (such as lying down or elevating your legs)
____ Physical therapy
____ Massage
____ Acupuncture
____ Rest
____ Psychological counseling
____ Talk to trusted friend, family, clergy
____ Prayer, meditation, guided imagery
____ Relaxation technique (hypnosis, biofeedback)
____ Creative technique (art or music therapy)
____ Other (e.g., specific chiropractic manipulation, osteopathic treatments):

_____

Check any of these common side effects that you've noticed after taking your pain medicine:
____ Drowsiness, sleepiness
____ Nausea, vomiting, upset stomach
____ Constipation
____ Lack of appetite
____ Other (describe):

_____

Did you sleep through the night? ____NO____YES

If not, how many times was your sleep disrupted? _____

How many hours did you sleep during the night? _____

COMMENTS AND MORE INFORMATION: Make notes for and about visits with your healthcare provider, side effects from treatments you may be experiencing, any problems you are having coping with your pain, and more about some of your previous answers or questions.

_____

_____

_____

1 DAILY DIARY

SATISFACTION CHART

DAY_____ DATE_____ WEIGHT_____

Connect the points on your Daily Satisfaction Chart so your medical team can see when and why your mental state changed.

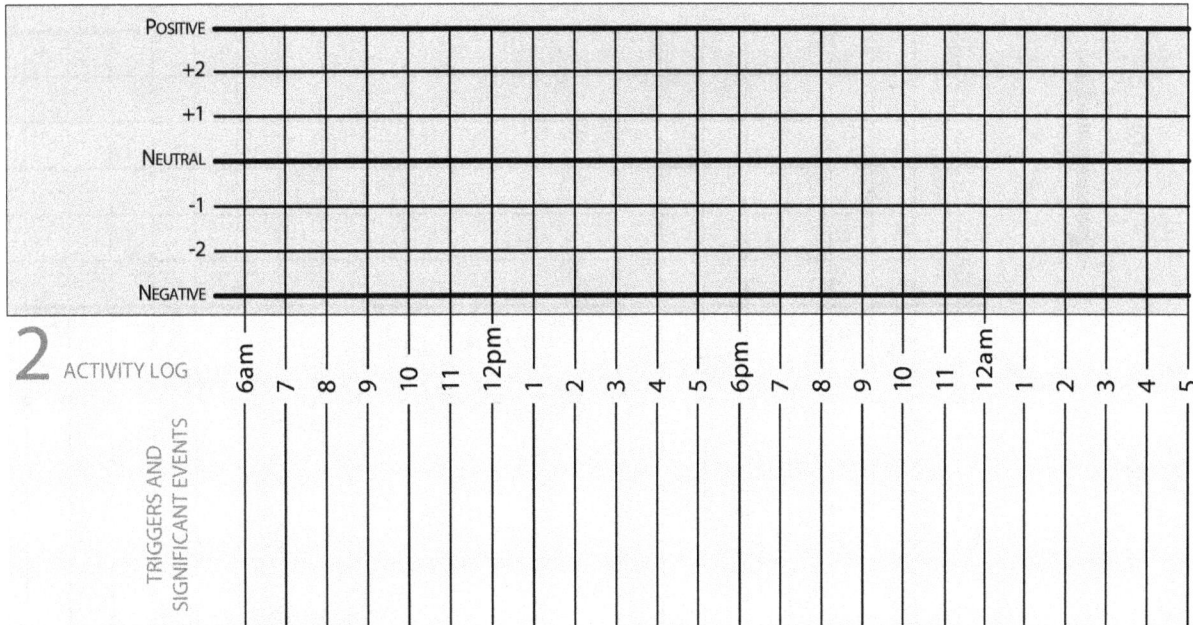

	POSITIVE
	+2
	+1
	NEUTRAL
	-1
	-2
	NEGATIVE

2 ACTIVITY LOG

TRIGGERS AND SIGNIFICANT EVENTS

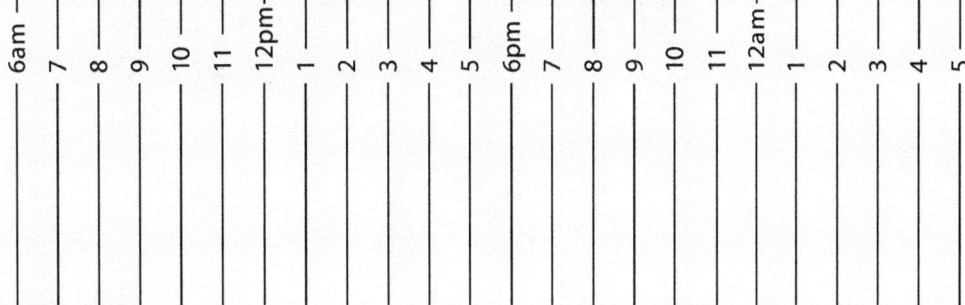

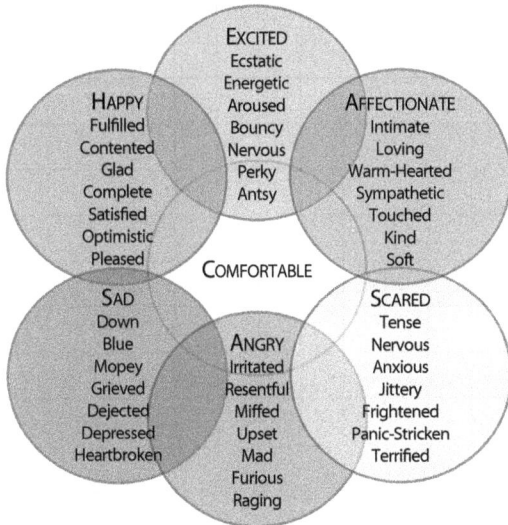

6am 7 8 9 10 11 12pm 1 2 3 4 5 6pm 7 8 9 10 11 12am 1 2 3 4 5

24

EXCITED
Ecstatic
Energetic
Aroused
Bouncy
Nervous
Perky
Antsy

HAPPY
Fulfilled
Contented
Glad
Complete
Satisfied
Optimistic
Pleased

AFFECTIONATE
Intimate
Loving
Warm-Hearted
Sympathetic
Touched
Kind
Soft

COMFORTABLE

SAD
Down
Blue
Mopey
Grieved
Dejected
Depressed
Heartbroken

ANGRY
Irritated
Resentful
Miffed
Upset
Mad
Furious
Raging

SCARED
Tense
Nervous
Anxious
Jittery
Frightened
Panic-Stricken
Terrified

Describe any changes in your pain today:

_____

_____

_____

_____

_____

Did anything unusual happen today?

_____

_____

_____

_____

_____

What did you spend the most time time thinking about today?

Positive Thoughts:

_____

Did your pain increase, decrease, or remain the same when you thought about it?

____ Increased

____ Decreased

____ Stayed the Same

Negative Thoughts:

_____

Did your pain increase, decrease, or remain the same when you thought about it?

____ Increased

____ Decreased

____ Stayed the Same

1 DAILY
MOOD CHART

DAY_____ DATE_____ WEIGHT_____

Connect the points on your Mood Satisfaction Chart so your medical team can see when and why your mental state changed.

HAPPY +3

MOOD   +2

       +1

        0

       -1

       -2

SAD   -3

2 ACTIVITY LOG

6am 7 8 9 10 11 12pm 1 2 3 4 5 6pm 7 8 9 10 11 12am 1 2 3 4 5

3 MEDICATION LOG
NAME/DOSE

1
2
3
4
5
6
7
8

4 PHYSIOLOGY

6am 7 8 9 10 11 12pm 1 2 3 4 5 6pm 7 8 9 10 11 12am 1 2 3 4 5

SLEEP

URINATION

DEFECATION

NAUSEA

EATING

EXERCISE

OTHER (LIST)

24

1 DAILY RESULTS
OF MEDICATIONS AND TREATMENTS

As you and your medical team develop new treatment plans, it will be especially helpful to record any side effects you experience as you add new treatments. This can help determine which types of treatments will work best for you.

Contact your care provider with any bad reactions or side effects to determine if you should discontinue the medication or treatment.

MEDICATION / TREATMENT	AMOUNT / TIME / COMMENTS

24

1 DAILY
TREATMENT PLAN

As you and your medical team develop new treatment plans, record your plan for the day including new medications, increases or decreases to medications, exercises, physical therapy, or any other treatment efforts.

MEDICATION / TREATMENT	AMOUNT / TIME / COMMENTS

25

1 DAILY
PAIN CHART

DAY_____ DATE_____ WEIGHT_____

Connect the points on your Daily Pain and Satisfaction Charts so your medical team can see when your status changed.

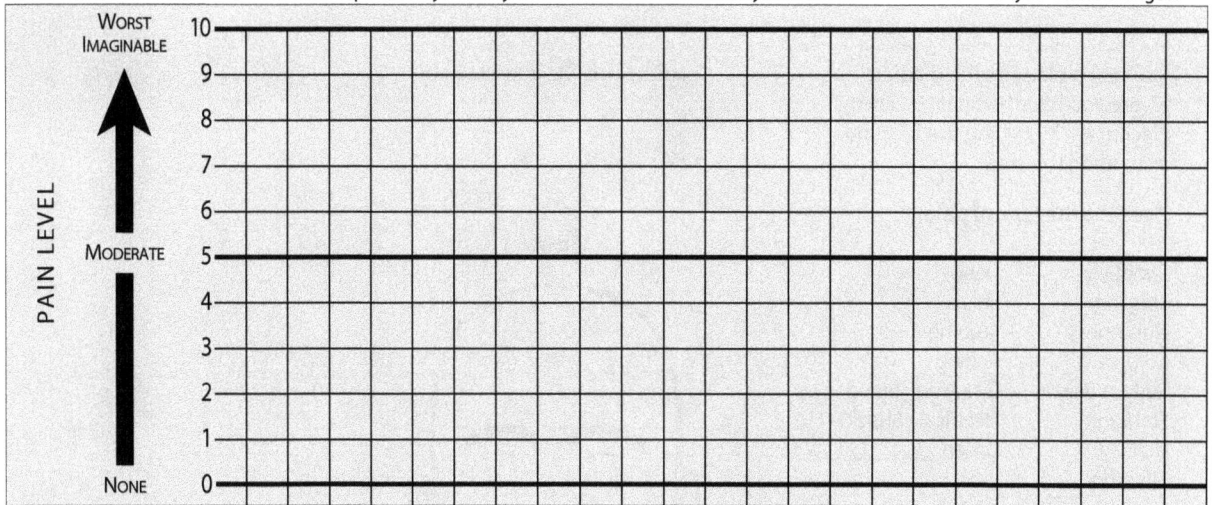

WORST IMAGINABLE

PAIN LEVEL

MODERATE

NONE

10
9
8
7
6
5
4
3
2
1
0

2 SATISFACTION

(HAPPY) POSITIVE

MOOD

(UNHAPPY) NEGATIVE

POSITIVE
+2
+1
NEUTRAL
-1
-2
NEGATIVE

6am 7 8 9 10 11 12pm 1 2 3 4 5 6pm 7 8 9 10 11 12am 1 2 3 4 5

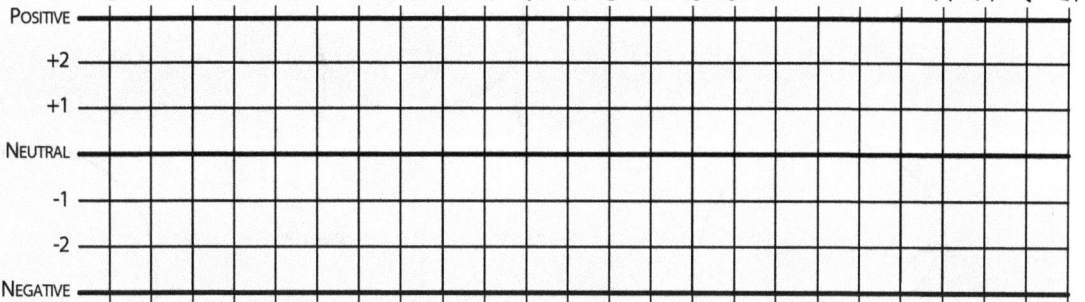

3 PHYSIOLOGY

6am 7 8 9 10 11 12pm 1 2 3 4 5 6pm 7 8 9 10 11 12am 1 2 3 4 5

SLEEP

RESTROOM

NAUSEA / DIZZINESS

MEAL / SNACK

EXERCISE

STRESS / ANXIETY

MEDICINE NAME / DOSE

1

2

3

BLOOD PRESSURE

PULSE

25

4 DAILY HEAD & FACE PAIN DIAGRAM

Mark each place on the diagram where you have had pain today by placing an 'X', circling the location, or shading the area .

Describe the type of pain:

Shooting	Deep
Tingling	Sharp
Numbness	Burning / Hot
Cold	Aching
Surface Pain	Gnawing / Biting
Stabbing	Electrical / Shocks
Dull	Other_____
Stinging	

COMMENTS AND MORE INFORMATION:

Front

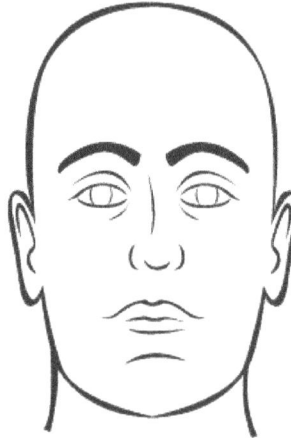

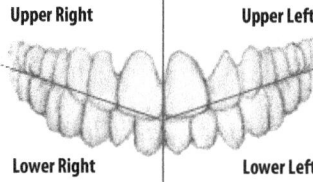

Upper Right   Upper Left

Lower Right   Lower Left

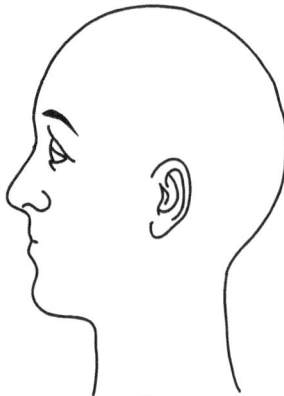

**Your
Right
Side**

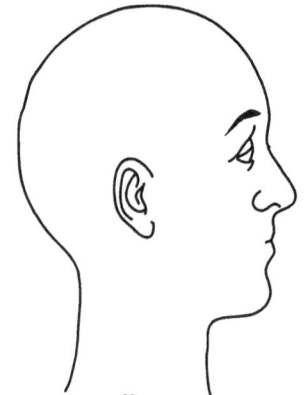

**Your
Right
Side**

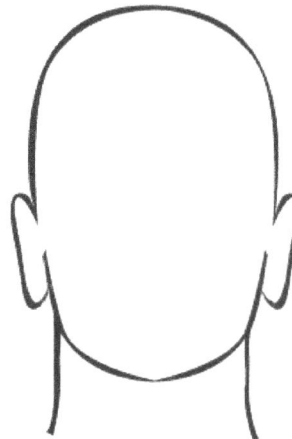

Back

25

5 DAILY BODY PAIN DIAGRAM

Mark each place on the diagram where you have had pain today by placing an 'X', circling the location, or shading the area .

Describe the type of pain:

Shooting	Deep
Tingling	Sharp
Numbness	Burning / Hot
Cold	Aching
Surface Pain	Gnawing / Biting
Stabbing	Electrical / Shocks
Dull	Other_____
Stinging	

COMMENTS AND MORE INFORMATION:

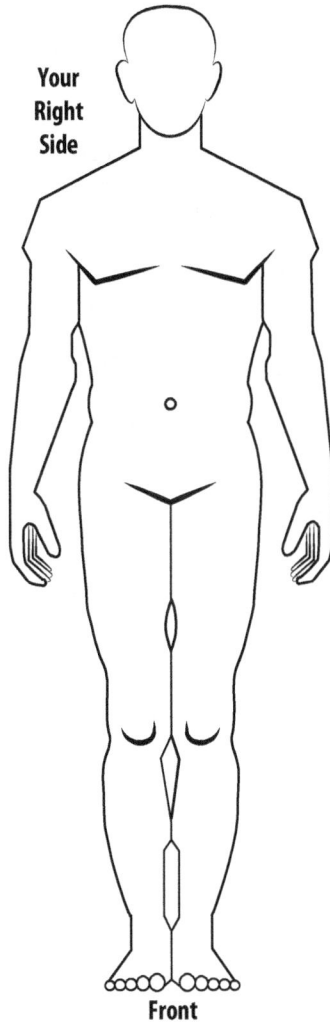

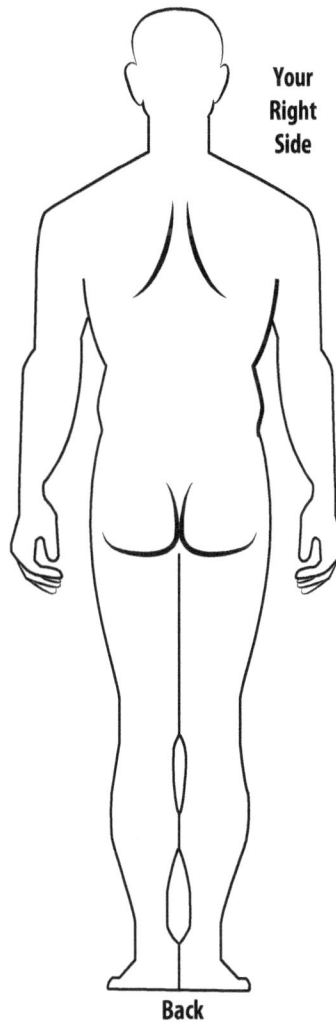

Your Right Side

Your Right Side

25

Front

Back

6 DAILY PAIN SUMMARY

Were there times during the day that you experienced unrelieved breakthrough pain? ____NO ____YES

How many times did this happen today?

   1 2 3 4   5 6 7 8 9 10   more than 10

Did any specific activity start your breakthrough pain?
____NO   ____YES: What activities?

_____

Put an "X" on the body diagram to show each place you've had **BREAKTHROUGH PAIN** today.

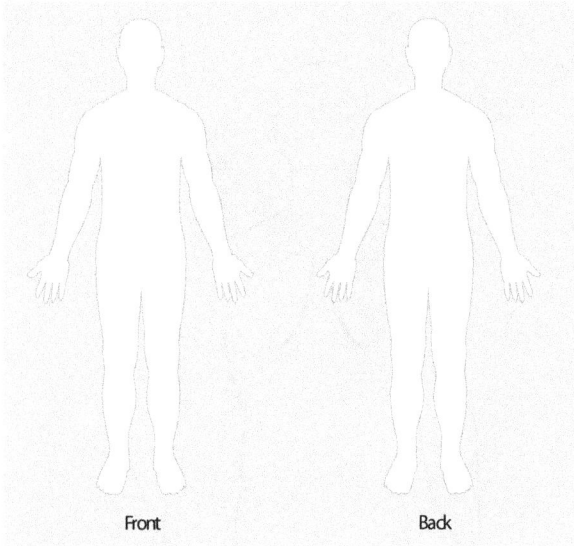

Front   Back

NON-DRUG THERAPIES
(other than prescription or other medicines)

_____

_____

ACTIVITIES/EXERCISE

_____

_____

What was your average level of pain today?

   0   1   2   3   4   5   6   7   8   9   10

Other than prescription medicine, did you do anything else today to relieve the pain? ____NO ____YES:
(Note any that you used.)
____ Non-prescription drugs (e.g., acetaminophen, ibuprofen)
____ Herbal remedies
____ Hot or cold packs
____ Exercise
____ Changing position (such as lying down or elevating your legs)
____ Physical therapy
____ Massage
____ Acupuncture
____ Rest
____ Psychological counseling
____ Talk to trusted friend, family, clergy
____ Prayer, meditation, guided imagery
____ Relaxation technique (hypnosis, biofeedback)
____ Creative technique (art or music therapy)
____ Other (e.g., specific chiropractic manipulation, osteopathic treatments):

_____

Check any of these common side effects that you've noticed after taking your pain medicine:
____ Drowsiness, sleepiness
____ Nausea, vomiting, upset stomach
____ Constipation
____ Lack of appetite
____ Other (describe):

_____

Did you sleep through the night? ____NO____YES

If not, how many times was your sleep disrupted? _____

How many hours did you sleep during the night? _____

COMMENTS AND MORE INFORMATION: Make notes for and about visits with your healthcare provider, side effects from treatments you may be experiencing, any problems you are having coping with your pain, and more about some of your previous answers or questions.

_____

_____

_____

25

1 DAILY DIARY

DAY_____ DATE_____ WEIGHT_____

SATISFACTION CHART Connect the points on your Daily Satisfaction Chart so your medical team can see when and why your mental state changed.

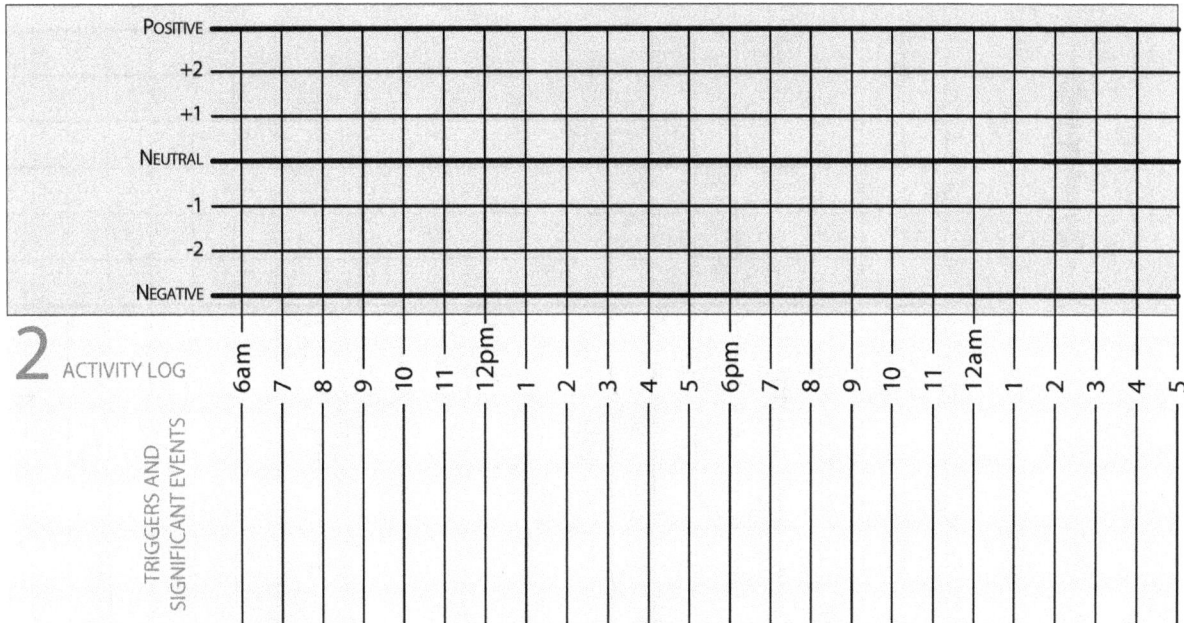

POSITIVE
+2
+1
NEUTRAL
-1
-2
NEGATIVE

2 ACTIVITY LOG

6am 7 8 9 10 11 12pm 1 2 3 4 5 6pm 7 8 9 10 11 12am 1 2 3 4 5

TRIGGERS AND SIGNIFICANT EVENTS

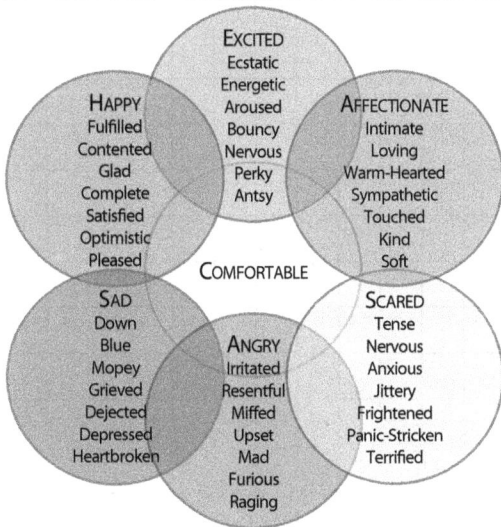

EXCITED
Ecstatic
Energetic
Aroused
Bouncy
Nervous
Perky
Antsy

HAPPY
Fulfilled
Contented
Glad
Complete
Satisfied
Optimistic
Pleased

AFFECTIONATE
Intimate
Loving
Warm-Hearted
Sympathetic
Touched
Kind
Soft

COMFORTABLE

SAD
Down
Blue
Mopey
Grieved
Dejected
Depressed
Heartbroken

ANGRY
Irritated
Resentful
Miffed
Upset
Mad
Furious
Raging

SCARED
Tense
Nervous
Anxious
Jittery
Frightened
Panic-Stricken
Terrified

Describe any changes in your pain today:

_____
_____
_____
_____

Did anything unusual happen today?

_____
_____
_____
_____

25

What did you spend the most time time thinking about today?

Positive Thoughts:

_____

Did your pain increase, decrease, or remain the same when you thought about it?
_____ Increased
_____ Decreased
_____ Stayed the Same

Negative Thoughts:

_____

Did your pain increase, decrease, or remain the same when you thought about it?
_____ Increased
_____ Decreased
_____ Stayed the Same

1 DAILY
MOOD CHART

Day_____ Date_____ Weight_____

Connect the points on your Mood Satisfaction Chart so your medical team can see when and why your mental state changed.

HAPPY +3

+2

+1

MOOD 0

-1

-2

SAD -3

2 ACTIVITY LOG

6am 7 8 9 10 11 12pm 1 2 3 4 5 6pm 7 8 9 10 11 12am 1 2 3 4 5

3 MEDICATION LOG
NAME/DOSE

1

2

3

4

5

6

7

8

4 PHYSIOLOGY

6am 7 8 9 10 11 12pm 1 2 3 4 5 6pm 7 8 9 10 11 12am 1 2 3 4 5

SLEEP

URINATION

DEFECATION

NAUSEA

EATING

EXERCISE

OTHER (LIST)

25

1 DAILY RESULTS
OF MEDICATIONS AND TREATMENTS

As you and your medical team develop new treatment plans, it will be especially helpful to record any side effects you experience as you add new treatments. This can help determine which types of treatments will work best for you.

Contact your care provider with any bad reactions or side effects to determine if you should discontinue the medication or treatment.

MEDICATION / TREATMENT	AMOUNT / TIME / COMMENTS

25

1 DAILY
TREATMENT PLAN

As you and your medical team develop new treatment plans, record your plan for the day including new medications, increases or decreases to medications, exercises, physical therapy, or any other treatment efforts.

MEDICATION / TREATMENT	AMOUNT / TIME / COMMENTS

26

1 DAILY
PAIN CHART

DAY_____ DATE_____ WEIGHT_____

Connect the points on your Daily Pain and Satisfaction Charts so your medical team can see when your status changed.

PAIN LEVEL

WORST IMAGINABLE — 10

9

8

7

6

MODERATE — 5

4

3

2

1

NONE — 0

6am 7 8 9 10 11 12pm 1 2 3 4 5 6pm 7 8 9 10 11 12am 1 2 3 4 5

2 SATISFACTION

MOOD

(HAPPY) POSITIVE

+2

+1

NEUTRAL

-1

-2

(UNHAPPY) NEGATIVE

6am 7 8 9 10 11 12pm 1 2 3 4 5 6pm 7 8 9 10 11 12am 1 2 3 4 5

3 PHYSIOLOGY

6am 7 8 9 10 11 12pm 1 2 3 4 5 6pm 7 8 9 10 11 12am 1 2 3 4 5

SLEEP

RESTROOM

NAUSEA / DIZZINESS

MEAL / SNACK

EXERCISE

STRESS / ANXIETY

MEDICINE NAME / DOSE

1

2

3

BLOOD PRESSURE

PULSE

26

4 DAILY HEAD & FACE PAIN DIAGRAM

Mark each place on the diagram where you have had pain today by placing an 'X', circling the location, or shading the area .

Describe the type of pain:

Shooting	Deep
Tingling	Sharp
Numbness	Burning / Hot
Cold	Aching
Surface Pain	Gnawing / Biting
Stabbing	Electrical / Shocks
Dull	Other_____
Stinging	

COMMENTS AND MORE INFORMATION:

Front

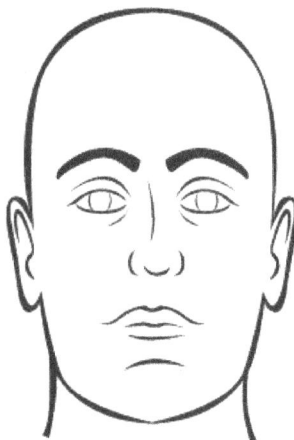

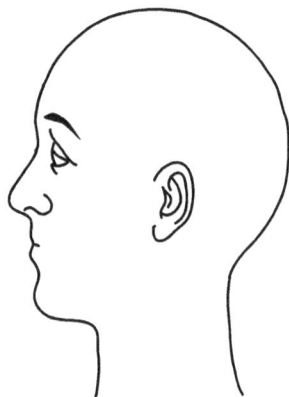

Your Right Side

Upper Right   Upper Left

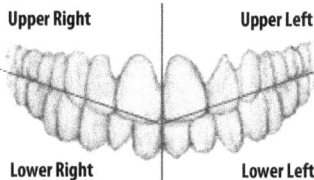

Lower Right   Lower Left

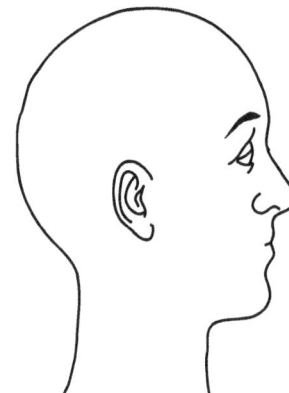

Your Right Side

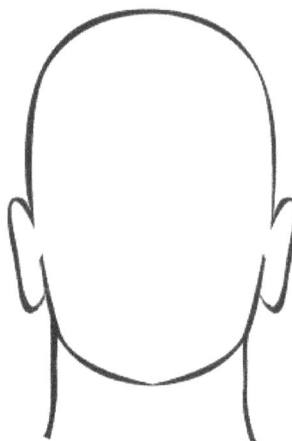

Back

26

5 DAILY BODY PAIN DIAGRAM

Mark each place on the diagram where you have had pain today by placing an 'X', circling the location, or shading the area .

Describe the type of pain:

Shooting	Deep
Tingling	Sharp
Numbness	Burning / Hot
Cold	Aching
Surface Pain	Gnawing / Biting
Stabbing	Electrical / Shocks
Dull	Other_____
Stinging	

COMMENTS AND MORE INFORMATION:

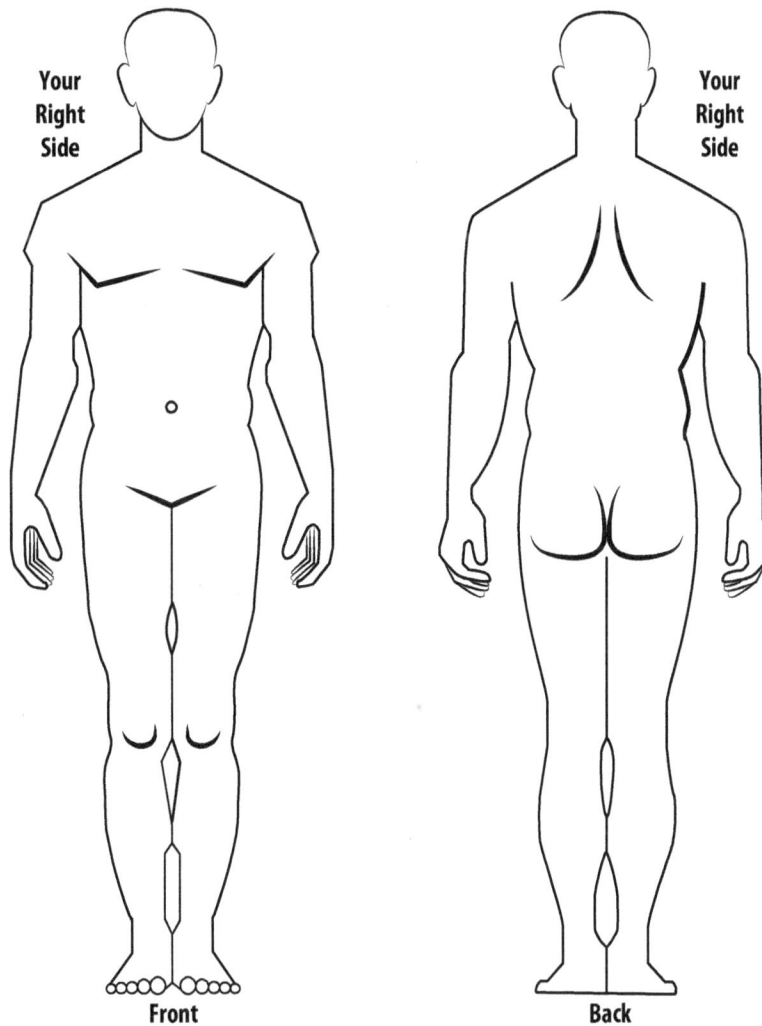

Your Right Side

Your Right Side

Front

Back

6 DAILY PAIN SUMMARY

Were there times during the day that you experienced unrelieved breakthrough pain? ____NO ____YES

How many times did this happen today?

1 2 3 4 5 6 7 8 9 10 more than 10

Did any specific activity start your breakthrough pain?
____NO ____YES: What activities?

_____

Put an "X" on the body diagram to show each place you've had **BREAKTHROUGH PAIN** today.

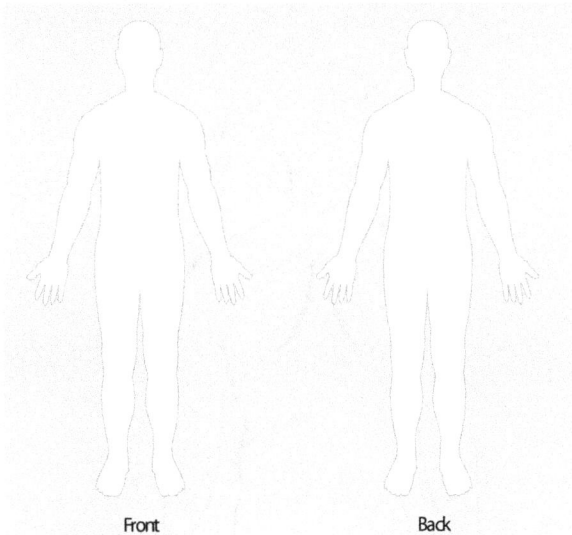

Front   Back

NON-DRUG THERAPIES
(other than prescription or other medicines)

_____

_____

ACTIVITIES/EXERCISE

_____

_____

What was your average level of pain today?

0 1 2 3 4 5 6 7 8 9 10

Other than prescription medicine, did you do anything else today to relieve the pain? ____NO ____YES:
(Note any that you used.)
____ Non-prescription drugs (e.g., acetaminophen, ibuprofen)
____ Herbal remedies
____ Hot or cold packs
____ Exercise
____ Changing position (such as lying down or elevating your legs)
____ Physical therapy
____ Massage
____ Acupuncture
____ Rest
____ Psychological counseling
____ Talk to trusted friend, family, clergy
____ Prayer, meditation, guided imagery
____ Relaxation technique (hypnosis, biofeedback)
____ Creative technique (art or music therapy)
____ Other (e.g., specific chiropractic manipulation, osteopathic treatments):

_____

Check any of these common side effects that you've noticed after taking your pain medicine:
____ Drowsiness, sleepiness
____ Nausea, vomiting, upset stomach
____ Constipation
____ Lack of appetite
____ Other (describe):

_____

Did you sleep through the night? ____NO____YES

If not, how many times was your sleep disrupted? _____

How many hours did you sleep during the night? _____

COMMENTS AND MORE INFORMATION: Make notes for and about visits with your healthcare provider, side effects from treatments you may be experiencing, any problems you are having coping with your pain, and more about some of your previous answers or questions.

_____

_____

_____

1 DAILY DIARY

SATISFACTION CHART   Connect the points on your Daily Satisfaction Chart so your medical team can see when and why your mental state changed.

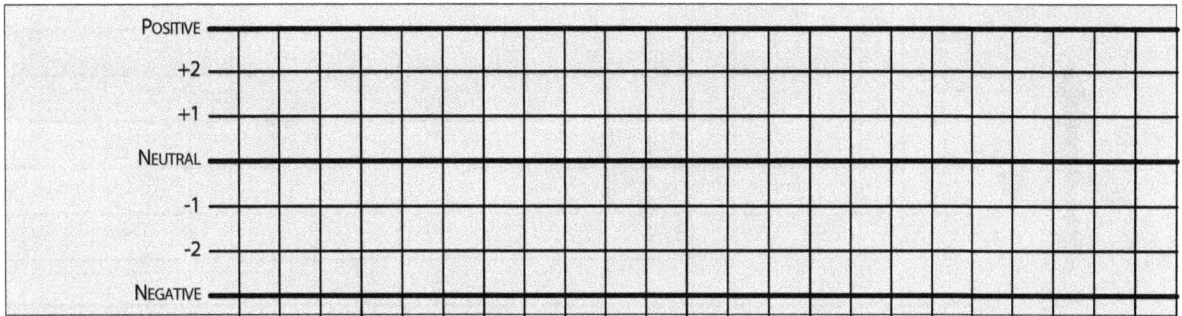

DAY_____   DATE_____   WEIGHT_____

| | | |
POSITIVE
+2
+1
NEUTRAL
-1
-2
NEGATIVE

2 ACTIVITY LOG

TRIGGERS AND SIGNIFICANT EVENTS

6am 7 8 9 10 11 12pm 1 2 3 4 5 6pm 7 8 9 10 11 12am 1 2 3 4 5

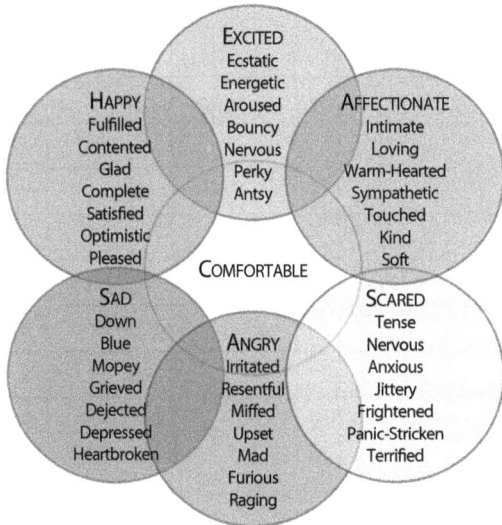

EXCITED
Ecstatic
Energetic
Aroused
Bouncy
Nervous
Perky
Antsy

HAPPY
Fulfilled
Contented
Glad
Complete
Satisfied
Optimistic
Pleased

AFFECTIONATE
Intimate
Loving
Warm-Hearted
Sympathetic
Touched
Kind
Soft

COMFORTABLE

SAD
Down
Blue
Mopey
Grieved
Dejected
Depressed
Heartbroken

ANGRY
Irritated
Resentful
Miffed
Upset
Mad
Furious
Raging

SCARED
Tense
Nervous
Anxious
Jittery
Frightened
Panic-Stricken
Terrified

Describe any changes in your pain today:

_____
_____
_____
_____

Did anything unusual happen today?

_____
_____
_____
_____

26

What did you spend the most time time thinking about today?

Positive Thoughts:

_____

Did your pain increase, decrease, or remain the same when you thought about it?
____ Increased
____ Decreased
____ Stayed the Same

Negative Thoughts:

_____

Did your pain increase, decrease, or remain the same when you thought about it?
____ Increased
____ Decreased
____ Stayed the Same

1 DAILY
MOOD CHART

DAY_____ DATE_____ WEIGHT_____

Connect the points on your Mood Satisfaction Chart so your medical team can see when and why your mental state changed.

MOOD	HAPPY	+3
		+2
		+1
		0
		-1
		-2
	SAD	-3

2 ACTIVITY LOG

6am 7 8 9 10 11 12pm 1 2 3 4 5 6pm 7 8 9 10 11 12am 1 2 3 4 5

3 MEDICATION LOG
NAME/DOSE

1
2
3
4
5
6
7
8

4 PHYSIOLOGY

6am 7 8 9 10 11 12pm 1 2 3 4 5 6pm 7 8 9 10 11 12am 1 2 3 4 5

SLEEP
URINATION
DEFECATION
NAUSEA
EATING
EXERCISE
OTHER (LIST)

26

1 DAILY RESULTS
OF MEDICATIONS AND TREATMENTS

As you and your medical team develop new treatment plans, it will be especially helpful to record any side effects you experience as you add new treatments. This can help determine which types of treatments will work best for you.

Contact your care provider with any bad reactions or side effects to determine if you should discontinue the medication or treatment.

MEDICATION / TREATMENT	AMOUNT / TIME / COMMENTS

26

1 DAILY
TREATMENT PLAN

As you and your medical team develop new treatment plans, record your plan for the day including new medications, increases or decreases to medications, exercises, physical therapy, or any other treatment efforts.

MEDICATION / TREATMENT	AMOUNT / TIME / COMMENTS

27

1 DAILY
PAIN CHART

DAY_____ DATE_____ WEIGHT_____

Connect the points on your Daily Pain and Satisfaction Charts so your medical team can see when your status changed.

PAIN LEVEL

WORST IMAGINABLE	10
	9
	8
	7
	6
MODERATE	5
	4
	3
	2
	1
NONE	0

2 SATISFACTION

Time axis: 6am 7 8 9 10 11 12pm 1 2 3 4 5 6pm 7 8 9 10 11 12am 1 2 3 4 5

MOOD

(HAPPY)	POSITIVE
	+2
	+1
	NEUTRAL
	-1
	-2
(UNHAPPY)	NEGATIVE

3 PHYSIOLOGY

Time axis: 6am 7 8 9 10 11 12pm 1 2 3 4 5 6pm 7 8 9 10 11 12am 1 2 3 4 5

SLEEP

RESTROOM

NAUSEA / DIZZINESS

MEAL / SNACK

EXERCISE

STRESS / ANXIETY

MEDICINE NAME / DOSE

1

2

3

BLOOD PRESSURE

PULSE

27

4 DAILY HEAD & FACE PAIN DIAGRAM

Mark each place on the diagram where you have had pain today by placing an 'X', circling the location, or shading the area .

Describe the type of pain:

Shooting	Deep
Tingling	Sharp
Numbness	Burning / Hot
Cold	Aching
Surface Pain	Gnawing / Biting
Stabbing	Electrical / Shocks
Dull	Other_____
Stinging	

COMMENTS AND MORE INFORMATION:

Front

Upper Right   **Upper Left**

Lower Right   **Lower Left**

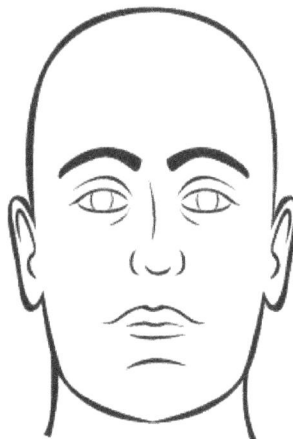

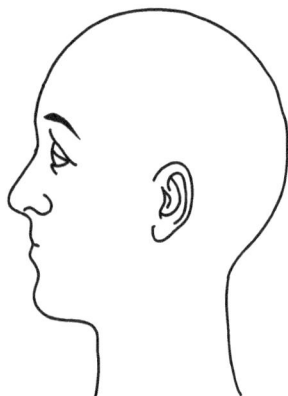

Your Right Side

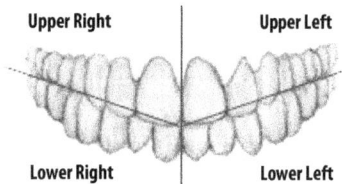

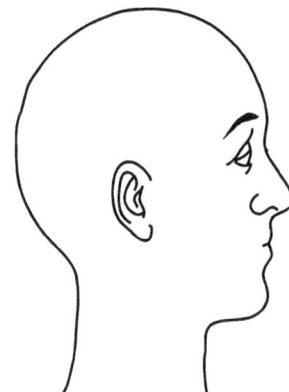

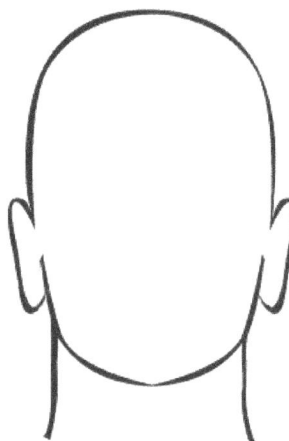

Your Right Side

Back

5 DAILY BODY PAIN DIAGRAM

Mark each place on the diagram where you have had pain today by placing an 'X', circling the location, or shading the area.

Describe the type of pain:

Shooting	Deep
Tingling	Sharp
Numbness	Burning / Hot
Cold	Aching
Surface Pain	Gnawing / Biting
Stabbing	Electrical / Shocks
Dull	Other_____
Stinging	

COMMENTS AND MORE INFORMATION:

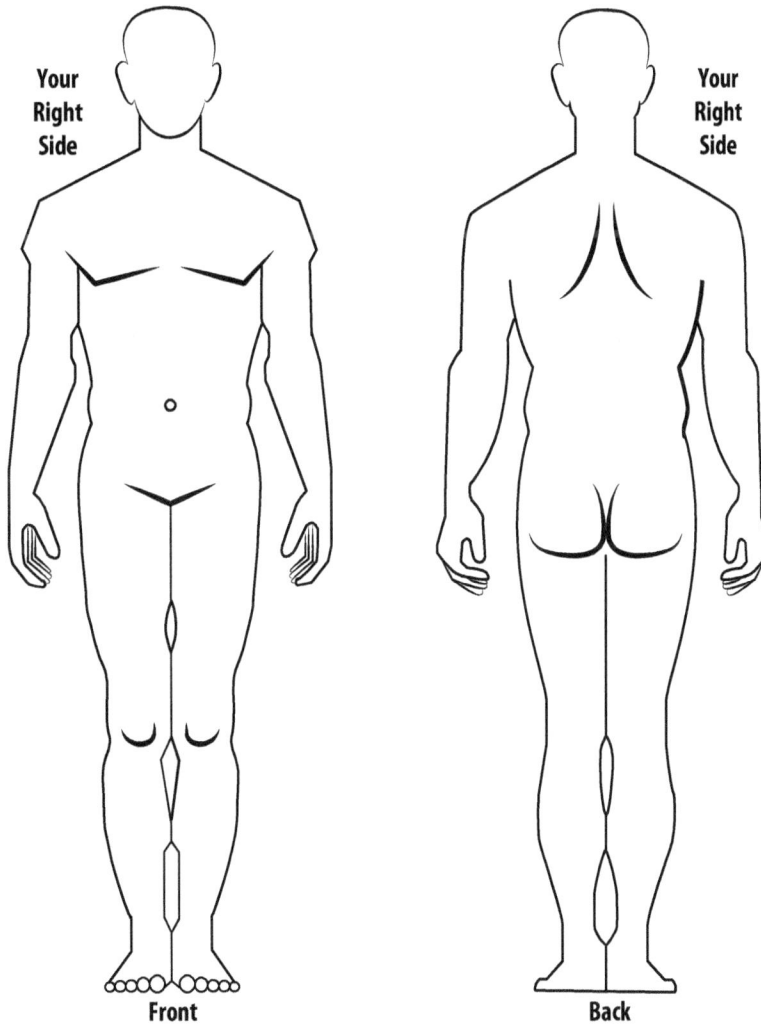

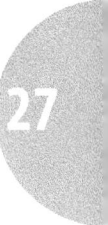

Your Right Side

Your Right Side

Front

Back

27

6 DAILY PAIN SUMMARY

Were there times during the day that you experienced unrelieved breakthrough pain? ____NO ____YES

How many times did this happen today?

1 2 3 4 5 6 7 8 9 10 more than 10

Did any specific activity start your breakthrough pain?
____NO ____YES: What activities?

_____

Put an "X" on the body diagram to show each place you've had **BREAKTHROUGH PAIN** today.

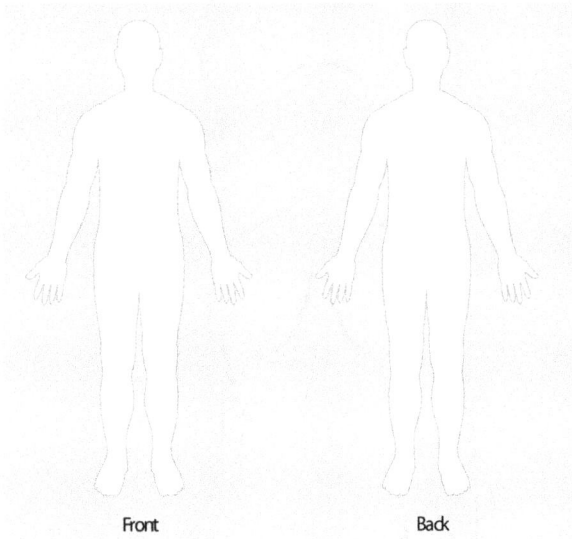

Front   Back

NON-DRUG THERAPIES
(other than prescription or other medicines)

_____

_____

ACTIVITIES/EXERCISE

_____

What was your average level of pain today?

0 1 2 3 4 5 6 7 8 9 10

Other than prescription medicine, did you do anything else today to relieve the pain? ____NO ____YES: (Note any that you used.)
____ Non-prescription drugs (e.g., acetaminophen, ibuprofen)
____ Herbal remedies
____ Hot or cold packs
____ Exercise
____ Changing position (such as lying down or elevating your legs)
____ Physical therapy
____ Massage
____ Acupuncture
____ Rest
____ Psychological counseling
____ Talk to trusted friend, family, clergy
____ Prayer, meditation, guided imagery
____ Relaxation technique (hypnosis, biofeedback)
____ Creative technique (art or music therapy)
____ Other (e.g., specific chiropractic manipulation, osteopathic treatments):

_____

Check any of these common side effects that you've noticed after taking your pain medicine:
____ Drowsiness, sleepiness
____ Nausea, vomiting, upset stomach
____ Constipation
____ Lack of appetite
____ Other (describe):

_____

Did you sleep through the night? ____NO____YES

If not, how many times was your sleep disrupted? _____

How many hours did you sleep during the night? _____

COMMENTS AND MORE INFORMATION: Make notes for and about visits with your healthcare provider, side effects from treatments you may be experiencing, any problems you are having coping with your pain, and more about some of your previous answers or questions.

1 DAILY DIARY

SATISFACTION CHART

DAY_____ DATE_____ WEIGHT_____

Connect the points on your Daily Satisfaction Chart so your medical team can see when and why your mental state changed.

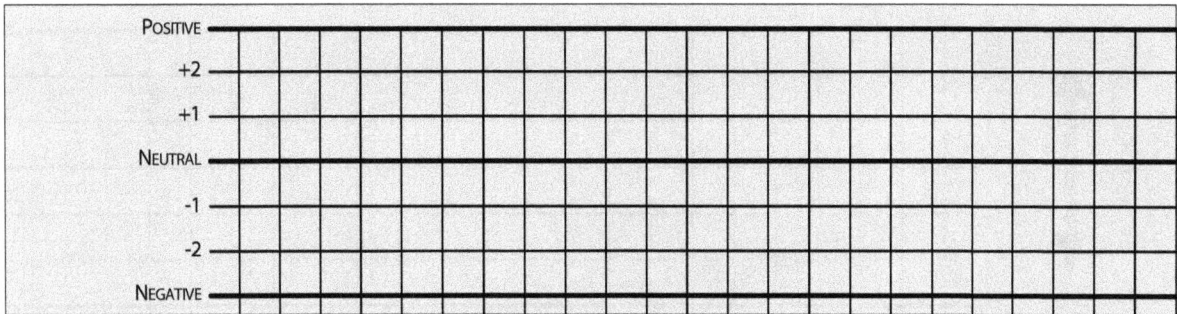

POSITIVE

+2

+1

NEUTRAL

-1

-2

NEGATIVE

2 ACTIVITY LOG

6am 7 8 9 10 11 12pm 1 2 3 4 5 6pm 7 8 9 10 11 12am 1 2 3 4 5

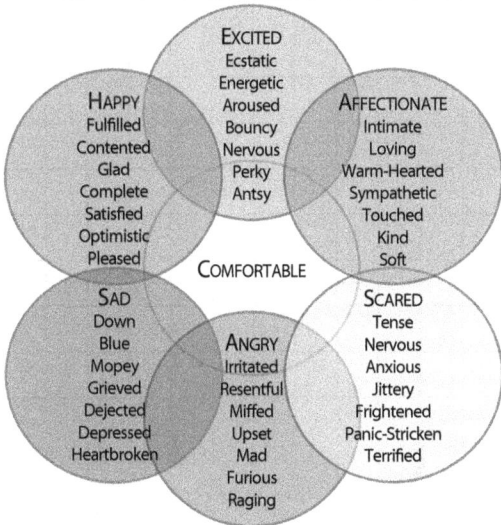

TRIGGERS AND SIGNIFICANT EVENTS

EXCITED
Ecstatic
Energetic
Aroused
Bouncy
Nervous
Perky
Antsy

HAPPY
Fulfilled
Contented
Glad
Complete
Satisfied
Optimistic
Pleased

AFFECTIONATE
Intimate
Loving
Warm-Hearted
Sympathetic
Touched
Kind
Soft

COMFORTABLE

SAD
Down
Blue
Mopey
Grieved
Dejected
Depressed
Heartbroken

ANGRY
Irritated
Resentful
Miffed
Upset
Mad
Furious
Raging

SCARED
Tense
Nervous
Anxious
Jittery
Frightened
Panic-Stricken
Terrified

Describe any changes in your pain today:

_____
_____
_____
_____

Did anything unusual happen today?

_____
_____
_____
_____

27

What did you spend the most time time thinking about today?

Positive Thoughts:

_____

Did your pain increase, decrease, or remain the same when you thought about it?
____ Increased
____ Decreased
____ Stayed the Same

Negative Thoughts:

_____

Did your pain increase, decrease, or remain the same when you thought about it?
____ Increased
____ Decreased
____ Stayed the Same

1 DAILY
MOOD CHART

DAY_____ DATE_____ WEIGHT_____

Connect the points on your Mood Satisfaction Chart so your medical team can see when and why your mental state changed.

MOOD

HAPPY	+3
	+2
	+1
	0
	-1
	-2
SAD	-3

2 ACTIVITY LOG

6am 7 8 9 10 11 12pm 1 2 3 4 5 6pm 7 8 9 10 11 12am 1 2 3 4 5

3 MEDICATION LOG
NAME/DOSE

1—
2—
3—
4—
5—
6—
7—
8—

4 PHYSIOLOGY

6am 7 8 9 10 11 12pm 1 2 3 4 5 6pm 7 8 9 10 11 12am 1 2 3 4 5

SLEEP
URINATION
DEFECATION
NAUSEA
EATING
EXERCISE
OTHER (LIST)

27

1 DAILY RESULTS
OF MEDICATIONS AND TREATMENTS

As you and your medical team develop new treatment plans, it will be especially helpful to record any side effects you experience as you add new treatments. This can help determine which types of treatments will work best for you.

Contact your care provider with any bad reactions or side effects to determine if you should discontinue the medication or treatment.

MEDICATION / TREATMENT	AMOUNT / TIME / COMMENTS

27

1 DAILY
TREATMENT PLAN

As you and your medical team develop new treatment plans, record your plan for the day including new medications, increases or decreases to medications, exercises, physical therapy, or any other treatment efforts.

MEDICATION / TREATMENT	AMOUNT / TIME / COMMENTS

1 DAILY
PAIN CHART

DAY_____ DATE_____ WEIGHT_____

Connect the points on your Daily Pain and Satisfaction Charts so your medical team can see when your status changed.

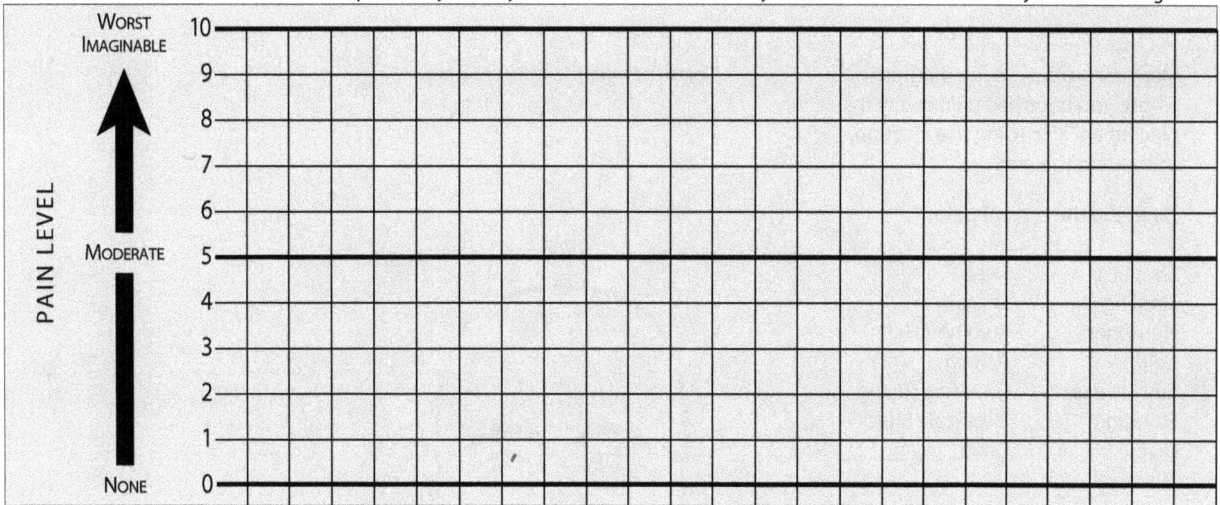

PAIN LEVEL

WORST IMAGINABLE — 10
9
8
7
6
MODERATE — 5
4
3
2
1
NONE — 0

2 SATISFACTION

MOOD

(HAPPY) POSITIVE
+2
+1
NEUTRAL
-1
-2
(UNHAPPY) NEGATIVE

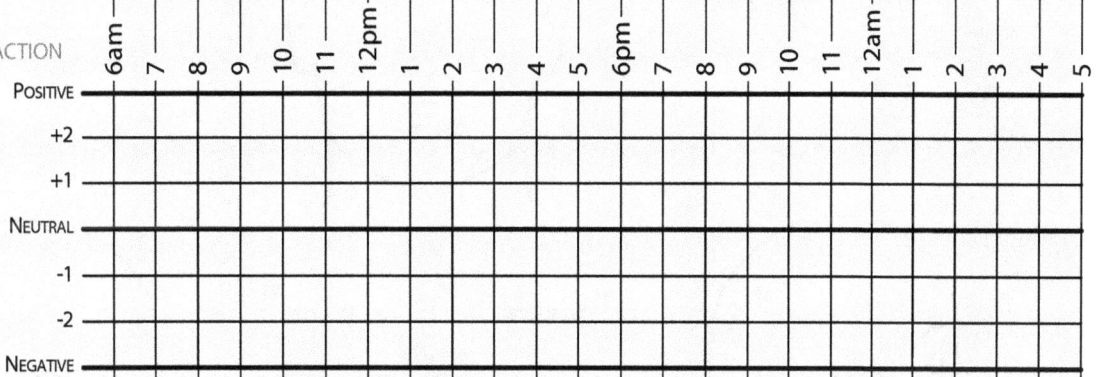

6am 7 8 9 10 11 12pm 1 2 3 4 5 6pm 7 8 9 10 11 12am 1 2 3 4 5

3 PHYSIOLOGY

6am 7 8 9 10 11 12pm 1 2 3 4 5 6pm 7 8 9 10 11 12am 1 2 3 4 5

SLEEP
RESTROOM
NAUSEA / DIZZINESS
MEAL / SNACK
EXERCISE
STRESS / ANXIETY
MEDICINE NAME / DOSE
1
2
3

BLOOD PRESSURE
PULSE

28

4 DAILY HEAD & FACE PAIN DIAGRAM

Mark each place on the diagram where you have had pain today by placing an 'X', circling the location, or shading the area .

Describe the type of pain:

Shooting	Deep
Tingling	Sharp
Numbness	Burning / Hot
Cold	Aching
Surface Pain	Gnawing / Biting
Stabbing	Electrical / Shocks
Dull	Other_____
Stinging	

COMMENTS AND MORE INFORMATION:

Front

Upper Right Upper Left

Lower Right Lower Left

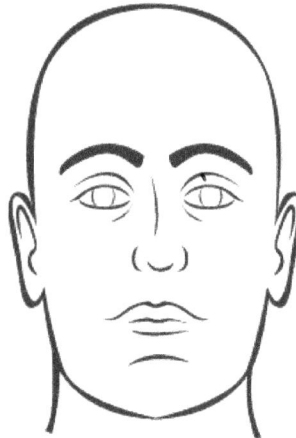

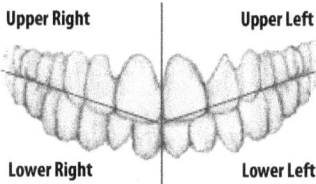

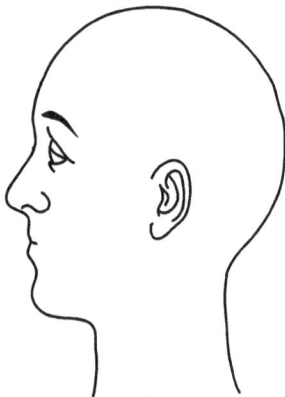

Your Right Side

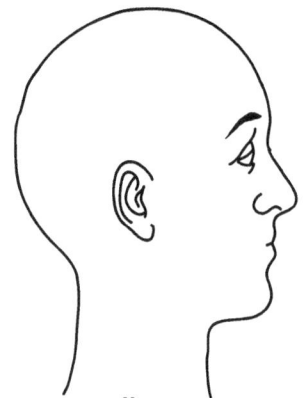

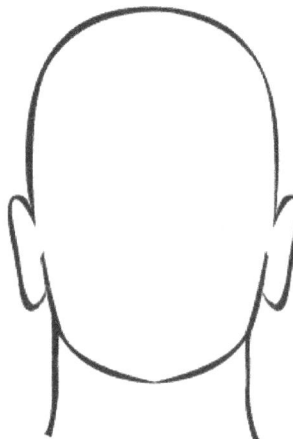

Your Right Side

Back

5 DAILY BODY PAIN DIAGRAM

Mark each place on the diagram where you have had pain today by placing an 'X', circling the location, or shading the area .

Describe the type of pain:

Shooting	Deep
Tingling	Sharp
Numbness	Burning / Hot
Cold	Aching
Surface Pain	Gnawing / Biting
Stabbing	Electrical / Shocks
Dull	Other_____
Stinging	

COMMENTS AND MORE INFORMATION:

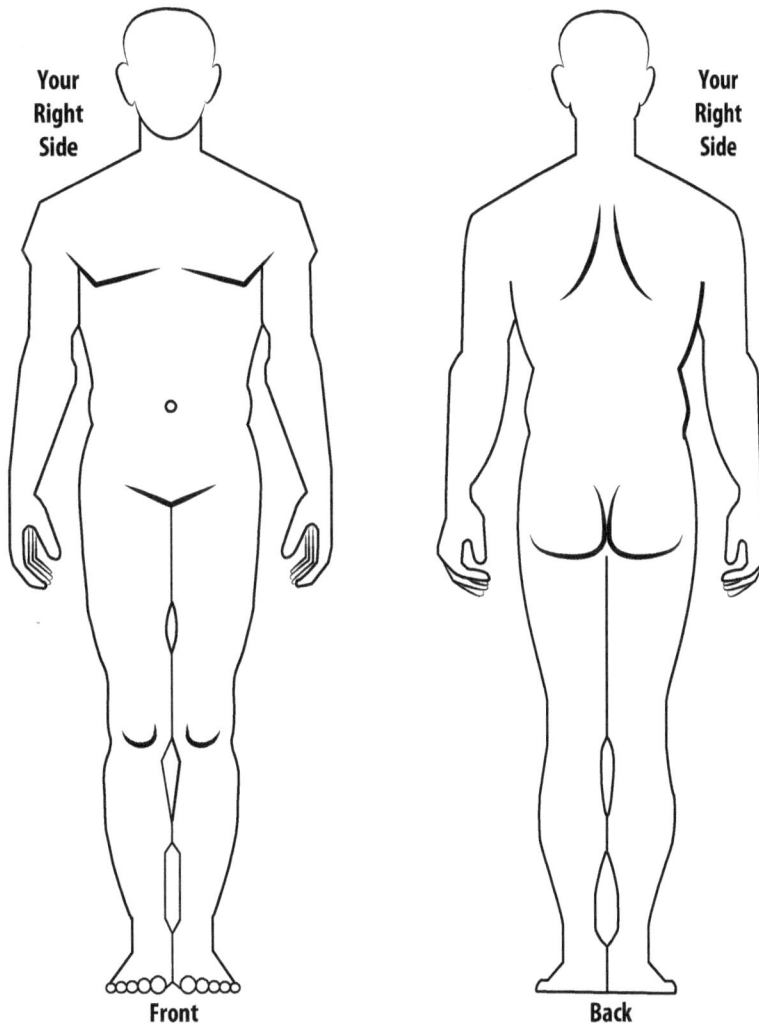

Your
Right
Side

Your
Right
Side

Front

Back

28

6 DAILY PAIN SUMMARY

Were there times during the day that you experienced unrelieved breakthrough pain? ____NO ____YES

How many times did this happen today?

1 2 3 4 5 6 7 8 9 10 more than 10

Did any specific activity start your breakthrough pain?
____NO ____YES: What activities?

_____

Put an "X" on the body diagram to show each place you've had *BREAKTHROUGH PAIN* today.

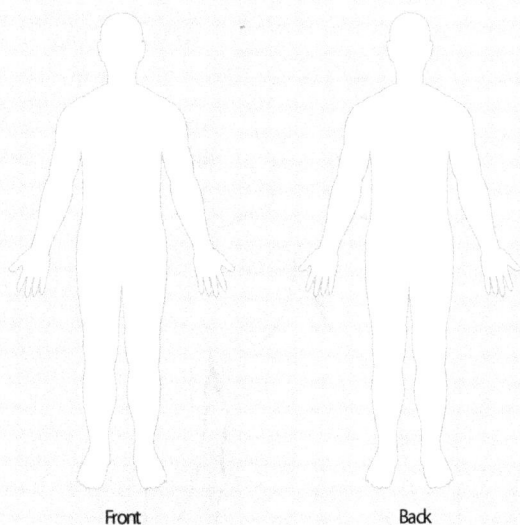

Front   Back

NON-DRUG THERAPIES
(other than prescription or other medicines)

_____

_____

ACTIVITIES/EXERCISE

_____

_____

What was your average level of pain today?

0   1   2   3   4   5   6   7   8   9   10

Other than prescription medicine, did you do anything else today to relieve the pain? ____NO ____YES:
(Note any that you used.)
____ Non-prescription drugs (e.g., acetaminophen, ibuprofen)
____ Herbal remedies
____ Hot or cold packs
____ Exercise
____ Changing position (such as lying down or elevating your legs)
____ Physical therapy
____ Massage
____ Acupuncture
____ Rest
____ Psychological counseling
____ Talk to trusted friend, family, clergy
____ Prayer, meditation, guided imagery
____ Relaxation technique (hypnosis, biofeedback)
____ Creative technique (art or music therapy)
____ Other (e.g., specific chiropractic manipulation, osteopathic treatments):

_____

Check any of these common side effects that you've noticed after taking your pain medicine:
____ Drowsiness, sleepiness
____ Nausea, vomiting, upset stomach
____ Constipation
____ Lack of appetite
____ Other (describe):

_____

Did you sleep through the night? ____NO____YES

If not, how many times was your sleep disrupted? _____

How many hours did you sleep during the night? _____

COMMENTS AND MORE INFORMATION: Make notes for and about visits with your healthcare provider, side effects from treatments you may be experiencing, any problems you are having coping with your pain, and more about some of your previous answers or questions.

_____

_____

_____

28

1 DAILY DIARY

SATISFACTION CHART

DAY_____ DATE_____ WEIGHT_____

Connect the points on your Daily Satisfaction Chart so your medical team can see when and why your mental state changed.

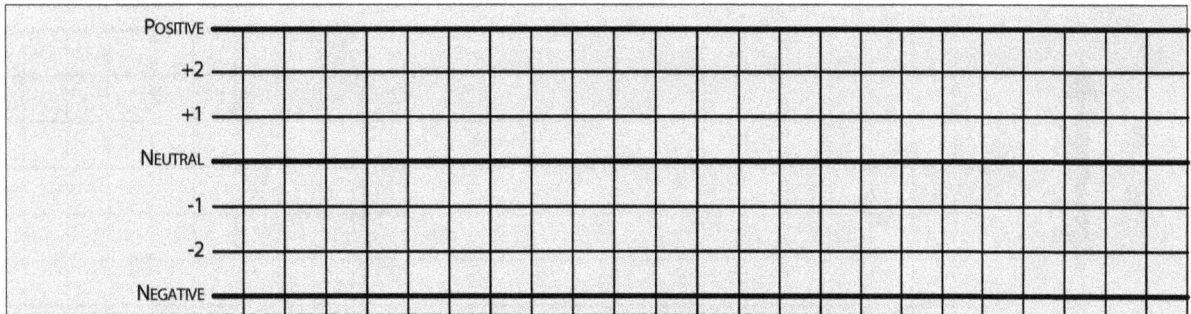

	POSITIVE
	+2
	+1
	NEUTRAL
	-1
	-2
	NEGATIVE

2 ACTIVITY LOG

6am 7 8 9 10 11 12pm 1 2 3 4 5 6pm 7 8 9 10 11 12am 1 2 3 4 5

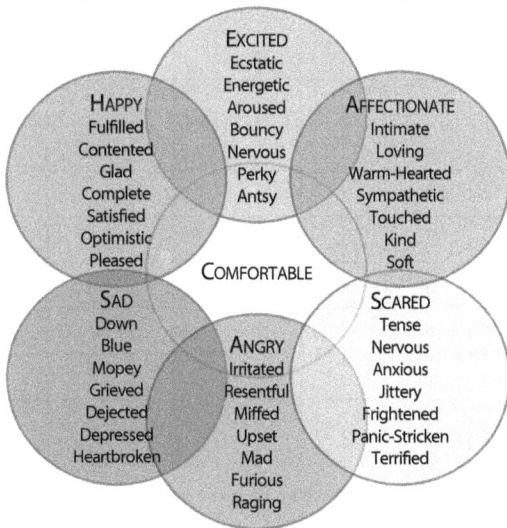

TRIGGERS AND SIGNIFICANT EVENTS

EXCITED
Ecstatic
Energetic
Aroused
Bouncy
Nervous
Perky
Antsy

HAPPY
Fulfilled
Contented
Glad
Complete
Satisfied
Optimistic
Pleased

AFFECTIONATE
Intimate
Loving
Warm-Hearted
Sympathetic
Touched
Kind
Soft

COMFORTABLE

SAD
Down
Blue
Mopey
Grieved
Dejected
Depressed
Heartbroken

ANGRY
Irritated
Resentful
Miffed
Upset
Mad
Furious
Raging

SCARED
Tense
Nervous
Anxious
Jittery
Frightened
Panic-Stricken
Terrified

Describe any changes in your pain today:

_____
_____
_____
_____
_____

Did anything unusual happen today?

_____
_____
_____
_____
_____

What did you spend the most time time thinking about today?

Positive Thoughts:

_____

Did your pain increase, decrease, or remain the same when you thought about it?
_____ Increased
_____ Decreased
_____ Stayed the Same

Negative Thoughts:

_____

Did your pain increase, decrease, or remain the same when you thought about it?
_____ Increased
_____ Decreased
_____ Stayed the Same

28

1 DAILY
MOOD CHART

DAY_____ DATE_____ WEIGHT_____

Connect the points on your Mood Satisfaction Chart so your medical team can see when and why your mental state changed.

HAPPY +3
+2
+1
MOOD 0
-1
-2
SAD -3

2 ACTIVITY LOG

6am 7 8 9 10 11 12pm 1 2 3 4 5 6pm 7 8 9 10 11 12am 1 2 3 4 5

3 MEDICATION LOG
NAME/DOSE

1
2
3
4
5
6
7
8

4 PHYSIOLOGY

6am 7 8 9 10 11 12pm 1 2 3 4 5 6pm 7 8 9 10 11 12am 1 2 3 4 5

SLEEP
URINATION
DEFECATION
NAUSEA
EATING
EXERCISE
OTHER (LIST)

1 DAILY RESULTS
OF MEDICATIONS AND TREATMENTS

As you and your medical team develop new treatment plans, it will be especially helpful to record any side effects you experience as you add new treatments. This can help determine which types of treatments will work best for you.

Contact your care provider with any bad reactions or side effects to determine if you should discontinue the medication or treatment.

MEDICATION / TREATMENT	AMOUNT / TIME / COMMENTS

29

1 DAILY
TREATMENT PLAN

As you and your medical team develop new treatment plans, record your plan for the day including new medications, increases or decreases to medications, exercises, physical therapy, or any other treatment efforts.

MEDICATION / TREATMENT	AMOUNT / TIME / COMMENTS

29

1 DAILY
PAIN CHART

DAY_____ DATE_____ WEIGHT_____

Connect the points on your Daily Pain and Satisfaction Charts so your medical team can see when your status changed.

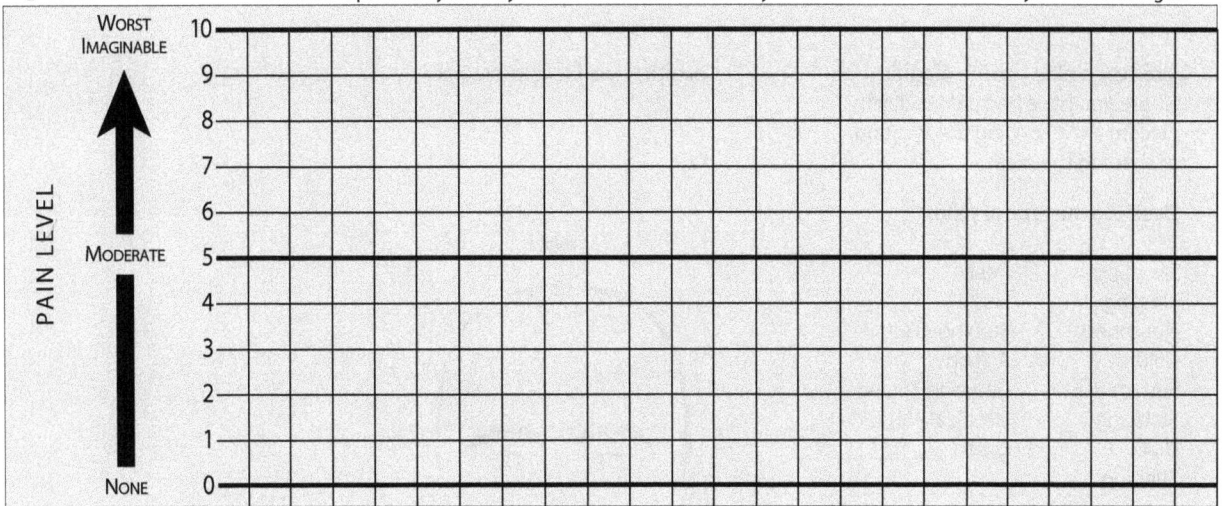

PAIN LEVEL

WORST IMAGINABLE — 10
9
8
7
6
MODERATE — 5
4
3
2
1
NONE — 0

6am 7 8 9 10 11 12pm 1 2 3 4 5 6pm 7 8 9 10 11 12am 1 2 3 4 5

2 SATISFACTION

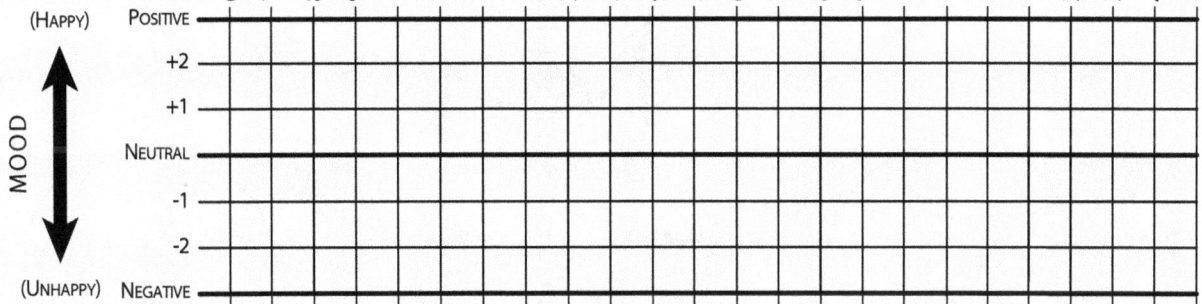

MOOD

(HAPPY) POSITIVE
+2
+1
NEUTRAL
-1
-2
(UNHAPPY) NEGATIVE

6am 7 8 9 10 11 12pm 1 2 3 4 5 6pm 7 8 9 10 11 12am 1 2 3 4 5

3 PHYSIOLOGY

6am 7 8 9 10 11 12pm 1 2 3 4 5 6pm 7 8 9 10 11 12am 1 2 3 4 5

SLEEP

RESTROOM

NAUSEA / DIZZINESS

MEAL / SNACK

EXERCISE

STRESS / ANXIETY

MEDICINE NAME / DOSE

1

2

3

BLOOD PRESSURE

PULSE

4 DAILY HEAD & FACE PAIN DIAGRAM

Mark each place on the diagram where you have had pain today by placing an 'X', circling the location, or shading the area .

Describe the type of pain:

Shooting	Deep
Tingling	Sharp
Numbness	Burning / Hot
Cold	Aching
Surface Pain	Gnawing / Biting
Stabbing	Electrical / Shocks
Dull	Other_____
Stinging	

COMMENTS AND MORE INFORMATION:

Front

Upper Right   **Upper Left**

Lower Right   **Lower Left**

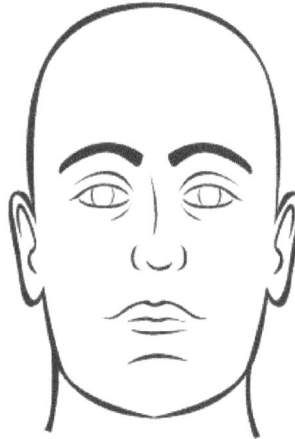

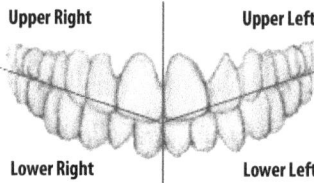

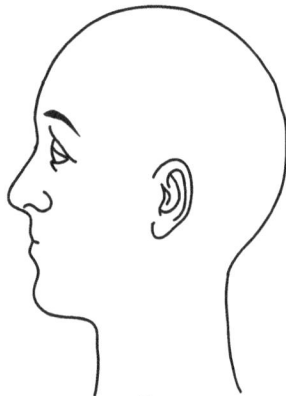

Your Right Side

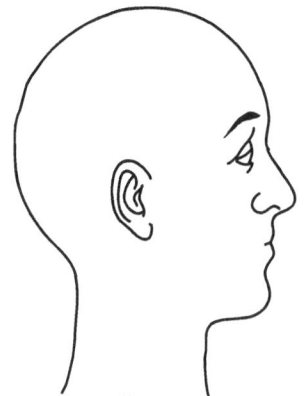

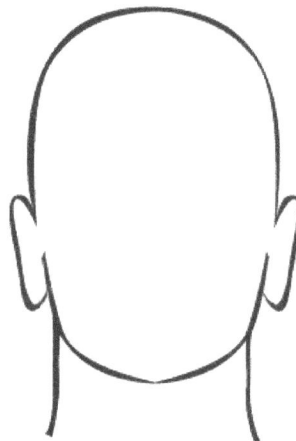

Your Right Side

Back

5 DAILY BODY PAIN DIAGRAM

Mark each place on the diagram where you have had pain today by placing an 'X', circling the location, or shading the area .

Describe the type of pain:

Shooting	Deep
Tingling	Sharp
Numbness	Burning / Hot
Cold	Aching
Surface Pain	Gnawing / Biting
Stabbing	Electrical / Shocks
Dull	Other_____
Stinging	

COMMENTS AND MORE INFORMATION:

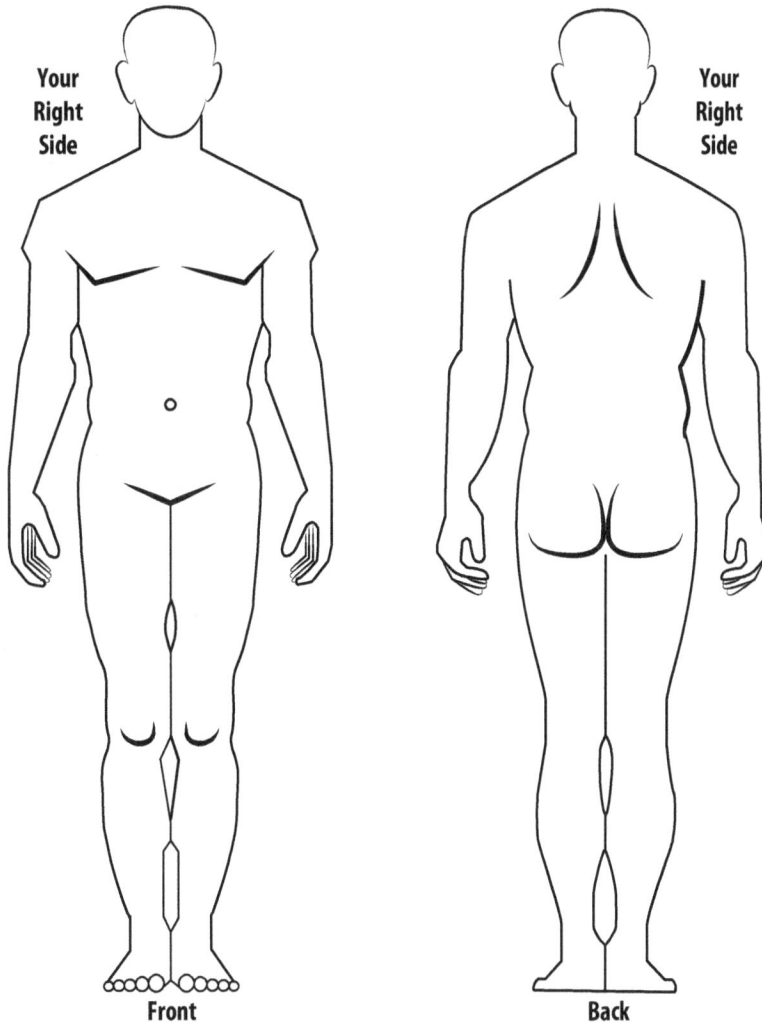

Your Right Side

Front

Your Right Side

Back

6 DAILY PAIN SUMMARY

Were there times during the day that you experienced unrelieved breakthrough pain? ____NO ____YES

How many times did this happen today?

1 2 3 4 5 6 7 8 9 10 more than 10

Did any specific activity start your breakthrough pain?
____NO ____YES: What activities?

_____

Put an "X" on the body diagram to show each place you've had **BREAKTHROUGH PAIN** today.

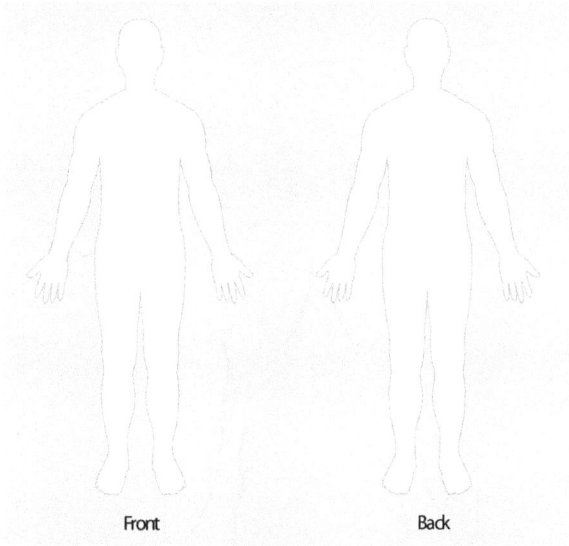

Front   Back

NON-DRUG THERAPIES
(other than prescription or other medicines)

_____

_____

ACTIVITIES/EXERCISE

_____

_____

What was your average level of pain today?

0 1 2 3 4 5 6 7 8 9 10

Other than prescription medicine, did you do anything else today to relieve the pain? ____NO ____YES:
(Note any that you used.)
____ Non-prescription drugs (e.g., acetaminophen, ibuprofen)
____ Herbal remedies
____ Hot or cold packs
____ Exercise
____ Changing position (such as lying down or elevating your legs)
____ Physical therapy
____ Massage
____ Acupuncture
____ Rest
____ Psychological counseling
____ Talk to trusted friend, family, clergy
____ Prayer, meditation, guided imagery
____ Relaxation technique (hypnosis, biofeedback)
____ Creative technique (art or music therapy)
____ Other (e.g., specific chiropractic manipulation, osteopathic treatments):

_____

Check any of these common side effects that you've noticed after taking your pain medicine:
____ Drowsiness, sleepiness
____ Nausea, vomiting, upset stomach
____ Constipation
____ Lack of appetite
____ Other (describe):

_____

Did you sleep through the night? ____NO____YES

If not, how many times was your sleep disrupted? _____

How many hours did you sleep during the night? _____

COMMENTS AND MORE INFORMATION: Make notes for and about visits with your healthcare provider, side effects from treatments you may be experiencing, any problems you are having coping with your pain, and more about some of your previous answers or questions.

1 DAILY DIARY

DAY_____ DATE_____ WEIGHT_____

SATISFACTION CHART Connect the points on your Daily Satisfaction Chart so your medical team can see when and why your mental state changed.

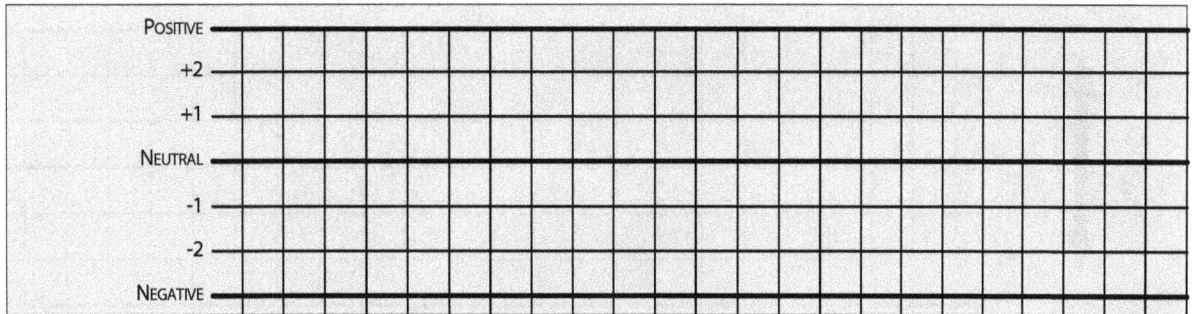

POSITIVE
+2
+1
NEUTRAL
-1
-2
NEGATIVE

2 ACTIVITY LOG

6am 7 8 9 10 11 12pm 1 2 3 4 5 6pm 7 8 9 10 11 12am 1 2 3 4 5

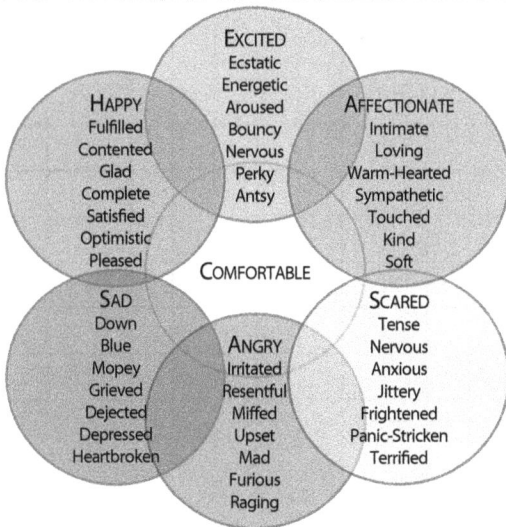

TRIGGERS AND SIGNIFICANT EVENTS

EXCITED Ecstatic Energetic Aroused Bouncy Nervous Perky Antsy

HAPPY Fulfilled Contented Glad Complete Satisfied Optimistic Pleased

AFFECTIONATE Intimate Loving Warm-Hearted Sympathetic Touched Kind Soft

COMFORTABLE

SAD Down Blue Mopey Grieved Dejected Depressed Heartbroken

ANGRY Irritated Resentful Miffed Upset Mad Furious Raging

SCARED Tense Nervous Anxious Jittery Frightened Panic-Stricken Terrified

Describe any changes in your pain today:

_____
_____
_____
_____
_____

Did anything unusual happen today?

_____
_____
_____
_____

What did you spend the most time time thinking about today?

Positive Thoughts:

_____

Did your pain increase, decrease, or remain the same when you thought about it?
____ Increased
____ Decreased
____ Stayed the Same

Negative Thoughts:

_____

Did your pain increase, decrease, or remain the same when you thought about it?
____ Increased
____ Decreased
____ Stayed the Same

29

1 DAILY
MOOD CHART

DAY_____ DATE_____ WEIGHT_____

Connect the points on your Mood Satisfaction Chart so your medical team can see when and why your mental state changed.

MOOD		
HAPPY	+3	
	+2	
	+1	
	0	
	-1	
	-2	
SAD	-3	

2 ACTIVITY LOG

6am 7 8 9 10 11 12pm 1 2 3 4 5 6pm 7 8 9 10 11 12am 1 2 3 4 5

3 MEDICATION LOG
NAME/DOSE

1————
2————
3————
4————
5————
6————
7————
8————

4 PHYSIOLOGY

6am 7 8 9 10 11 12pm 1 2 3 4 5 6pm 7 8 9 10 11 12am 1 2 3 4 5

SLEEP ————
URINATION ————
DEFECATION ————
NAUSEA ————
EATING ————
EXERCISE ————
OTHER (LIST) ————

1 DAILY RESULTS
OF MEDICATIONS AND TREATMENTS

As you and your medical team develop new treatment plans, it will be especially helpful to record any side effects you experience as you add new treatments. This can help determine which types of treatments will work best for you.

Contact your care provider with any bad reactions or side effects to determine if you should discontinue the medication or treatment.

MEDICATION / TREATMENT	AMOUNT / TIME / COMMENTS

1 DAILY
TREATMENT PLAN

As you and your medical team develop new treatment plans, record your plan for the day including new medications, increases or decreases to medications, exercises, physical therapy, or any other treatment efforts.

30

MEDICATION / TREATMENT	AMOUNT / TIME / COMMENTS

1 DAILY
PAIN CHART

DAY_____ DATE_____ WEIGHT_____

Connect the points on your Daily Pain and Satisfaction Charts so your medical team can see when your status changed.

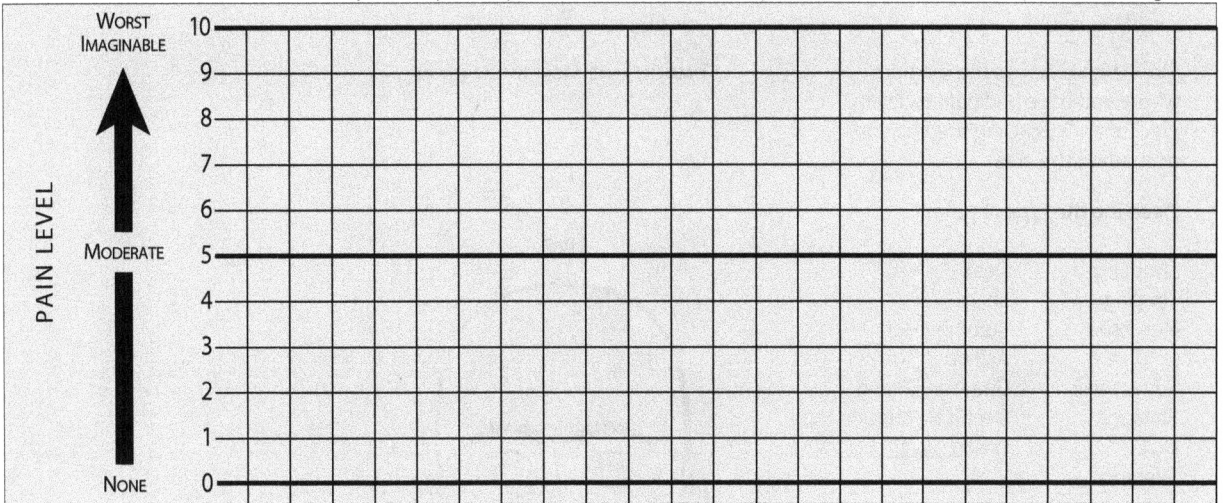

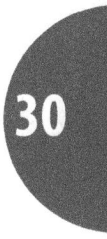

30

2 SATISFACTION

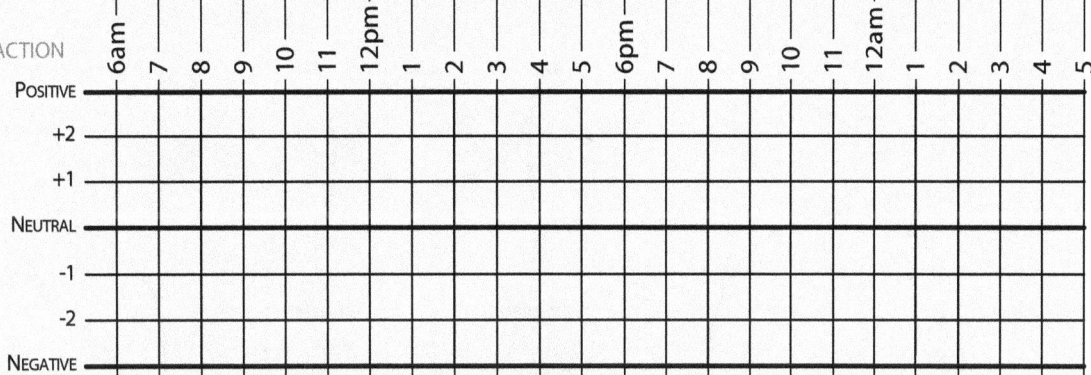

3 PHYSIOLOGY

SLEEP

RESTROOM

NAUSEA / DIZZINESS

MEAL / SNACK

EXERCISE

STRESS / ANXIETY

MEDICINE NAME / DOSE

1

2

3

BLOOD PRESSURE

PULSE

4 DAILY HEAD & FACE PAIN DIAGRAM

Mark each place on the diagram where you have had pain today by placing an 'X', circling the location, or shading the area .

30

Describe the type of pain:

Shooting	Deep
Tingling	Sharp
Numbness	Burning / Hot
Cold	Aching
Surface Pain	Gnawing / Biting
Stabbing	Electrical / Shocks
Dull	Other_____
Stinging	

COMMENTS AND MORE INFORMATION:

Front

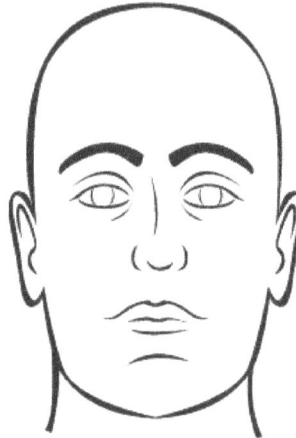

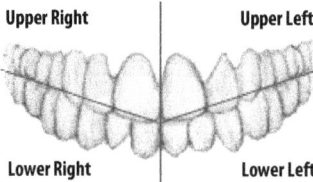

Upper Right   Upper Left

Lower Right   Lower Left

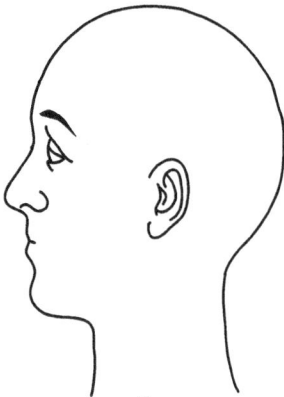

Your Right Side

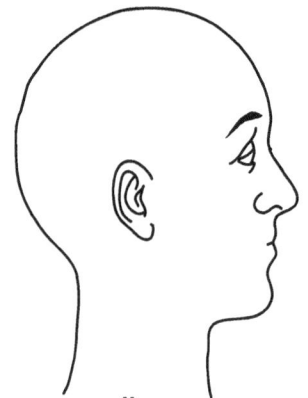

Your Right Side

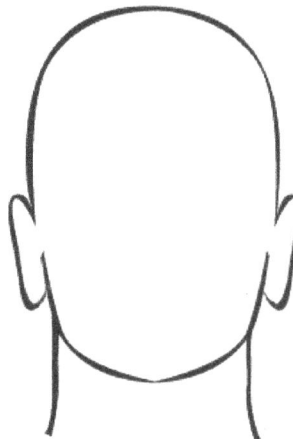

Back

5 DAILY BODY PAIN DIAGRAM

Mark each place on the diagram where you have had pain today by placing an 'X', circling the location, or shading the area .

Describe the type of pain:

Shooting   Deep
Tingling   Sharp
Numbness   Burning / Hot
Cold   Aching
Surface Pain   Gnawing / Biting
Stabbing   Electrical / Shocks
Dull   Other_____
Stinging

COMMENTS AND MORE INFORMATION:

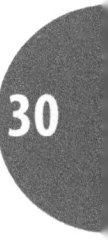

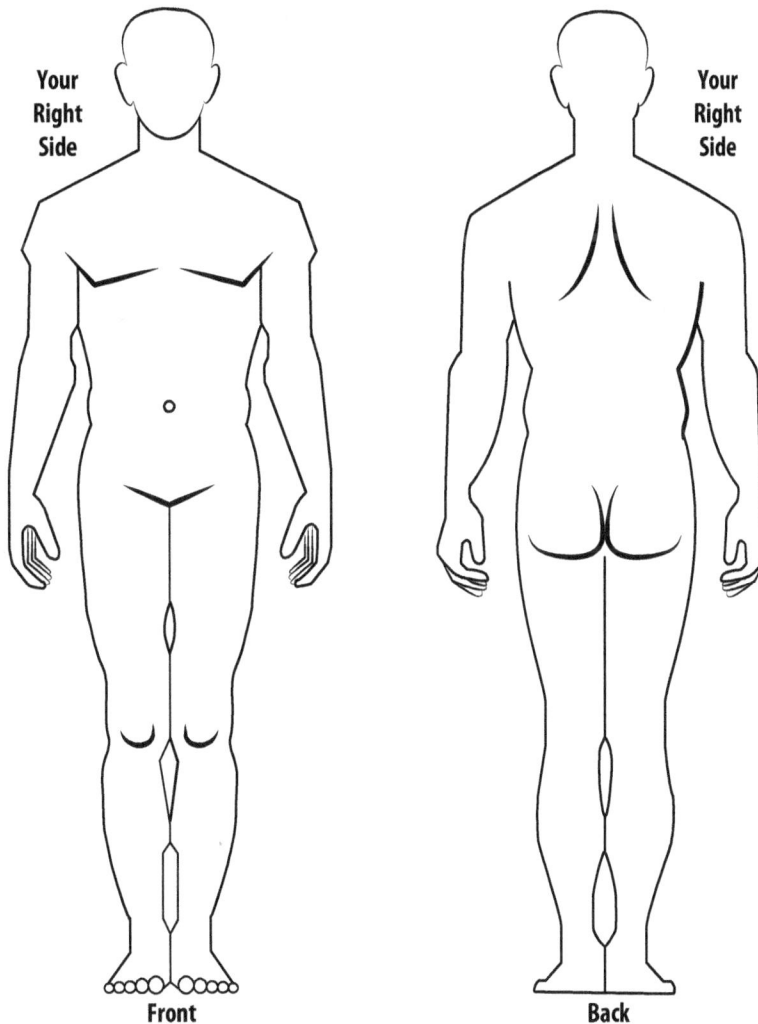

30

Your Right Side

Your Right Side

Front

Back

6 DAILY PAIN SUMMARY

Were there times during the day that you experienced unrelieved breakthrough pain? ____NO ____YES

How many times did this happen today?

   1 2 3 4 5 6 7 8 9 10   more than 10

Did any specific activity start your breakthrough pain?
____NO   ____YES: What activities?

_____

Put an "X" on the body diagram to show each place you've had **BREAKTHROUGH PAIN** today.

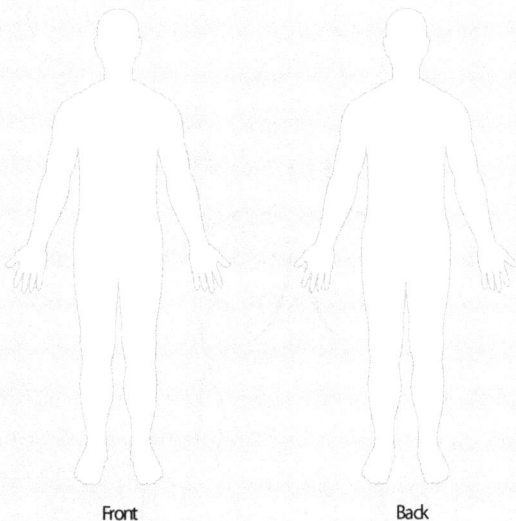

Front   Back

NON-DRUG THERAPIES
(other than prescription or other medicines)

_____

_____

ACTIVITIES/EXERCISE

_____

What was your average level of pain today?

   0   1   2   3   4   5   6   7   8   9   10

Other than prescription medicine, did you do anything else today to relieve the pain? ____NO ____YES:
(Note any that you used.)
____ Non-prescription drugs (e.g., acetaminophen, ibuprofen)
____ Herbal remedies
____ Hot or cold packs
____ Exercise
____ Changing position (such as lying down or elevating your legs)
____ Physical therapy
____ Massage
____ Acupuncture
____ Rest
____ Psychological counseling
____ Talk to trusted friend, family, clergy
____ Prayer, meditation, guided imagery
____ Relaxation technique (hypnosis, biofeedback)
____ Creative technique (art or music therapy)
____ Other (e.g., specific chiropractic manipulation, osteopathic treatments):

_____

Check any of these common side effects that you've noticed after taking your pain medicine:
____ Drowsiness, sleepiness
____ Nausea, vomiting, upset stomach
____ Constipation
____ Lack of appetite
____ Other (describe):

_____

Did you sleep through the night? ____NO____YES

If not, how many times was your sleep disrupted? _____

How many hours did you sleep during the night? _____

COMMENTS AND MORE INFORMATION: Make notes for and about visits with your healthcare provider, side effects from treatments you may be experiencing, any problems you are having coping with your pain, and more about some of your previous answers or questions.

_____

_____

_____

1 DAILY DIARY

SATISFACTION CHART   Connect the points on your Daily Satisfaction Chart so your medical team can see when and why your mental state changed.

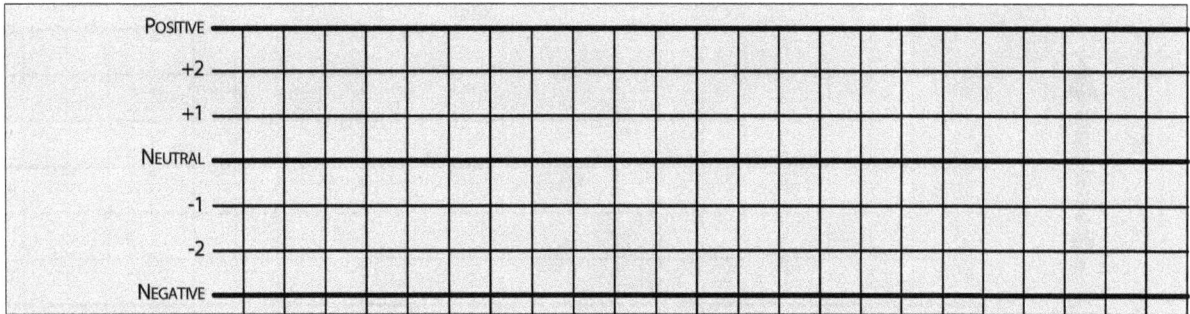

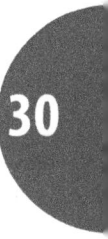

DAY_____   DATE_____   WEIGHT_____

30

	POSITIVE
	+2
	+1
	NEUTRAL
	-1
	-2
	NEGATIVE

2 ACTIVITY LOG

TRIGGERS AND SIGNIFICANT EVENTS

6am 7 8 9 10 11 12pm 1 2 3 4 5 6pm 7 8 9 10 11 12am 1 2 3 4 5

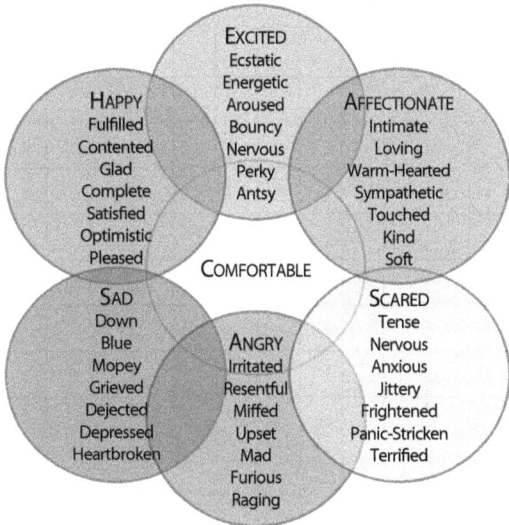

EXCITED
Ecstatic
Energetic
Aroused
Bouncy
Nervous
Perky
Antsy

HAPPY
Fulfilled
Contented
Glad
Complete
Satisfied
Optimistic
Pleased

AFFECTIONATE
Intimate
Loving
Warm-Hearted
Sympathetic
Touched
Kind
Soft

COMFORTABLE

SAD
Down
Blue
Mopey
Grieved
Dejected
Depressed
Heartbroken

ANGRY
Irritated
Resentful
Miffed
Upset
Mad
Furious
Raging

SCARED
Tense
Nervous
Anxious
Jittery
Frightened
Panic-Stricken
Terrified

Describe any changes in your pain today:

_____

_____

_____

_____

_____

Did anything unusual happen today?

_____

_____

_____

_____

_____

What did you spend the most time time thinking about today?

Positive Thoughts:

_____

Did your pain increase, decrease, or remain the same when you thought about it?
____ Increased
____ Decreased
____ Stayed the Same

Negative Thoughts:

_____

Did your pain increase, decrease, or remain the same when you thought about it?
____ Increased
____ Decreased
____ Stayed the Same

1 DAILY
MOOD CHART

DAY_____ DATE_____ WEIGHT_____

Connect the points on your Mood Satisfaction Chart so your medical team can see when and why your mental state changed.

MOOD

HAPPY	+3
	+2
	+1
	0
	-1
	-2
SAD	-3

30

2 ACTIVITY LOG

6am 7 8 9 10 11 12pm 1 2 3 4 5 6pm 7 8 9 10 11 12am 1 2 3 4 5

3 MEDICATION LOG
NAME/DOSE

1
2
3
4
5
6
7
8

4 PHYSIOLOGY

6am 7 8 9 10 11 12pm 1 2 3 4 5 6pm 7 8 9 10 11 12am 1 2 3 4 5

SLEEP
URINATION
DEFECATION
NAUSEA
EATING
EXERCISE
OTHER (LIST)

1 DAILY RESULTS
OF MEDICATIONS AND TREATMENTS

As you and your medical team develop new treatment plans, it will be especially helpful to record any side effects you experience as you add new treatments. This can help determine which types of treatments will work best for you.

Contact your care provider with any bad reactions or side effects to determine if you should discontinue the medication or treatment.

30

MEDICATION / TREATMENT	AMOUNT / TIME / COMMENTS

1 DAILY
TREATMENT PLAN

As you and your medical team develop new treatment plans, record your plan for the day including new medications, increases or decreases to medications, exercises, physical therapy, or any other treatment efforts.

MEDICATION / TREATMENT	AMOUNT / TIME / COMMENTS

31

1 DAILY
PAIN CHART

Day_____ Date_____ Weight_____

Connect the points on your Daily Pain and Satisfaction Charts so your medical team can see when your status changed.

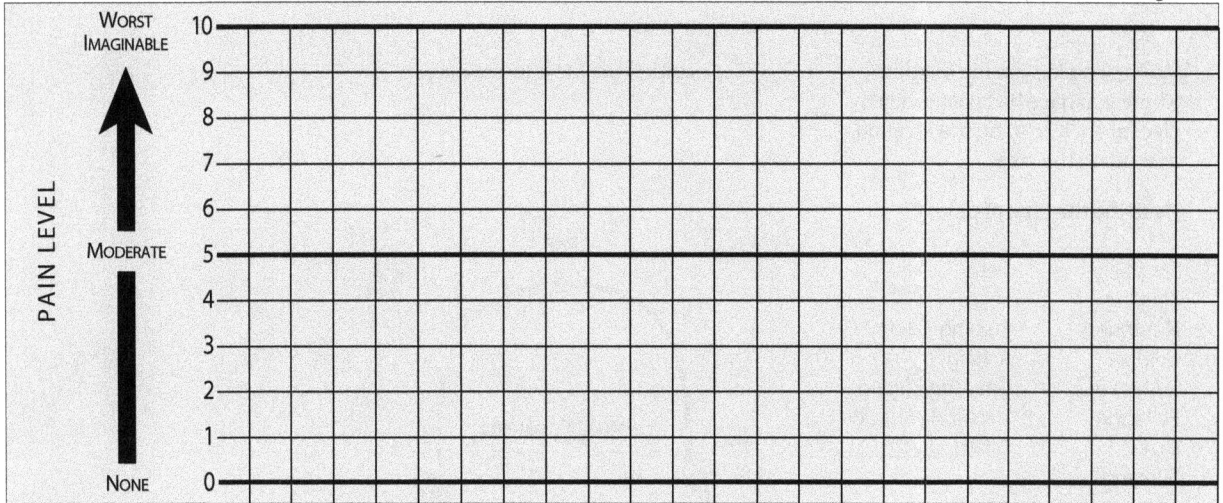

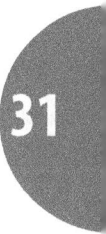

31

2 SATISFACTION

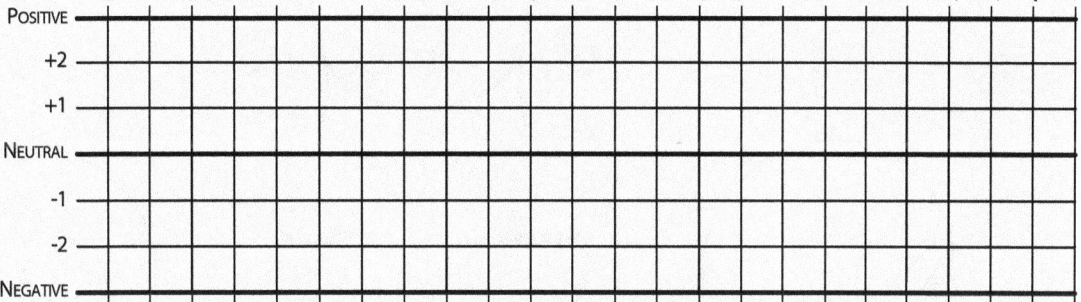

3 PHYSIOLOGY

SLEEP

RESTROOM

NAUSEA / DIZZINESS

MEAL / SNACK

EXERCISE

STRESS / ANXIETY

MEDICINE NAME / DOSE

1

2

3

BLOOD PRESSURE

PULSE

4 DAILY HEAD & FACE PAIN DIAGRAM

Mark each place on the diagram where you have had pain today by placing an 'X', circling the location, or shading the area .

Describe the type of pain:

Shooting	Deep
Tingling	Sharp
Numbness	Burning / Hot
Cold	Aching
Surface Pain	Gnawing / Biting
Stabbing	Electrical / Shocks
Dull	Other_____
Stinging	

31

COMMENTS AND MORE INFORMATION:

Front

Upper Right   Upper Left

Lower Right   Lower Left

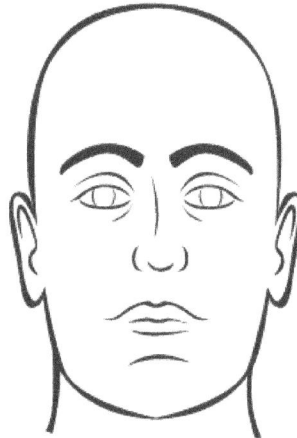

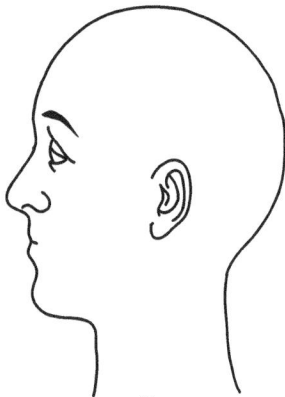

**Your
Right
Side**

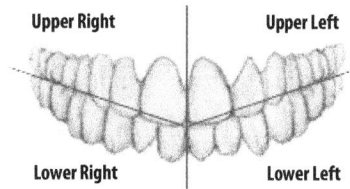

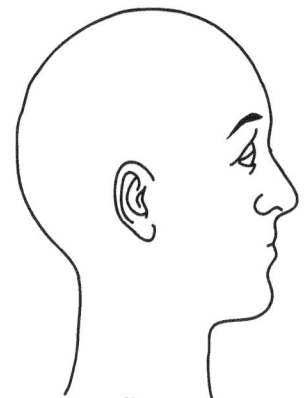

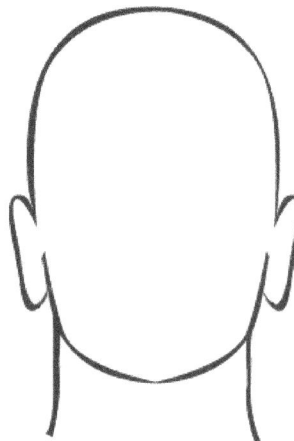

**Your
Right
Side**

Back

5 DAILY BODY PAIN DIAGRAM

Mark each place on the diagram where you have had pain today by placing an 'X', circling the location, or shading the area .

Describe the type of pain:

Shooting	Deep
Tingling	Sharp
Numbness	Burning / Hot
Cold	Aching
Surface Pain	Gnawing / Biting
Stabbing	Electrical / Shocks
Dull	Other_____
Stinging	

COMMENTS AND MORE INFORMATION:

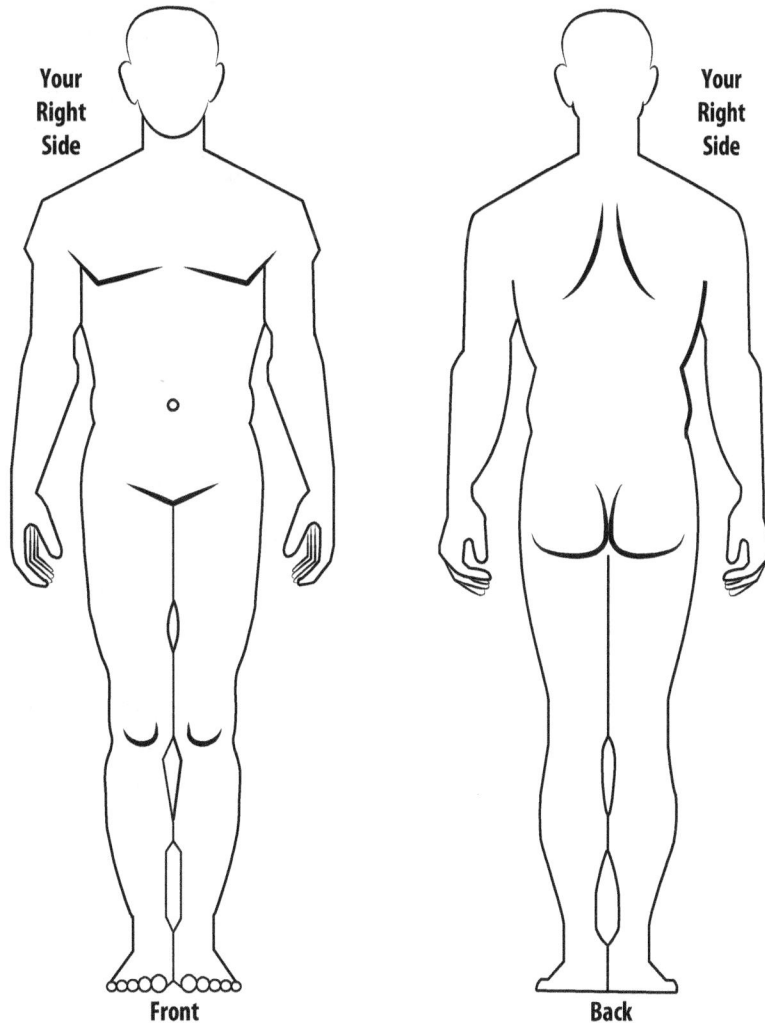

31

Your
Right
Side

Your
Right
Side

Front

Back

6 DAILY PAIN SUMMARY

Were there times during the day that you experienced unrelieved breakthrough pain? ____NO ____YES

How many times did this happen today?

1 2 3 4 5 6 7 8 9 10   more than 10

Did any specific activity start your breakthrough pain?
____NO   ____YES: What activities?

_____

Put an "X" on the body diagram to show each place you've had *BREAKTHROUGH PAIN* today.

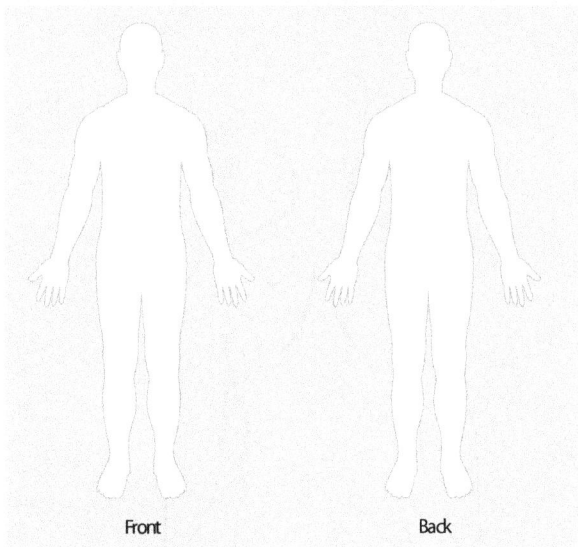

Front   Back

NON-DRUG THERAPIES
(other than prescription or other medicines)

_____

ACTIVITIES/EXERCISE

_____

What was your average level of pain today?

0 1 2 3 4 5 6 7 8 9 10

Other than prescription medicine, did you do anything else today to relieve the pain? ____NO ____YES:
(Note any that you used.)
____ Non-prescription drugs (e.g., acetaminophen, ibuprofen)
____ Herbal remedies
____ Hot or cold packs
____ Exercise
____ Changing position (such as lying down or elevating your legs)
____ Physical therapy
____ Massage
____ Acupuncture
____ Rest
____ Psychological counseling
____ Talk to trusted friend, family, clergy
____ Prayer, meditation, guided imagery
____ Relaxation technique (hypnosis, biofeedback)
____ Creative technique (art or music therapy)
____ Other (e.g., specific chiropractic manipulation, osteopathic treatments):

_____

Check any of these common side effects that you've noticed after taking your pain medicine:
____ Drowsiness, sleepiness
____ Nausea, vomiting, upset stomach
____ Constipation
____ Lack of appetite
____ Other (describe):

_____

Did you sleep through the night? ____NO____YES

If not, how many times was your sleep disrupted? _____

How many hours did you sleep during the night? _____

COMMENTS AND MORE INFORMATION: Make notes for and about visits with your healthcare provider, side effects from treatments you may be experiencing, any problems you are having coping with your pain, and more about some of your previous answers or questions.

1 DAILY DIARY

DAY_____ DATE_____ WEIGHT_____

SATISFACTION CHART Connect the points on your Daily Satisfaction Chart so your medical team can see when and why your mental state changed.

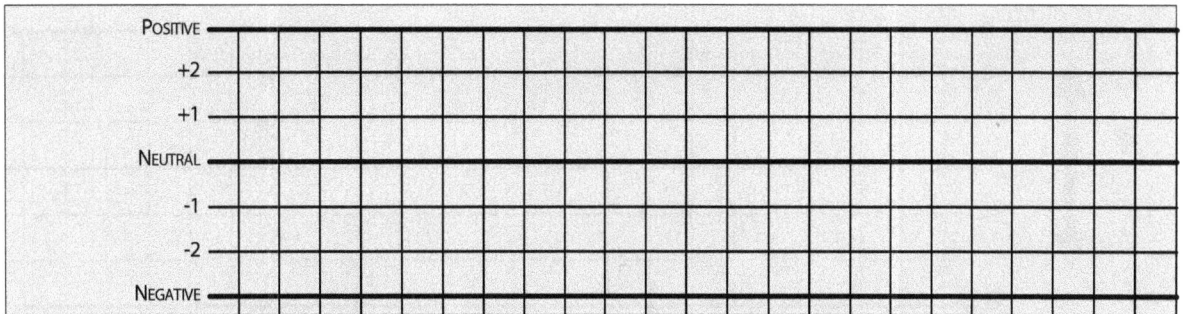

POSITIVE

+2

+1

NEUTRAL

-1

-2

NEGATIVE

2 ACTIVITY LOG

6am 7 8 9 10 11 12pm 1 2 3 4 5 6pm 7 8 9 10 11 12am 1 2 3 4 5

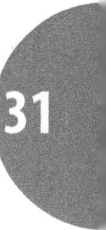

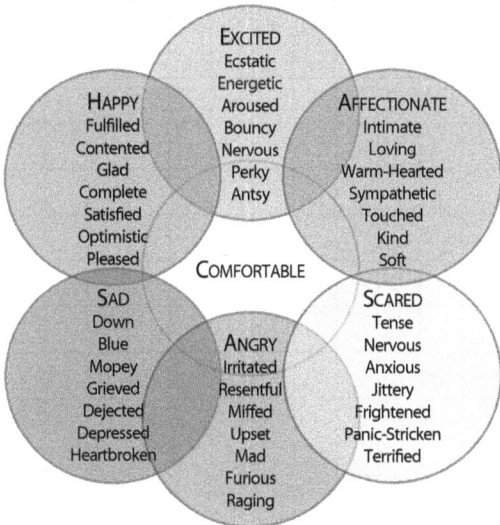

TRIGGERS AND SIGNIFICANT EVENTS

31

EXCITED
Ecstatic
Energetic
Aroused
Bouncy
Nervous
Perky
Antsy

HAPPY
Fulfilled
Contented
Glad
Complete
Satisfied
Optimistic
Pleased

AFFECTIONATE
Intimate
Loving
Warm-Hearted
Sympathetic
Touched
Kind
Soft

COMFORTABLE

SAD
Down
Blue
Mopey
Grieved
Dejected
Depressed
Heartbroken

ANGRY
Irritated
Resentful
Miffed
Upset
Mad
Furious
Raging

SCARED
Tense
Nervous
Anxious
Jittery
Frightened
Panic-Stricken
Terrified

Describe any changes in your pain today:

_____
_____
_____
_____
_____

Did anything unusual happen today?

_____
_____
_____
_____

What did you spend the most time time thinking about today?

Positive Thoughts:

_____

Did your pain increase, decrease, or remain the same when you thought about it?
____ Increased
____ Decreased
____ Stayed the Same

Negative Thoughts:

_____

Did your pain increase, decrease, or remain the same when you thought about it?
____ Increased
____ Decreased
____ Stayed the Same

1 DAILY
MOOD CHART

DAY_____ DATE_____ WEIGHT_____

Connect the points on your Mood Satisfaction Chart so your medical team can see when and why your mental state changed.

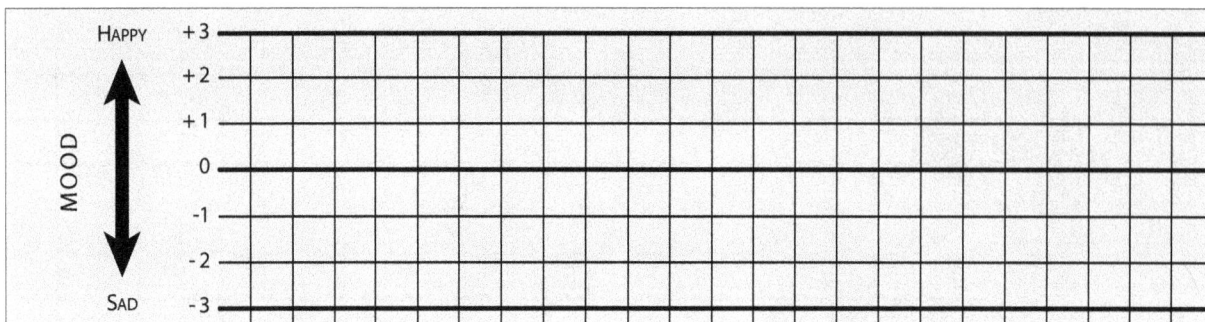

MOOD		HAPPY	+3	
			+2	
			+1	
			0	
			-1	
			-2	
		SAD	-3	

2 ACTIVITY LOG

6am 7 8 9 10 11 12pm 1 2 3 4 5 6pm 7 8 9 10 11 12am 1 2 3 4 5

3 MEDICATION LOG
NAME/DOSE

1 —
2 —
3 —
4 —
5 —
6 —
7 —
8 —

4 PHYSIOLOGY

6am 7 8 9 10 11 12pm 1 2 3 4 5 6pm 7 8 9 10 11 12am 1 2 3 4 5

SLEEP

URINATION

DEFECATION

NAUSEA

EATING

EXERCISE

OTHER (LIST)

31

1 DAILY RESULTS
OF MEDICATIONS AND TREATMENTS

As you and your medical team develop new treatment plans, it will be especially helpful to record any side effects you experience as you add new treatments. This can help determine which types of treatments will work best for you.

Contact your care provider with any bad reactions or side effects to determine if you should discontinue the medication or treatment.

MEDICATION / TREATMENT	AMOUNT / TIME / COMMENTS

31

www.ingramcontent.com/pod-product-compliance
Lightning Source LLC
Chambersburg PA
CBHW080231270326
41926CB00020B/4206